Copyright 2020 by Philip Guzman -All rights reserved.

No part of this book may be reproduced or transmitted in any form or by any means, electronic or mechanical, including photocopying and recording, or by any information storage and retrieval system, without permission in writing from the publisher. This is a work of fiction. Names, places, characters and incidents are either the product of the author's imagination or are used fictitiously, and any resemblance to any actual persons, living or dead, organizations, events or locales is entirely coincidental. The unauthorized reproduction or distribution of this copyrighted work is ilegal.

Disclaimer Notice:

Please note the information contained within this document is for educational and entertainment purposes only. All effort has been executed to present accurate, up to date, reliable, complete information. No warranties of any kind are declared or implied. Readers acknowledge that the author is not engaged in the rendering of legal, financial, medical, or professional advice. The content within this book has been derived from various sources. Please consult a licensed professional before attempting any techniques outlined in this book.

By reading this document, the reader agrees that under no circumstances is the author responsible for any losses, direct or indirect, that are incurred as a result of the use of the information contained within this document, including, but not limited to, errors, omissions, or inaccuracies.

CONTENTS

- Introduction 6
  - Dash Diet 6
- Breakfast 9
  - Breakfast Fruit Pizzas 9
  - Peanut Butter Overnight Oats 9
  - Wedge Salad Skewers 9
  - Low Sodium Sheet Pan Chicken Fajitas 9
  - Pineapple Protein Smoothie 10
  - Spinach Sunshine Smoothie Bowl 10
  - Almond Butter Berry Smoothie 10
  - Pomegranate And Peaches Avocado Toast 10
  - Breakfast In a Jar 10
  - Avocado Egg Cups 10
  - Sugar Break Apple And Peanut Butter Oatmeal 11
  - Sweet Potato Toast 11
  - Ulli'Sgranelli 11
  - Tofu Turmeric Scramble 11
  - Whole Grain Cheese Pancakes 11
  - Red Pepper, Kale, And Cheddar Frittata 12
  - Scrambled Eggs With Bell Pepper And Feta 12
  - Devilled Egg Toast 12
  - Basic Scrambled Eggs 12
  - Baked Butternut-Squash Rigatoni 13
  - Yogurt With Almonds & Honey 13
  - Quick Buffalo Chicken Salad 13
  - All American Tuna 13
  - Pimento Cheese Sandwich 14
  - Coconut Oil Fat Bombs 14
  - Apricot Jam And Almond Butter Sandwich 14
  - Peanut Butter And Honey Toast 14
  - Cucumber & Hummus 14
  - Carrot And Hummus Snack 14
  - Yogurt With Walnuts & Honey 14
  - Simple Caprese Sandwich 14
  - Cottage Cheese Honey Toast 15
  - Pimento Cheese Sandwich 15
  - Tomato Salad 15
  - Tomato And Cheese Wrap 15
  - Peanut Butter Yogurt 15
  - Peanut Butter & Carrots 15
  - Cucumber Tomato Salad With Tuna 15
  - Peanut Butter And Jelly 15
  - Chicken Scampi Pasta 16
- DINNER 17
  - Chicken & Goat Cheese Skillet 17
  - Green Curry Salmon With Green Beans 17
  - Chicken Veggie Packets 17
  - Sweet Onion & Sausage Spaghetti 17
  - Beef And Blue Cheese Penne With Pesto 18
  - Asparagus Turkey Stir-Fry 18
  - Chicken With Celery Root Puree 18
  - Apple-Cherry Pork Medallions 18
  - Butternut Turkey Soup 19
  - Black Bean & Sweet Potato Rice Bowls 19
  - Pepper Ricotta Primavera 19
  - Bow Ties With Sausage & Asparagus 19
  - Pork And Balsamic Strawberry Salad 19
  - Peppered Tuna Kabobs 20
  - Weeknight Chicken Chop Suey 20
  - Thai Chicken Pasta Skillet 20
  - Spinach-Orzo Salad With Chickpeas 21
  - Roasted Chicken Thighs With Peppers & Potatoes 21
  - Spiced Split Pea Soup 21
  - Escarole And Bean Soup 21
- Snacks 22
  - Chili-Lime Grilled Pineapple 22
  - Spicy Almonds 22
  - Italian Sausage-Stuffed Zucchini 22
  - Mimi's Lentil Medley 22
  - Tomato Green Bean Soup 22
  - Shrimp Orzo With Feta 23
  - Garden Vegetable Beef Soup 23
  - Layered Hummus Dip 23
  - Mango Rice Pudding 23
  - Fruit & Almond Bites 24
  - Peppered Tuna Kabobs 24
  - Asparagus With Horseradish Dip 24
  - California Quinoa 24
  - Raspberry Peach Puff Pancake 24
  - Turkey Medallions With Tomato Salad 25
  - Skinny Quinoa Veggie Dip 25
  - Simple Asparagus Soup 25
  - Brunch Banana Splits 26
  - Citrus-Herb Pork Roast 26
  - Macaroni And Cheese 26
  - Bacon In The Microwave 26
  - Strawberry Microwave Breakfast Bowl 26
  - Microwavecinnamonmaple Breakfast Quinoa 27
  - Mug Banana Bread 27
  - Second English Muffin 27
  - Chocolate Chip Pecan Mug Cake 27
  - Spiced Pumpkin Molten Mug Cake 27
  - Minute Microwave Cheesecake 28
  - Granola Cereal Bars 28
  - Bart's Black Bean Soup For Two 28
  - Microwave Egg Sandwich 28
  - Microwave Parmesan Chicken 28
  - Salmon With Tarragon Sauce 28
  - Coconut Acorn Squash 28
  - Microwave Peanut Butter And Jam Brownies 29
  - Sweet & Spicy Popcorn 29
  - Fastest Ever Lemon Pudding 29
  - Almond And Apricot Biscotti 29
  - Ambrosia With Coconut And Toasted Almonds 30
  - Apple-Berry Cobbler 30
  - Apple-Blueberry Cobbler 30
  - Baked Apples With Cherries And Almonds 30
  - Grilled Angel Food Cake 31
  - Grilled Fruit With Balsamic Vinegar Syrup 31
  - Grilled Pineapple 31
  - Mixed Berry Whole-Grain Coffeecake 32
  - Orange Dream Smoothie 32
  - Orange Slices With Citrus Syrup 32
  - Peach Crumble 33

- Pumpkin-Hazelnut Tea Cake 33
- Rainbow Ice Pops 33
- Sautéed Bananas 33
- Summer Fruit Gratin 34
- Warm Chocolate Souffles 34
- Watermelon-Cranberry Agua Fresca 35
- Skillet Apple-Ginger Crisp 35
- Cast-Iron Cornmeal Cake With Buttermilk Cream 35

Recipes by type of food 36
Vegan and vegetarian recipes 36
- Quick And Easy Vegetarian Biryani Recipe 36
- Whole Roasted Cauliflower With Tahini Sauce 36
- Vegan Ramen With Miso Shiitake Broth 36
- Chipotle Portobello Tacos (Vegan!) 37
- Chinese Eggplant With Spicy Szechuan Sauce 37
- Crispy Vegan Quinoa Cakes With Tomato-Chickpea Relish 38
- Spicy Mexicanoaxacan Bowl 38
- Instant Pot Mujadara 39
- Black Pepper Tofu With Bok Choy 39
- Spicy Miso Portobello Mushroom Burger (Vegan) 40
- Simple Baked Sheet-Pan Ratatouille! 40
- Blackened Tempeh With Avocado, Kale, Vegan Cajun Ranch 41
- Veggie Lo Mien 41
- Szechuan Tofu And Veggies 41
- How To Make Tlayudas 42
- Middle Eastern Salad Tacos 42
- Roasted Chiles Rellenos With Black Beans 43
- Roasted Portobello Mushrooms With Walnut Coffee Sauce 43
- Roasted Spaghetti Squash w/ Eggplant Puttanesca 44
- Bali Bowls With Peanut Tofu 44
- Jade Noodles 45
- Vegan Mushroom Pasta With Roasted Sun Chokes 45
- Roasted Eggplant With Zaatar 45
- Fresh Spring Rolls With Peanut Sauce 46
- Bucatini Pasta With Arugula Pesto & Heirloom Tomatoes 46
- Middle Eastern Eggplant Wrap 46
- Chili Garlic Tofu With Sesame Broccolini 47
- Crispy Sheet Pan Jackfruit Tacos 47
- Lentil Dal With Sweet Potatoes 47
- Zaatar Roasted Cauliflower Steaks With Sauce 48
- Tofu Stir-Fry With Broccoli And Mushrooms 48
- Sesame Brussel Sprouts, Mushrooms & Tofu 49
- Make Life Simple Instant Pot Lentil Soup 49
- Vegan Stuffed Poblanos With Avocado Crema 49
- Vegan Lentil Cakes With Zhoug Sauce 50
- Vegan Tikka Masala With Cauliflower 51
- Smoky Chipotle Black Bean Burger Recipe 51
- Hemp Crusted Tofu With Celeriac Puree 51
- Vegan Collard Green Wraps 52
- Vegan Mashed Potatoes 52

Poultry and Meat Recipes 53
- Oven-Roasted Whole Chicken 53
- Cauliflower Rice Bowls With Grilled Asparagus And Chicken Sausage 53
- Baked Lemon-Pepper Chicken 53
- Antipasto Baked Smothered Chicken 54
- Lemon & Dill Chicken 54
- Balsamic Marinated Chicken 54
- Asian-Style Chicken Salad Bowls 54
- Moroccan Chicken Tagine With Apricots & Olives 55
- Baked Lemon-Pepper Chicken 55
- Slow-Cooker Honey-Orange Chicken Drumsticks 56
- Buffalo-Style Bistro Lunch Box 56
- Chicken Breasts With Mushroom Cream Sauce 56
- Cauliflower Chicken Fried "Rice" 56
- Chicken Club Wraps 57
- Southwest Black-Bean Pasta Salad Bowls 57
- Chicken & Shiitake Dumplings In Tangy Chile-Oil Sauce 57
- Filipino Pancitbihon 58
- Creamy Mushroom, Chicken & Asparagus Bake 58
- Chicken Kurma 59
- Skillet Lemon Chicken & Potatoes With Kale .59
- Crock-Pot Pineapple Chicken 59
- Chicken Cutlets And Zucchini Noodles With Creamy Tomato Sauce 60
- Chicken Paillards With Blood Orange Pan Sauce 60
- Creamy Lemon Chicken Parmesan 60
- Instant Pot Brisket 61
- Lola Beef Kebabs 61
- Instant Pot "Corned" Beef & Cabbage 62
- Shepherd's Pie With Cauliflower Topping 62
- Instant Pot Goulash 63
- Beef Tenderloin With Pomegranate Sauce &Farro Pilaf 63
- Slow-Cooker Ropavieja 64
- Afghan Beef Dumplings(Mantu) 64
- Beef Rib Roast With Mushrooms & Fennel 65
- Slow-Cooker Flank Steak Au Jus Sandwiches 65
- Irish Beef Stew 66
- Slow-Cooker Barbecue Brisket Sliders 66
- Spaghetti Squash Casserole 67
- Sausage-Spiked Meatloaves 67
- Braised Brisket With Dried Fruit 67
- Orange Dream Smoothie 68
- Strawberry Banana Milkshak 68
- Watermelon-Cranberry Agua Fresca 68
- Chocolate Berry Smoothies 68
- Ginger Carrot And Turmeric Smoothie 68
- Raspberry Green Smoothie 69
- Avocado Smoothie 69
- Peanut Butter & Banana Breakfast Smoothie 69
- Oatmeal Smoothie For The Dash Diet Breakfast 69
- Kale And Banana Smoothie 69

Strawberry Banana Smoothie 69
Banana, Avocado, And Spinach Smoothie 69
Strawberry Oatmeal Breakfast Smoothie........ 70
Orange Banana Smoothie.................................. 70
Kiwi Banana Apple Smoothie 70
Spinach And Kale Smoothie 70
Banana Pina Coladasmoothie............................ 70
Power Drink ***The Orange*** 70
Sissy's Frozen Banana And Pumpkin
Smoothie 70
Broccolicious 71
Green Power Mojito Smoothie 71
Pumpkin Smoothie.. 71
Grapefruit Smoothie... 71
Almond Butter And Blueberry Smoothie 71
Groovy Green Smoothie 71
Green Slime Smoothie 71
Strawberry Blueberry Smoothies 71
Red, White, And Blue Fruit Smoothie............... 72
Triple Threat Fruit Smoothie 72
Super Healthy Fruit Smoothie 72
Blueberry Mint Smoothie.................................. 72
All-Fruit Smoothies 72
Lemon Berry Smoothie 72
Zucchini Chocolate Banana Nut Milkshake 72
Heavenly Blueberry Smoothie 72
Orange Smoothie.. 73
Mongolian Strawberry-Orange Juice
Smoothie 73
Mango Pineapple Green Smoothie 73
Orange Snowman 73

SOUPS 74
Pumpkin Soup.. 74
Summer Vegetable Soup.................................... 74
Tuscan White Bean Stew 74
Chicken Noodle Soup 75
Steak And Vegetable Soup 75
Thai Red Curry Chicken Soup............................ 75
Ham And Split Pea Soup Recipe - A Great
Soup.. 75
Vegan Red Lentil Soup....................................... 76
Slow-Cooker Chicken Tortilla Soup 76
Quick And Easy Chicken Noodle Soup 76
Delicious Ham And Potato Soup....................... 76
Butternut Squash Soup 77
Geneva's Ultimate Hungarian Mushroom
Soup.. 77
Super-Delicious Zuppa Toscana 77
California Italian Soup 77
Soup Hamburger... 78
Broccoli Cheese Soup 78
Beef Noodle Soup... 78
Soup Lentil... 78
Absolutely Ultimate Potato Soup 78
Slow Cooker Taco Soup...................................... 79
Moroccan Lentil Soup 79
Baked Potato Soup... 79
Turkish Red Lentil 'Bride' Soup 79
Chicken Tortilla Soup V...................................... 80
Clam Chowder... 80
Classic Minestrone 80
Creamy Italian White Bean Soup 80
Spicy Chicken Soup 81
Split Pea And Ham Soup I.................................. 81
Spinach And Leek White Bean Soup 81
Spicy Black Bean Vegetable Soup 81
Pumpkin Black Bean Soup 82
Spicy Slow Cooker Black Bean Soup 82
Black Bean And Salsa Soup 82
Split Pea Soup With Rosemary 82
Split Pea Soup... 82
Bean Soup 83
Sweet Potato, Carrot, Apple, And Red Lentil
Soup.. 83

SALADS 84
Ambrosia With Coconut And Almonds............ 84
Quick Bean And Tuna Salad 84
Couscous Salad 84
Steak Salad With Roasted Corn Vinaigrette ... 84
Greek Salad.. 85
Warm Coleslaw With Honey Dressing............. 85
Yellow Pear And Cherry Tomato Salad 85
Chunky Spicy Egg Salad 86
Pasta Salad With Mixed Vegetables 86
Chicken Broccoli Salad 86
Blue Cheese Broccoli Salad 86
Curry Broccoli Salad 87
Broccoli Coleslaw.. 87
Broccoli Buffet Salad 87
Bodacious Broccoli Salad 87
Minnesota Broccoli Salad 87
Loaded Egg Salad 88
Crunchy Egg Salad 88
Fresh Broccoli Salad 88
Egg Salad I... 88
Broccoli And Tortellini Salad 89
Shrimp Egg Salad 89
Broccoli And Ramen Noodle Salad 89
Delicious Egg Salad For Sandwiches 89
Easy Egg Salad.. 89
Crisp Apples With Citrus Dressing.................... 89
Green Grape Salad 89
Colorful Winter Fruitsalad................................. 90
Egg Salad With Chopped Gherkins 90
Smoked Salmon And Egg Salad 90
Pistachio Fluff Fruit Salad 90
Delicious Egg Salad For Sandwiches 90
Mango Cashew Salad... 91
Salad Frog Eye... 91
Almost Eggless Egg Salad 91
Peach And Berry Salad 91
Layered Deviled Egg Pasta Salad 91
Strawberry Spinach Salad 92
Cranberry And Cilantro Quinoa Salad.............. 92

FISH RECIPES 93
Healthier Broiled Tilapia Parmesan 93
Grilled Salmon... 93
Veracruz-Style Red Snapper 93
Avocado And Tuna Tapas.................................. 93
Quick Fish Tacos 93

- Classic Fish And Chips 94
- Grilled Fish Tacos With Chipotle-Lime Dressing 94
- Hudson's Baked Tilapia With Dill Sauce 95
- Spanish Moroccan Fish 95
- Cedar Planked Salmon 95
- Blackened Tuna 95
- Baked Dijon Salmon 95
- Ginger Glazed Mahi Mahi 96
- Pretzel Coated Fried Fish 96
- Spanish Cod 96
- Baked Cod In Foil 96
- Coast Cod And Shrimp 97
- Perfect Ten Baked Cod 97
- Moroccan Fish Tagine 97
- Crispy Beer Batter Fish & Chips 98
- Cod Grilled 98
- Crispy Fish 98
- Sardines With Sun-Dried Tomato And Capers 98
- Fresh Sardines 99
- Pasta Con Sarde (Pasta with Sardines) 99
- Quick Sardine Curry 99
- Island-Style Sardines and Rice 99
- Pasta Sardine 99
- Miso & Tofu 100
- MediterraneanCasserole 100
- Avocado Salsa and Sardine Frenchy 100
- Vegetale Sardina 100
- Bagna Calda 101
- Solo Spaghetti Dinner 101
- Sandwich Toast (Sardines and Pineapple) .. 101
- Iana's Pasta con le Sarde 101
- Crab Stuffed Flounder 101
- Italian Style Flounder 102
- Blueberry Sauce 102
- EZ Red Pesto Sauce 102
- Easy Pesto 102
- Quick Alfredo Sauce 102
- Cilantro-Lime Dressing 103
- Yummy Honey Mustard Dipping Sauce 103
- Bill's Blue Cheese Dressing 103
- Proper Pesto 103
- Cilantro Jalapeno Pesto with Lime 103
- Garlic Scape Pesto 103
- Cranberry, Apple, and Fresh Ginger Chutney 104
- Alfredo Sauce 104
- Homemade Mayonnaise 104
- Spinach Basil Pesto 104
- Spiced Apple Chutney 104
- Sweet Tamarind Chutney 105
- Hot Pepper Jelly 105
- Chimichurri Sauce 105
- Bar-B-Q Sauce 105
- Spicy Cranberry Chutney 105
- MINI BELL PEPPER TURKEY "NACHOS" 106
- ROAST CHICKPEAS 106
- Strawberry Corn Salsa 106
- Balsamic-Goat Cheese Grilled Plums 106
- Berry White Ice Pops 107
- Strawberry Lime Smoothies 107
- Mixed Fruit with Lemon-Basil Dressing 107
- Crunchy Peanut Butter Apple Dip 107
- Citrusy Fruit Kabobs 107
- Frozen Pops (Pineapple-Kiwi) 108
- Grilled Stone Fruits with Balsamic Syrup 108
- Avocado Fruit Salad with Tangerine Vinaigrette 108
- Chili-Lime Grilled Pineapple 108
- Italian Sausage-Stuffed Zucchini 108
- Frozen Berry & Yogurt Swirls 109
- Tomato Green Bean Soup 109
- Avocado Fruit Salad 109
- Double-Nut Stuffed Figs 109
- Frosty Watermelon Ice 109
- Apple-Nut Blue Cheese Tartlets 110
- Dessert Recipes 111
  - Ambrosia With Coconut And Toasted Almonds 111
  - Apple-Berry Cobbler 111
  - Apple-Blueberry Cobbler 111
  - Baked Apples, Cherries And Almonds 112
  - Grilled Food Cake 112
  - Balls Buckeye 112
  - Toffee Honeycomb 112
  - Peanut Brittle 113
  - Caramel 113
  - Pineapple Grilled 113
  - Mixed Berry Whole-Grain Coffee-Cake 113
  - Orange Smoothie 114
  - Orange Slices 114
  - Crumble Peach 114
  - Pumpkin-Hazelnut Cake 115
  - Marshmallows 115
  - Oreo Truffles 115
  - Chocolate Fudge 115
  - Easiest Peanut Butter Fudge 116
  - Ice Pops Like Rainbow 116
  - Bananas Sautéed 116
  - Fruit Gratin For Summer 116
  - Chocolate Souffles 117
  - Decadent Truffles 117
  - Cookie Ball 117
- Appendix : Recipes Index 118

Introduction
Dash Diet

DASH diet is the abbreviation of Dietary Approaches to Stop Hypertension. The DASH diet is used to live a healthy lifestyle and prevent diseases like high blood pressure, which is known as hypertension. If you want to lower your blood pressure, reduces the risk of heart attacks, you should follow the DASH diet.

The variety of foods rich in nutrients included in the DASH diet will lower your blood pressure and prevent diseases. If you follow the DASH diet, you will see a big difference in your blood pressure in just two weeks. Besides lowering blood pressure, it will also help to prevent osteoporosis, cancer, diabetes, and strokes.

DASH diet: Sodium levels

The DASH diet mainly includes vegetables, fruits, low-fat foods, whole grains, fish, nuts, and poultry.

Standard DASH diet: : In the DASH diet, you are allowed to consume up to 2,300 mg of sodium daily..

Lower sodium DASH diet: In this diet, you are only allowed to consume up to 1,500 mg of sodium a day.

DASH diet: What to eat

The DASH diet includes a variety of fruits, vegetables, fish, legumes, poultry, and nuts and seeds a few timesa week. You can eat beef, sweets, and fats in small amounts. Overall, the DASH diet includes low amounts of saturated fat.

DASH diet: Alcohol and caffeine

When you drink too much alcohol and caffeine, it will drastically increase your blood pressure. The DASH diet will help you to limit alcohol, since you will only be allowed to have two or less drinks a day.

DASH diet and weight loss

Although the DASH diet is not a weight-loss program, you may unintentionally lose weight as this diet includes healthy foods.

You can consume 2000 calories daily by following this diet, so you will maintain or lose weight because you will eat fewer calories

Strategies to start the DASH

Change gradually. If you want to follow this diet, add things to your diet slowly. If you eat only one or two servings of fruits or vegetables a day, then add one more serving at lunch and one at dinner. It is not advised to change your entire diet plan. With these gradual changes, you will not get bloating or diarrhea that may occur if you are not used to eating a lot of fiber at once. Beans and vegetables also help you to reduce gas.

Reward successes. Reward yourself with your favorite food for your achievements. Lease a movie, buy a book, or get together with a friend. Everyone slips, especially when learning something new. Remember that changing your lifestyle is a time-consuming process. Determine the problems which are becoming hurdles, and pick up where you left off with the DASH diet.

Add a physical activity. If you want to notice a positive change in your lifestyle, you should include physical activities in your schedule. Doing exercise daily and following the DASH diet will help you to live a longer and healthier life.

Get support. If you are facing difficulty, stick to your diet. Talk to your doctor, dietitian, or close friend about it. You can get help from your friends – they will motivate you and help you to stick to your diet.

Health benefits

High blood pressure, or hypertension, can increase the risk of heart attacks, heart failure, stroke, and kidney disease. If people with high blood pressure follow the DASH diet strictly, this could prevent around 400,000 deaths from cardiovascular disease over ten years.

The DASH diet can reduce levels of:

Blood pressure

Blood sugar

Triglycerides, or fat, in the blood

Low-density lipoprotein (LDL), or "bad" cholesterol

Insulin resistance

These are all the features of metabolic syndrome, a condition that also involves obesity, type 2-diabetes, and a higher risk of cardiovascular disease.

Results showed that on average:

In people with metabolic syndrome, the systolic pressure fell by 4.9 millimeters of mercury (mm Hg), and the diastolic fell by 1.9 mm Hg.

In people without metabolic syndrome, the systolic pressure fell by 5.2 mm Hg, and the diastolic fell by 2.9 mm Hg.

In other words, DASH can be effective at lowering blood pressure in people with or without metabolic syndrome. There is also proof that it may decrease the risk of colorectal cancer and improve overall life expectancy. The National Kidney Foundation recommends DASH for people with kidney disease.

Understanding blood pressure

Systolic pressure is the blood pressure while the heart is pumping blood, while diastolic is the pressure when the heart is resting between beats. A person with a systolic pressure of 120 mm Hg and a diastolic pressure of 80 mm Hg will have a reading of 120/80 mm Hg.

Current guidelines from the American College of Cardiology describe blood pressure as follows:

Normal: Below 120/80 mm Hg.
Elevated: Systolic 120–129, and diastolic is below 80.
Stage 1 hypertension: Systolic is 130–139, and diastolic is 80–89.
Stage 2 hypertension: Systolic is 140 or above; diastolic is 90 or above.
Hypertensive crisis: Systolic is over 180; diastolic is over 120.

Proven Benefits of the DASH Diet

These include:

Lower blood pressure

The primary benefit of the DASH diet is that it lowers blood pressure. For anyone who currently takes medication to control their blood pressure or individuals who are hoping to manage symptoms of pre-hypertension better, this diet is a great option.

The DASH diet can decrease your blood pressure by a few points after only two weeks – and over time, you could see your systolic blood pressure drop by eight to 14 points. This is a significant improvement to your overall health and wellness.

More nutritious meals

To get results will require a bit of adaptation, especially for people who have never spent much time in the kitchen.

Spend some time trying new fruits and vegetables and experimenting with different salt-free seasonings to create some healthy meals that will suit your tastes – and that your family can enjoy with you. Instead of grabbing a quick sandwich or fast food burger, a little planning and a focus on DASH means you'll be enjoying much more nutritious foods.

Healthier cholesterol levels

Thanks to the fiber you'll be getting from fruits and vegetables, whole grains, and nuts and beans, along with lean cuts of meat and fish and your limited intake of sweets and refined carbohydrates, the DASH diet has been shown to improve cholesterol levels. This improvement continues even with a higher fat version of the diet, which also increases "good" cholesterol.

Stick with it

Because this diet is designed to include readily available, delicious foods, it's very easy for dieters to maintain. Once you've committed to the DASH diet, you'll be able to enjoy a long-term lifestyle change that will be a huge benefit to your overall health and wellness.

The DASH diet is even easy to follow while you're eating out – just be aware of any foods that could sabotage your efforts. There are lots of methods to make the DASH diet work for you, which is a massive benefit for anyone looking to improve their well-being.

Healthy weight maintenance

Whether you're looking to lose weight or not, the DASH diet is a great option to ensure you can maintain your goal weight once you've reached it. You can follow a customized version of the DASH diet to achieve your weight loss goals, then stick to a higher calorie count to maintain your new weight – and with the healthy options included in this diet, you won't have to deal with any weight gain after working so hard to lose it.

The DASH plan provides plenty of protein without overloading on carbs, meaning you'll enjoy building muscle and boosting your metabolism while keeping yourself from ever feeling heavy. And it's not a short-term diet – this is a new, healthy lifestyle.

Lower risk of developing osteoporosis

Most dietary strategies for the prevention and treatment of osteoporosis include the increased intake of vitamin D and calcium – which are both found in plenty of the foods included in the DASH diet. Research has also revealed that sodium reduction can be another effective option, proving that the DASH diet may also benefit bone health.

Studies showed that following the DASH diet resulted in "significantly reduced bone turnover," which may eventually improve bone mineral status if sustained over a longer period of time. The diet is also rich in other nutrients – magnesium, vitamin C, antioxidants, and polyphenols – that have been associated with improved bone health.

Healthier kidneys

This diet has proven to lower one's risk of kidney disease and kidney stones, thanks to all the potassium, magnesium, fiber, and calcium found in the foods encouraged in the DASH eating plan. The diet's focus on reduced sodium intake is also recommended for those who are at risk of developing kidney disease.

However, the diet should not be followed by patients who have already been diagnosed with chronic kidney disease or those on dialysis without the guidance of a healthcare professional, as there may be special restrictions for these individuals.

Protected from certain cancers
Researchers have examined the correlation between the DASH diet and various types of cancer. They have uncovered a positive association relating to reduced salt intake and monitoring consumption of dietary fat. The diet is also low in red meat, which has been linked to cancers of the colon, rectum, esophagus, stomach, lung, prostate, and kidney.
The focus on fresh produce helps prevent several cancers, and the emphasis on low-fat dairy products can also contribute to a decreased risk of colon cancer.

Prevent diabetes
The DASH diet has been proven to be effective in helping prevent insulin resistance, which is shown to be linked to high blood pressure and cardiovascular health risks. By helping dieters manage their sodium intake, eat more fiber and potassium, and maintain a healthy weight, the DASH eating plan helps those who are predisposed to diabetes avoid or delay the onset of this condition.
According to some studies, this impact is even more significant when the DASH plan is implemented as a component of a more comprehensive healthy lifestyle – including diet, exercise, and weight control.

Improved mental health
The boost to your mood and decreased symptoms of disorders like depression or anxiety can be attributed to the lifestyle impacts of the DASH diet – like exercise, moderate alcohol consumption, and avoiding cigarettes. However, the nutrient-rich foods recommended by this eating plan are all helpful in balancing the chemicals and hormones in your brain and in your body, contributing to improved mental health and wellbeing.

Healthier lifestyle
The DASH plan isn't just about diet – it's about taking manageable steps to control your own health and wellness. By incorporating the elements of nutrition, exercise, and healthy living into your lifestyle, you'll see a wider range of valuable benefits along with the wellness that comes with DASH eating.
It's also an easy lifestyle to maintain. Start slowly and train yourself to eat DASH-recommended options and get used to the flavor of food without so much added salt. Work up to exercising multiple times each week, and try to limit your intake of alcohol and sweets. Soon, you'll notice that following the DASH diet is second nature – and maintaining your healthy lifestyle doesn't require any effort at all.

Foods for a Longer and Healthy Life
Some of the foods which are good for health and help you to live a healthy and longer life are as follows:
Broccoli, grapes, and salad
Berries
Garlic
Olive oil
Bok Choy
Avocadoes
Tomatoes
Beans
Grains and seeds
Less red meat
White meat
More nuts
Bananas
Fish
DASH diet

Foods to avoid
Foods you should avoid in order to live a longer and healthy life include:
Sugary drinks
Junk/Fast food
White bread
Sweetened breakfast cereals
Fried, grilled, broiled food
Pastries, cookies, and cakes
Gluten-free junk food
Agave nectar
Low-fat yogurt
Candy bars
Processed meat
Processed cheese

Breakfast

Breakfast Fruit Pizzas

Ingredients
- Two whole-wheat pita flatbreads
- 7 ounces Arla Original Cream Cheese
- 1-2 teaspoons honey
- 1/2 teaspoon pure vanilla extract
- Three kiwi skin removed and sliced
- 1/2 cup sliced strawberries
- 1/2 cup blackberries
- 1/4 cup blueberries
- Two raspberries for the center

Instructions
1. Preheat the oven to broil. Put the whole wheat pita flatbreads in the oven. Broil for 1 minute and turn over. Broil for one minute more. You can also toast the whole pita bread in a toaster oven. Set the dough aside to cool.
2. Take a bowl and mix the cream cheese, honey, and vanilla. Spread the cream cheese on the pita bread.
3. Decorate the fruit on top of the cream cheese. Cut into slices and serve immediately.
4. Note-you can use your favorite fruit. Bananas, peaches, pineapple, oranges, nectarines would also be good!

Peanut Butter Overnight Oats

Ingredients
OATS
- Half of cup unsweetened plain almond milk (or sub other dairy-free milk, such as coconut, soy, or hemp!)
- 3/4 Tbsp of chia seed
- 2 Tbsp of natural salted peanut butter or almond butter (creamy or crunchy // or sub other nut or seed butter)
- 1 Tbsp of maple syrup (or sub coconut sugar, natural brown sugar, or stevia to taste)
- half of cup gluten-loose rolled oats (rolled oats are best, vs. Steel-cut or quick-cooking)

TOPPINGS optional
- Sliced banana, strawberries, or raspberries
- Flaxseed meal or additional chia seed
- *Granola*

Instructions
1. Take a small bowl with a lid, add almond milk, chia seeds, peanut butter, and maple syrup (or every other sweetener) and stir with a spoon to combine. The peanut butter doesn't need to be very well blended with the almond milk (doing so leaves swirls of peanut butter to revel in the subsequent day).
2. Add oats and stir a few extra times. Then press down with a spoon to make sure all oats were moistened and are immersed in almond milk.
3. Cover tightly with a lid or seal and set within the fridge overnight (or for at least 6 hours) to place/soak.
4. The subsequent day, open and experience as is or garnish with preferred toppings.
5. Overnight oats will preserve within the refrigerator for 2-three days, though high-quality within the first 12-24 hours in our experience. Not freezer friendly.

Nutrition
● Calories: 452, Fat: 22.8g, Saturatedfat: 4.1g, Sodium: 229mgPotassium: 479mgCarbohydrates: 51.7g Fiber: 8.3gSugar: 15.8g Protein: 14.6g

Wedge Salad Skewers

Ingredients
- One head of iceberg lettuce *(cut into wedge pieces)*
- Four Roma tomatoes cut in half
- One red onion *(cut into 1-inch pieces)*
- Two avocados cut into 1-inch pieces
- Five slices of bacon cooked and cut into thirds
- One cucumber *(sliced (peeled or unpeeled))*
- Eight wooden skewers
- Two green onions *(diced)*
- 1 5 oz container blue cheese crumbles
- One bottle blue cheese dressing

Instructions
One skewer at a time adds an iceberg wedge, tomato, onion, avocado, two pieces of bacon, every other iceberg wedge, and then cucumber.
Continue till all skewers have been made, then garnish with crumbled blue cheese, blue cheese dressing, and diced leafy green onions.

Nutrition
Calories: 238kcal, Fat: 19g, Saturated fat: 6g Cholesterol: 25mg Sodium: 401mgPotassium: 573mgCarbohydrates: 10gFiber: 5g Sugar: 3g Protein: 8gVitamin A: 890%Vitamin C: 13.9%Calcium: 144%Iron: 0.9%

Low Sodium Sheet Pan Chicken Fajitas

Ingredients
- Two lbs chicken breast tenderloin each sliced in half lengthwise
- One green pepper sliced
- One red bell pepper sliced
- One Vidalia onion sliced
- Olive oil spray
- One tablespoon olive oil

Seasoning:
- One teaspoon chili powder
- 1/2 teaspoon smoked paprika
- 1/2 teaspoon garlic powder
- 1/2 teaspoon onion powder

- 1/2 teaspoon dried oregano
- 1/2 teaspoon dried cilantro
- 1/2 teaspoon cumin
- 1/4 teaspoon cayenne pepper

Instructions
1. Preheat oven to 350 degrees F.
2. Apply a coat on a sheet pan with olive oil spray.
3. Spread pepper and onion slices onto a prepared sheet pan.
4. Place chicken slices on top of vegetables.
5. Combine seasoning ingredients and stir to combine.
6. Drizzle seasoning mixture over chicken, peppers, and onion.
7. Sprinkle 1 tbsp of olive oil over chicken, peppers, and onion.
8. Gently toss ingredients to distribute seasoning and oil evenly. (make sure chicken strips are not overlapping)
9. Bake for 20 min or until chicken reaches 165 deg F.
10. Serve in warm low sodium tortillas.
11. Top with your favorite toppings! I love cheddar cheese and sour cream.

Nutrition Facts
Calories 168Calories from Fat 36 Fat 4g6% Sodium 140mg6% Potassium 531mg15% Carbohydrates 5g2% Fiber 1g4% Sugar 3g3% Protein 24g48% Vitamin C 34.3mg42% Calcium 17mg2% Iron 0.8mg4%

Pineapple Protein Smoothie

Ingredients
- 3/4 cup milk
- 3/4 cup pineapple chunks
- 1/2 cup ice
- 3/4 cup canned chickpeas (rinsed and drained)
- 2 tbsp almond butter
- Two pitted dates
- 2 tsp ground turmeric

Directions
1. Blend all ingredients until smooth.

Nutrients CALORIES: 461

Spinach Sunshine Smoothie Bowl

Ingredients
- One packed cup baby spinach
- One banana
- 1 cup of orange juice
- 1/2 avocado
- 1/2 cup ice cubes
- Blueberries (optional)
- diced pineapple (optional)
- ground flaxseeds (optional)

Directions
1. Process the spinach, banana, orange juice, avocado, and ice in a blender until very smooth.
2. Serve topped with blueberries, diced pineapple, and ground flaxseeds.

Almond Butter Berry Smoothie

Ingredients
- 1/4 cup 1% low-fat milk
- 1/2 medium ripe banana
- 1 tbsp creamy almond butter
- 1 cup fresh or frozen raspberries
- 1/2 cup crushed ice

Directions
Blend all ingredients until smooth and enjoy!

Pomegranate And Peaches Avocado Toast

Ingredients
- one slice whole-grain bread
- 1/2 avocado
- 1 tbsp ricotta
- Pomegranate seeds, a small amount like one handful
- Drizzle honey

Directions
1. Toast the whole grain bread within the oven or toaster.
2. Spread avocado onto the toast, as smooth or coarse as you prefer.
3. Spread a dollop of ricotta across the avocado.
4. Drizzle a chunk of honey over the avocado mixture.
5. Sprinkle pomegranate seeds on top and enjoy.

Breakfast In a Jar

Ingredients
- 1/4 cup of oatmeal
- 3/4 cup of kefir
- 1 tbsp of chia seeds
- 2 tbsp of raisins
- 1 tbsp of unsweetened coconut flakes

Instructions
Make Layers of elements in a 16-ounce mason jar, close the lid and refrigerate overnight.
2. When it is ready to eat, remove the jar from the fridge and give it a quick stir.

Avocado Egg Cups

Ingredients
- Two avocados, ripe
- 1/4 tsp coarse salt
- 1/4 tsp pepper
- 1/2 tsp olive oil
- Four medium eggs
- 1 tbsp grated cheese, such as Parmesan, cheddar, or Swiss
- assorted toppings: herbs, scallions, salsa, diced tomato, crumbled bacon, Sriracha, paprika, crumbled feta

Directions
1. Heat oven to 375°F. Halve avocados lengthwise and pit. Cut a skinny slice from bottom of each avocado half so that it sits level. Where the pit was, scoop out just enough of the flesh (about ½ tbsp) to make room for an egg.
2. Place avocados on a foil-lined rimmed baking sheet. Season each with salt and pepper, and rub with olive oil.

3. Crack an egg into each cavity (some of the egg white will run over the side, but don't worry about it). Sprinkle with cheese, if using. Cover loosely with foil.
4. Bake almost 20 to 25 min, or until eggs are set to your liking. Sprinkle with toppings.

Sugar Break Apple And Peanut Butter Oatmeal

Ingredients
- 1 cup steel-cut oats
- Three medium-large Granny Smith apples, cored and sliced into 1-2" chunks
- a swirl of peanut butter
- pinch ground cinnamon
- 1 tbsp butter (optional)
- 4 cups of water
- pinch salt

Directions
Cook the oats till they reach the desired texture and creaminess.
Cut apples, toss them into the oats, and stir.
Then add peanut butter into it and stir until melted and spread throughout.
Top with a dash of cinnamon and butter (optional) and enjoy!
Nutrient CALORIES: 453

Sweet Potato Toast

Ingredients
- One potato (sweet)

Instructions
1. Divide the sweet potato into 1/4-inch slices and pop into the toaster.
2. Top with anything you choose. Popular combinations include nut butter with fruit, avocado, hummus, eggs, cheese, and tuna salad.
Nutrient CALORIES: 112

Ulli'Sgranelli

Ingredients
- 4 cups rolled oats
- 2 cups raw cashews
- 2 cups raw walnuts
- 2 cups of raw almonds
- 2 cups of fresh sunflower seed
- 2 cups of raw pumpkin seeds
- 3 cups unsweetened coconut flakes
- 1/2 cup of maple liquid syrup
- 1/4 cup of unrefined coconut oil, plus 2 tsp for oiling the baking sheet
- pinch of sea salt
- 1/3 cup of pure orange oil
- 2 cups of organic raisins
- 2 cups of dried cherries or cranberries

Directions
1. Set the oven to 300°F.
2. In a considerable bowl, mix the oats, nuts, seeds, and coconut flakes.
3. Take a small bowl, stir together the maple syrup, coconut oil, salt, and orange oil till well combined, then pour over the oat-nut combination and mix nicely.
4. Spread granola on a large oiled baking sheet (coat in batches if needed) and bake for 35-forty minutes until golden brown (rotate the baking sheet halfway via for even baking).
5. Remove from oven and permit refreshing absolutely earlier than mixing with raisins and dried cherries or cranberries.
6. Store in airtight place in the fridge to keep extra crispiness.

Tofu Turmeric Scramble

Ingredients
- One 8-ounce block of firm or extra-firm tofu, drained
- 1 tbsp extra virgin olive oil
- ¼ red onion, chopped
- One green or purple bell pepper, chopped
- 2 cups of clean spinach, loosely chopped
- ½ cup sliced button mushrooms
- ½ tsp every salt and pepper
- 1 tsp garlic powder
- ½ tbsp turmeric
- ¼ cup nutritional yeast

Directions
1. Drain the tofu and squeeze lightly to do away with extra water. Crumble tofu right into a bowl with the aid of hand - the smaller the pieces, the better.
2. Prep vegetables and region a large skillet at medium temperature. Once ready, then add olive oil, onions, and bell peppers. Mix in a pinch of the salt and pepper and prepare dinner for about five minutes to melt the vegetables. Then add mushrooms and sauté for 2 mins. Then upload tofu. Sauté for about three minutes, a little more if the tofu is watery.
3. Add the rest of the salt, pepper, garlic turmeric, and nutritional yeast and blend with a spatula, ensuring the spices combo well. Cook for another 5 to 8 mins till tofu is lightly browned.
4. Add the spinach and cover the pan in order to steam for two minutes. Serve immediately with facets of your choice.
Nutrient CALORIES: 158

Whole Grain Cheese Pancakes

Ingredients
- 1 cup of oat flour
- 1/2 cup of sorghum flour
- 2 tbsp of teff flour
- 1/3 cup of plus 1 tbsp, tapioca starch
- 1 tbsp of baking powder
- 1/2 of tsp salt
- 3 1/2 of tsp sugar
- 1/2 tsp of flax meal
- 3/4 cup of buttermilk
- 1/3 cup of cottage cheese
- Three eggs
- half tsp vanilla extract

- 4 tsp canola oil
- 1-pint blueberries
- 1/2 cup maple syrup
- 3 tbsp water
- 1 tsp lemon juice
- pinch of salt

Instructions
1. Combine all of your dry elements in a huge mixing bowl and stir to mix evenly.
2. Whisk all of your wet ingredients in another bowl collectively.
3. Make a hole in the center of your dry substances and begin to slowly pour in the wet materials, about a quarter cup at a time. This will make sure that no lumps form when whisking.
4. Continue including your wet components to the flour base till a smooth batter forms. Let the batter relax for 15 minutes at the same time as you preheat your grill.
5. While the grill is warming up, make a warm maple blueberry compote. Mix blueberries, maple syrup, water, lemon juice, and a pinch salt in a small pot. Stir frivolously to mix.
6. Gently heat the pot over medium-low warmth till the blueberries start to pop and release their natural juices. Set aside, but maintain heat.
7. Once the grill is preheated to a medium-hot temperature, lightly oil the restaurant using a nonstick spray or a small amount of neutral-flavored oil.
8. Ladle the batter on to the skillet, making sure you do not overload it.
9. Give time to the pancakes to cook undisturbed until the appearance of the edges dry and bubbles come to the surface without breaking. This has to take roughly minutes.
10. Flip the pancakes over and cook at the other facet for another two minutes.
11. Keep heat or serve straight away with the sweet and cozy maple-blueberry compote.

Nutrient CALORIES: 511

Red Pepper, Kale, And Cheddar Frittata

Ingredients
- 1 tsp olive oil
- 5 oz baby kale and spinach
- One red pepper, diced
- 1/3 cup sliced scallions
- 12 eggs
- 3/4 cup milk
- 1 cup sharp shredded cheddar cheese
- 1/4 tsp salt
- 1/4 tsp pepper

Directions
1. Preheat oven to 375°F.
2. Spray an eight 1/2-inch by using 12-inch glass or casserole dish with olive oil or nonstick spray.
3. Heat oil in a large frying pan. Add crimson peppers on low and cook until tender. Add kale and spinach, on occasion stirring till vegetables are wilted, or for about three min.
4. Transfer peppers and greens to the plate, spreading evenly. Add sliced scallions.
5. Beat eggs with milk, salt, and pepper. Pour the egg aggregate over the pan. Sprinkle cheese on top.
6. Bake about 35-40 mins or till the aggregate is completely set and beginning to lightly brown. For extra color, place under broiler for a further 1 to three minutes, looking at to ensure the top doesn't burn. Let cool about five mins before cutting it.
7. Serve it as warm or refrigerate for a quick breakfast all through the week — microwave for 1-2 minutes to reheat.

Nutrient CALORIES: 77

Scrambled Eggs With Bell Pepper And Feta

Ingredients
- Olive oil-Salad or cooking-1 tsp-4.5 grams
- Green bell pepper-Sweet, green, raw-2 medium (approx 2-3/4" long, 2-1/2" dia)-238 grams
- Egg-Whole, fresh eggs-Four large-200 grams
- Feta cheese-1 oz-28.4 grams

Directions
eatureHeat the oil in a skillet on medium heat. Add chopped peppers and cook till tender.
Stir the eggs and add to the skillet with the peppers. Stir slowly over medium-low heat till they attain your preferred doneness. Sprinkle inside the feta cheese and stir to mix and soften the cheese. Serve right away and enjoy it!

Nutrient
Calories 448 Carbs 14g Fat 30g Protein 31g Fiber 4g Net carbs 10g Sodium 551mg Cholesterol 769mg

Devilled Egg Toast

Ingredients
- Egg-Whole, fresh eggs-Two large-100 grams
- Mustard-Prepared, yellow-2 tbsp-30 grams
- Light mayonnaise-Salad dressing, Kraft brand-2 tbsp-30 grams
- Whole-wheat bread-Commercially prepared-Four slice-112 grams

Directions
Place egg in a bowl and cover with water. Boil the water, remove from heat, cover, and let sit 10 minutes. Drain under cold water, peel, and mash. Combine egg with the mustard and mayonnaise. Mix well.
Toast bread and top with egg mixture. Enjoy!

Nutrition
Calories 543 Carbs 53g Fat 24g Protein 28g Fiber 8g Net carbs 45g Sodium 1173mg Cholesterol 382mg

Basic Scrambled Eggs

Ingredients
- Egg-Whole, fresh eggs-Six large-300 grams
- Butter-Unsalted-1 tbsp-14.2 grams
- Chives-Raw-1 tbsp chopped-3 grams

- Tarragon-Spices, dried-1 tbsp, ground-4.8 grams
- Salt-Table-One dash-0.40 grams
- Pepper-Spices, black-One dash-0.10 grams

Directions
- Beat the eggs in a bowl and till damaged up. Sprinkle with a pinch each of salt and pepper and beat to incorporate. Place tablespoons of the eggs in a small bowl; set aside.
- Heat a 10-inch nonstick frying pan over medium-low warmth until hot, approximately 2 minutes. Add butter to the pan and the usage of a rubber spatula, swirl until it's melted and foamy, and the box is flippantly coated. Pour in the massive part of the eggs, sprinkle with chives and tarragon (if the usage of), and let sit down undisturbed till eggs just start to set around the edges, about 1 to 2 minutes. Using the rubber spatula, push the eggs from the sides into the middle. After 30 seconds repeat pushing the eggs from the perimeters into the center every 30 seconds till simply set, for a total cooking time of about 5 minutes.
- Add the ultimate tablespoons raw egg and stir till eggs not look wet. Remove from warmness and season with salt and pepper as needed. Serve immediately.

Nutrition
Calories 546 Carbs 5g Fat 40g Protein 39g Fiber 0g Net carbs 4g Sodium 586mg Cholesterol 1147mg

Baked Butternut-Squash Rigatoni

Ingredients
One large butternut squash
Three clove garlic
2 tbsp. olive oil
1 lb. rigatoni
1/2 c. heavy cream
3 c. shredded fontina
2 tbsp. chopped fresh sage
1 tbsp. salt
1 tsp. freshly ground pepper
1 c. panko breadcrumbs

Directions
1. Set oven at 425 degrees. At the same time, take a large bowl and toss garlic, squash, and olive oil for coating. Take a baking sheet and roast for about 60 minutes. Then cool it for 20 minutes. Reduce oven to 350 degrees.
2. Then, boil the salted water and cook rigatoni according to package directions. Drain and set aside.
3. Using a blender, purée reserved squash with heavy cream until smooth.
4. Take a large bowl and mix squash puree with reserved rigatoni, 2 cups fontina, sage, salt, and pepper. Apply olive oil on the sides of the baking pan. Transfer rigatoni-squash mixture to plate.
5. Take a small bowl, combine the remaining fontina and panko. Sprinkle over pasta and bake until golden brown, 20 to 25 minutes.

LUNCH Recipes
1. Veggie Quesadillas with Cilantro Yogurt Dip

Ingredients
- 1 cup beans, black or pinto
- 2 Tablespoons cilantro, chopped
- ½ bell pepper, finely chopped
- ½ cup corn kernels
- 1 cup low-fat shredded cheese
- Six soft corn tortillas
- One medium carrot, shredded
- ½ jalapeno pepper, finely minced (optional)
- CILANTRO YOGURT DIP
- 1 cup plain nonfat yogurt
- 2 Tablespoons cilantro, finely chopped
- Juice from ½ of a lime

Instructions
1. Preheat large skillet over low heat.
2. Line up three tortillas. Spread cheese, corn, beans, cilantro, shredded carrots, and peppers over the tortillas.
3. Cover each side with a 2nd tortilla.
4. Place a tortilla on a dry plate and heat until cheese is melted and tortilla is slightly golden after 3 minutes.
5. Flip and cook another side until golden, about 1 minute.
6. In a small bowl, mix the nonfat yogurt, cilantro, and lime juice.
7. Cut each quesadilla into four wedges (12 wedges total) and serve three wedges per person with about ¼ cup of the dip.
8. Refrigerate leftovers within 2 hours.

Yogurt With Almonds & Honey

Ingredients
Non-fat greek yoghurt-Nonfat, plain-16 oz-453 grams
Almonds-Nuts, raw-1/4 cup, whole-35.8 grams
Honey-2 tsp-14.1 grams

Directions
Rough-chop almonds and mix into yogurt and honey. Enjoy!

Nutrition
Calories 517 Carbs 36g Fat 20g Protein 54g Fiber 5g Net carbs 31g Sodium 164mg Cholesterol 23mg

Quick Buffalo Chicken Salad

Ingredients
Pepper or hot sauce-Ready-to-serve-4 tbsp-57.6 grams
Canned chicken-No broth-1 cup-205 grams
Spinach-Raw-2 cup-60 grams
Tomatoes-Green, raw-Two medium-246 grams

Directions
Mix hot sauce with chicken. Spread spinach and tomatoes on the top. Toss together and enjoy it!

Nutrition
Calorie 456 Carbs 18g Fat 18g Protein 57g Fiber 4g Net carbs 13g Sodium 2590mg Cholesterol 103mg

All American Tuna

Ingredients
Tuna-Fish, light, canned in water, drained solids-Two can-330 grams
Light mayonnaise-Salad dressing, light-2 tbsp-30 grams
Celery-Cooked, boiled, drained, without a salt-1/4 cup, diced-37.5 grams
Pickles-Cucumber, dill or kosher dill-One large (4" long)-135 grams
Wheat bread-Two slice-50 grams
Directions
Mix all ingredients in a bowl.
Serve with bread.
Nutrition
Calories 512 Carbs 32g Fat 12g Protein 71g Fiber 4g Net carbs 28g Sodium 2443mg
Cholesterol 124mg

Pimento Cheese Sandwich
Ingredients
Pimento cheese-Pasteurized process-2 oz-56.7 grams
Multi-grain bread-Four slices regular-104 grams
Directions
Spread the pimento cheese over the bread.
Then, a slice of bread to form a sandwich. Enjoy!
Nutrition
Calories 488 Carbs 46g Fat 22g Protein 26g Fiber 8g Net carbs 38g Sodium 915mg
Cholesterol 53mg

Coconut Oil Fat Bombs
Ingredients
Coconut oil-1 1/2 tbsp-20.8 grams
Cocoa-Dry powder, unsweetened-3/4 tbsp-4.1 grams
Honey-5/16 tsp-2 grams
Salt-Table-1/8 tsp-0.57 grams
Directions
Mix all the ingredients in a processor until the mixture is smooth and creamy.
Pour into small-sized ice cube trays or silicone moulds and freeze.
Once frozen, pop the coconut oil fat bombs out of the images and store them in a freezer zip-top bag or jar. Enjoy!
Nutrition
Calories 194 Carbs 4g Fat 21g Protein 1g Fiber 2g Net carbs 3g Sodium 222mg Cholesterol 0mg

Apricot Jam And Almond Butter Sandwich
Ingredients
Multi-grain bread-Two slices regular-52 grams
Jams and preserves-1 tbsp-20 grams
Almond butter-Nuts, every day, without salt, added-1 tbsp-16 grams
Directions
Toast the bread optionally.
Spread almond butter on one side and jam on another side.
Nutrition
Calories 292 Carbs 39g Fat 11g Protein 10g Fiber 6g Net carbs 34g Sodium 206mg
Cholesterol 0mg

Peanut Butter And Honey Toast
Ingredients
Multi-grain bread-Two slices regular-52 grams
Peanut butter-Smooth style, without salt-3 tbsp-48 grams
Honey-2 tbsp-42 grams
Directions
Toast the bread, and it is optionally.
Spread peanut butter on the bread and sprinkle with honey. Enjoy!
Nutrition
Calories 553 Carbs 68g Fat 27g Protein 18g Fiber 6g Net carbs 62g Sodium 208mg
Cholesterol 0mg

Cucumber & Hummus
Ingredients
Hummus-Commercial-1/4 cup-61.5 grams
Cucumber-With peel, raw-1 cup slices-104 grams
Directions
Cut the cucumber into round slices and eat with hummus.
Nutrition
Calories 118 Carbs13gFat6g Protein6gFiber4gNet carbs8g Sodium235mg Cholesterol0mg

Carrot And Hummus Snack
Ingredients
Hummus-Commercial-2 tbsp-30 grams
Baby carrots-Baby, raw-1 cup-246 grams
Directions
Dip carrots into hummus and enjoy!
Nutrition
Calories136Carbs25gFat3g Protein4gFiber9gNet carbs16g Sodium306mg Cholesterol0mg

Yogurt With Walnuts & Honey
Ingredients
Walnuts-Nuts, black, dried-1/4 cup, chopped-31.3 grams
Non-fat greek yoghurt-Nonfat, plain-480cup-480 grams
Honey-2 tsp-14.1 gram
Directions
Rough-chop walnuts and mix into yogurt.
Top with honey and enjoy!
Nutrition
Calories520Carbs32gFat20g Protein56gFiber2gNet carbs30g Sodium174mg Cholesterol24mg

Simple Caprese Sandwich
Ingredients
● Sourdough bread
French or Vienna
Two slices
192 grams

- Mozzarella cheese
Whole milk
2 oz
56.7 grams
- Tomatoes
Red, ripe, raw, year-round average
Four slices, medium (1/4" thick)
80 grams
Cut a large slice of sourdough in half (or use two small slices). Top one slice with 1oz of sliced mozzarella and then two slices of tomatoes. The flavor is mild, so season with salt pepper if desired.
Calories707Carbs104gFat17g Protein34gFiber5gNet carbs99g Sodium1515mg Cholesterol45mg

Cottage Cheese Honey Toast

Ingredients
Whole-wheat bread-Commercially prepared-Two slice-56 grams
Cottage cheese- 1% milkfat-1 cup, (not packed)-226 grams
Honey-2 tbsp-42 grams
Directions
Toast bread to your liking. Spread with cottage cheese and drizzle with honey. Enjoy
Nutrition
Calories432Carbs65gFat4g Protein35gFiber3gNet carbs61g Sodium1174mg Cholesterol9mg

Pimento Cheese Sandwich

Ingredients
Pimento cheese-Pasteurized process-2 oz-56.7 grams
Multi-grain bread-Four slices regular-104 grams
Directions
Spread the pimento cheese on each side of bread. And then on the other slice of bread to form a sandwich. Enjoy!
Nutrition
Calories488Carbs46gFat22g Protein26gFiber8gNet carbs38g Sodium915mg Cholesterol53mg

Tomato Salad

Ingredients
Vinegar-Cider-2 2/3 tbsp-39.4 grams
Cucumber-Peeled, raw-Two medium-402 grams
Onions-Raw-1/2 large-75 grams
Tomatoes-Red, ripe, fresh, year-round average
Three medium whole (2-3/5" dia)-369 grams
Water-Plain, clean water-1/2 cup-118 grams
Directions
Peel and slice cucumbers into coins. Cut tomatoes into pieces. Dice red onion. Add vinegar and water and mix well.
Nutrition
Calories153Carbs31gFat1g Protein6gFiber9gNet carbs22g Sodium32mg Cholesterol0mg

Tomato And Cheese Wrap

Ingredients
Tortillas-2 tortilla -92 grams
mayonnaise-like dressing-Regular, with salt-2 tbsp-29.4 grams
Tomatoes-Two medium whole -246 grams
Lettuce-2 cup shredded-144 grams
Cheddar cheese-2 oz-56.7 grams
Directions
Lightly spread mayo on tortilla shell.
Cut tomatoes however you like them.
Layer ingredients, spreading them over the tortilla. Tuck up about an inch the side of the shell you've decided is the bottom and roll up the wrap. Enjoy!
Nutrition
Calories638Carbs66gFat32g Protein25gFiber7gNet carbs59g Sodium1236mg Cholesterol63mg

Peanut Butter Yogurt

Ingredients
Nonfat greek yogurt-1 cup-240 grams
Peanut butter-2 tbsp-32 grams
Vanilla extract-1 tsp-2.2 grams
Directions
Combine ingredients and enjoy it!
Nutrition
Calories345Carbs16gFat17g Protein32gFiber2gNet carbs15g Sodium223mg Cholesterol12mg

Peanut Butter & Carrots

Ingredients
Peanut butter-4 tbsp-64 grams
Carrots-2 cup chopped-256 grams
Directions
Spread peanut butter on carrots and enjoy!
Nutrition
Calories482Carbs38gFat33g Protein18gFiber12gNet carbs26g Sodium188mg Cholesterol0mg

Cucumber Tomato Salad With Tuna

Ingredients
Tomatoes-Two medium whole -246 grams
Lettuce-1 cup shredded-36 grams
Cucumber-With peel, raw-One cucumber-301 grams
Tuna-One can-165 grams
Directions
Chop vegetables and lettuce.
Toss together with the tuna and enjoy it!
Calories237Carbs22gFat2g Protein37gFiber5gNet carbs17g Sodium436mg Cholesterol59mg

Peanut Butter And Jelly

Ingredients
Multi-grain bread-Four slices regular-104 grams
Butter-Unsalted-2 tsp-9.5 grams
Peanut butter-Smooth style, without salt-3 tbsp-48 grams
Jams and preserves-2 tbsp-40 grams
Directions
Toast the bread, and it is optionally. Drizzle1/2 teaspoon of butter on each side of the bread.
Spread butter on one side and jam on another side.
Nutrition

Calories742Carbs83gFat37g Protein25gFiber11gNet carbs73g Sodium418mg Cholesterol20mg

Chicken Scampi Pasta

Ingredients
1 pound of thinly-sliced chicken cutlets, cut into 1/2-inch-thick strips
Three tablespoons olive oil
Eight tablespoons unsalted butter, cubed
Six cloves garlic, sliced
1/2 teaspoon crushed red pepper flakes
1/2 cup dry white wine
12 ounces angel hair pasta
One teaspoon lemon zest plus the juice of 1 large lemon
1/2 cup freshly grated Parmesan
1/2 cup chopped fresh Italian parsley

Directions
Take a massive pot of salted water to a boil for the pasta. Sprinkle the chook with a few salts. Heat a massive skillet over medium-high warmth until hot, and then upload the oil. Working in 2 batches, brown the chook until golden however no longer cooked through, 2 to a few minutes in keeping with batch. Remove the chicken to a plate.

Melt four tablespoons of the butter within the skillet. Add the garlic and crimson pepper flakes and cook dinner until the garlic begins to turn golden at the edges, 30 seconds to 1 minute. Add the wine, deliver to a simmer, and cook dinner till reduced by using half, approximately 2 minutes. Remove from the warmth.

Meanwhile, cook dinner the pasta till very al dente, reserving 1 cup of the pasta water. Add the pasta and 3/four cup pasta water to the skillet alongside the hen, lemon zest and juice, and the last four tablespoons butter. Return the skillet to medium-low warmness and gently stir the pasta until the butter is melted, including the ultimate 1/four pasta water if the pasta appears too dry. Remove the skillet from the warmth, sprinkle with the grated cheese and parsley and toss before serving.

DINNER

Chicken & Goat Cheese Skillet

Ingredients
- 1/2 pound of boneless skinless chicken breasts, cut into 1-inch pieces
- 1/4 teaspoon salt
- 1/8 teaspoon pepper
- Two teaspoons olive oil
- 1 cup sliced fresh asparagus (1-inch pieces)
- One garlic clove, minced
- Three plum tomatoes, chopped
- Three tablespoons 2% milk
- Two tablespoons herbed fresh goat cheese, crumbled
- Hot cooked rice or pasta
- Additional goat cheese, optional

Directions
- Toss chicken with salt and pepper. Heat oil at medium heat; saute chicken until no longer pink, 4-6 minutes. Remove from pan; keep warm.
- Add asparagus to skillet; cook and mix at medium-high heat 1 minute. Add garlic; cook and stir 30 seconds. Stir in tomatoes, milk, and two tablespoons cheese; cook, covered, over medium heat until cheese begins to melt, 2-3 minutes. Stir in chicken. Serve with rice. If desired, top with additional cheese.

Nutrition
251 calories, 11g fat, 74mg cholesterol, 447mg sodium, 8g carbohydrate (5g sugars, 3g fiber), 29g protein. Diabetic Exchanges: 4 lean meat, two fat, one vegetable.

Green Curry Salmon With Green Beans

Ingredients
- Four salmon fillets (4 ounces each)
- 1 cup light coconut milk
- Two tablespoons green curry paste
- 1 cup uncooked instant brown rice
- 1 cup reduced-sodium chicken broth
- 1/8 teaspoon pepper
- 3/4 pound fresh green beans, trimmed
- One teaspoon sesame oil
- One teaspoon sesame seeds, toasted
- Lime wedges

Directions
Preheat oven to 400°. Place salmon in an 8-in. Square baking dish. Mix together coconut milk and curry paste; pour over salmon. Bake, uncovered, till fish simply starts offevolved to flake effortlessly with a fork, 15-20 minutes.
Meanwhile, in a small saucepan, integrate rice, broth and pepper; convey to a boil. Reduce warmth; simmer, covered, 5 minutes. Remove from heat; let stand five minutes.
In a big saucepan, area steamer basket over 1 in. Of water. Place inexperienced beans inside the basket; convey water to a boil. Reduce heat to maintain a simmer; steam, covered, till beans are crisp-tender, 7-10 minutes. Toss with sesame oil and sesame seeds. Serve salmon with rice, beans and lime wedges. Spoon coconut sauce over the salmon.

Nutrition Facts
366 calories, 17g fat (5g saturated fat), 57mg cholesterol, 340mg sodium, 29g carbohydrate (5g sugars, 4g fibre), 24g protein.

Chicken Veggie Packets

Ingredients
- Four boneless and skinless chicken breast halves (4 ounces each)
- 1/2 pound sliced fresh mushrooms
- 1-1/2 cups fresh baby carrots
- 1 cup pearl onions
- 1/2 cup julienned sweet red pepper
- 1/4 teaspoon pepper
- Three teaspoons minced fresh thyme
- 1/2 teaspoon salt, optional
- Lemon wedges, optional

Directions
Flatten bird breasts to 1/2-in. Thickness; vicinity every on a bit of heavy-duty foil (about 12 in. Square). Layer the mushrooms, carrots, onions and pink pepper over bird; sprinkle with pepper, thyme and salt if desired.
Fold foil around hen and greens and seal tightly. Place on a baking sheet. Bake at 375° for a half-hour or until chook juices run clear. If desired, serve with lemon wedges.

Nutrition Facts
175 calories, 3g fat (1g saturated fat), 63mg cholesterol, 100mg sodium, 11g carbohydrate (6g sugars, 2g fibre), 25g protein.

Sweet Onion & Sausage Spaghetti

Ingredients
- 6 ounces uncooked whole-wheat spaghetti
- 3/4 pound Italian turkey sausage links, casings removed
- Two teaspoons olive oil
- One sweet onion, thinly sliced
- 1-pint cherry tomatoes halved
- One and a half cup of fresh basil leaves (sliced)
- 1/2 cup half-and-half cream
- Shaved Parmesan cheese, optional

Directions
Cook spaghetti according to directions given. At the same time, in a large nonstick skillet over medium heat, cook sausage in oil for 5 minutes. Add onion; bake 8-10 minutes longer or until meat is no longer pink and onion is tender.
Stir in tomatoes and basil; heat through. Add cream; bring to a boil. Drain spaghetti; toss with sausage mixture. Garnish with cheese if desired.

Nutrition Facts

334 calories, 12g fat (4g saturated fat), 46mg cholesterol, 378mg sodium, 41g carbohydrate (8g sugars, 6g fibre), 17g protein.

Beef And Blue Cheese Penne With Pesto

Ingredients
- 2 cups uncooked whole wheat penne pasta
- Two beef tenderloin steaks (6 ounces each)
- 1/4 teaspoon salt
- 1/4 teaspoon pepper
- 5 ounces of fresh baby spinach (about 6 cups), coarsely chopped
- 2 cups grape tomatoes, halved
- 1/3 cup prepared pesto
- 1/4 cup chopped walnuts
- 1/4 cup crumbled Gorgonzola cheese

Directions
Cook pasta according to package directions. Meanwhile, sprinkle steaks with salt and pepper. Grill steaks, covered, over medium heat. Heat for 5-7 mins on each side or until meat reaches desired doneness.

Drain pasta; transfer to a large bowl. Add spinach, tomatoes, pesto and walnuts; toss to coat. Cut steak into thin slices. Serve pasta mixture with beef; sprinkle with cheese.

Nutrition Facts
532 calories, 22g fat (6g saturated fat), 50mg cholesterol, 434mg sodium, 49g carbohydrate (3g sugars, 9g fibre), 35g protein.

Asparagus Turkey Stir-Fry

Ingredients
- Two teaspoons cornstarch
- 1/4 cup chicken broth
- One tablespoon lemon juice
- One teaspoon soy sauce
- 1 pound of turkey breast tenderloins, cut into 1/2-inch strips
- One garlic clove, minced
- Two tablespoons canola oil, divided
- 1 pound of asparagus, cut into 1-1/2-inch pieces
- One jar (2 ounces) sliced pimientos, drained
- In a small bowl, mix the cornstarch, broth, lemon juice and soy sauce until smooth; set aside. In a large skillet or wok, stir-fry turkey and garlic in 1 tablespoon oil until meat is no longer pink; remove and keep warm.
- Stir-fry asparagus in remaining oil until crisp-tender. Add pimientos. Stir the mixture and add to the pan; cook and stir for 1 minute or until thickened. Return turkey to the pan; heat through.

Nutrition Facts
205 calories, 9g fat (1g saturated fat), 56mg cholesterol, 204mg sodium, 5g carbohydrate (1g sugars, 1g fibre), 28g protein.

Chicken With Celery Root Puree

Ingredients
- Four boneless skinless chicken breast halves (6 ounces each)
- 1/2 teaspoon pepper
- 1/4 teaspoon salt
- Three teaspoons canola oil, divided
- One large celery root, peeled and chopped (about 3 cups)
- 2 cups diced peeled butternut squash
- One small onion, chopped
- Two garlic cloves, minced
- 2/3 cup unsweetened apple juice

Sprinkle chicken with pepper and salt. Take a large skillet and coat with cooking spray, heat two teaspoons oil over medium heat. Brown chicken on both sides. Remove chicken from pan.

Heat the remaining oil over medium-high in the same pan. Add celery root, squash and onion; cook and stir until squash is crisp-tender. Add garlic; cook 1 minute longer.

Return chicken to pan; add apple juice. Bring to a boil. Reduce heat; simmer, covered, 12-15 minutes or until a thermometer inserted in chicken reads 165°. Remove chicken; keep warm. Cool vegetable mixture slightly. Process in a food processor until smooth. Return to pan and heat through. Serve with chicken.

Nutrition Facts
328 calories, 8g fat (1g saturated fat), 94mg cholesterol, 348mg sodium, 28g carbohydrate (10g sugars, 5g fibre), 37g protein.

Apple-Cherry Pork Medallions

Ingredients
- One pork tenderloin (1 pound)
- One teaspoon minced fresh rosemary or 1/4 teaspoon dried rosemary, crushed
- One teaspoon minced fresh thyme or 1/4 teaspoon dried thyme
- 1/2 teaspoon celery salt
- One tablespoon olive oil
- One large apple, sliced
- 2/3 cup unsweetened apple juice
- Three tablespoons dried tart cherries
- One tablespoon honey
- One tablespoon cider vinegar
- One package (8.8 ounces) ready-to-serve brown rice

Cut tenderloin crosswise into 12 slices; sprinkle with rosemary, thyme and celery salt. In a huge skillet, heat oil over medium-excessive heat. Brown pork on both sides; do away with from pan.

In the equal skillet, combine apple, apple juice, cherries, honey and vinegar. Boil it and stirring to loosen browned bits from pan. Reduce warmness; simmer, uncovered, 3-four minutes or just till apple is tender.

Return red meat to the pan, turning to coat with sauce; cook, covered, 3-4 minutes or till red meat is tender. Meanwhile, put together rice in keeping with package deal directions; serve with red meat mixture.

Nutrition Facts

349 calories, 9g fat (2g saturated fat), 64mg cholesterol, 179mg sodium, 37g carbohydrate (16g sugars, 4g fibre), and 25g protein.

Butternut Turkey Soup

Ingredients
- Three shallots, thinly sliced
- One tsp of olive oil
- 3 cups of reduced-sodium chicken broth
- 3 cups of cubed peeled butternut squash (3/4-inch cubes)
- Two medium-sized red potatoes, cut into 1/2-inch cubes
- 1-1/2 cups of water
- Two teaspoons of minced fresh thyme
- 1/2 teaspoon pepper
- Two whole cloves
- 3 cups cubed cooked turkey breast

In a large-size saucepan coated with cooking spray, cook dinner shallots in oil over medium heat till tender. Stir within the broth, squash, potatoes, water, thyme and pepper.

Place spices on a double thickness of cheesecloth; carry up corners of the fabric and tie with string to shape a bag. Stir into soup. Bring to a boil. Reduce warmness; cowl and simmer for 10-15 mins or till vegetables are tender. Stir in turkey; warmth through. Discard spice bag.

Nutrition
192 calories, 2g fat (0 saturated fat), 50mg cholesterol, 332mg sodium, 20g carbohydrate (3g sugars, 3g fibre), 25g protein.

Black Bean & Sweet Potato Rice Bowls

Ingredients
- 3/4 cup uncooked long-grain rice
- 1/4 teaspoon garlic salt
- 1-1/2 cups water
- Three tablespoons olive oil, divided
- One large sweet potato, peeled and diced
- One medium red onion, finely chopped
- 4 cups chopped fresh kale (sturdy stems removed)
- One can (15 ounces) black beans, rinsed and drained
- Two tablespoons sweet chilli sauce
- Lime wedges, optional
- Additional sweet chilli sauce, optional

Place rice, garlic salt and water in a large saucepan; bring to a boil. Reduce heat; simmer, covered until liquid is absorbed and rice is tender 15-20 minutes. Remove from heat; let stand 5 minutes.

At the same time take a large pan and heat two tablespoons oil over medium-high heat; saute sweet potato 8 minutes. Add onion; cook and stir until potato is tender 4-6 minutes. Add kale; cook and stir until tender, 3-5 minutes. Stir in beans; heat through. Gently stir two tablespoons chilli sauce and remaining oil into rice; add to potato mixture. If you want, serve with lime wedges and additional chilli sauce.

Nutrition
435 calories, 11g fat (2g saturated fat), 0 cholesterol, 405mg sodium, 74g carbohydrate (15g sugars, 8g fibre), 10g protein.

Pepper Ricotta Primavera

Ingredients
- 1 cup part-skim ricotta cheese
- 1/2 cup fat-free milk
- Four teaspoons olive oil
- One garlic clove, minced
- 1/2 teaspoon crushed red pepper flakes
- One medium green pepper, julienned
- One medium sweet red pepper, julienned
- One medium fresh yellow pepper, julienned
- One medium zucchini, sliced
- 1 cup frozen peas, thawed
- 1/4 teaspoon dried oregano
- 1/4 teaspoon dried basil
- 6 ounces fettuccine, cooked and drained

Whisk together ricotta cheese and milk; set aside Take a large skillet, heat oil over medium heat. Add garlic and pepper; saute 1 minute. Add the next seven ingredients. Cook and mix over medium heat until vegetables are crisp-tender, about 5 minutes. Add cheese mixture to fettuccine; top with vegetables. Toss to coat. Serve immediately.

Nutrition
229 calories, 7g fat (3g saturated fat), 13mg cholesterol, 88mg sodium, 31g carbohydrate (6g sugars, 4g fibre), 11g protein.

Bow Ties With Sausage & Asparagus

Ingredients
- 3 cups of uncooked whole wheat bow tie pasta (about 8 ounces)
- 1 pound of asparagus, cut into 1-1/2-inch pieces
- One package (19-1/2 ounces) Italian turkey sausage links, casings removed
- One medium onion, chopped
- Three garlic cloves, minced
- 1/4 cup shredded Parmesan cheese
- Additional shredded Parmesan cheese, optional

In a 6-qt. Stockpot, prepare dinner pasta in line with package directions, including asparagus over the last 2-three minutes of cooking. Drain, reserving half cup pasta water; go back pasta and asparagus to the pot. Meanwhile, in a big skillet, cook sausage, onion and garlic over medium heat until no pink, 6-8 minutes, breaking sausage into large crumbles. Add to stockpot. Stir in 1/four cup cheese and reserved pasta water as desired. Serve with additional cheese if desired.

Nutrition
247 calories, 7g fat (2g saturated fat), 36mg cholesterol, 441mg sodium, 28g carbohydrate (2g sugars, 4g fibre), 17g protein

Pork And Balsamic Strawberry Salad

Ingredients

- One pork tenderloin (1 pound)
- 1/2 cup Italian salad dressing
- 1-1/2 cups halved fresh strawberries
- Two tablespoons balsamic vinegar
- Two teaspoons sugar
- 1/4 teaspoon salt
- 1/4 teaspoon pepper
- Two tablespoons olive oil
- 1/4 cup chicken broth
- One package about 5 ounces spring mix salad greens
- 1/2 cup crumbled goat cheese

Place pork in a shallow dish. Add salad dressing; flip for coating. Refrigerate and cover for at least eight hours. Mix strawberries, vinegar and sugar; cover and refrigerate.

Preheat oven to 425°. Drain and wipe off red meat, discarding marinade. Sprinkle with salt and pepper. In a large cast-iron or every other ovenproof skillet, warmness oil over medium-high warmness. Add beef; brown on all sides.

Bake until a thermometer reads 145°, 15-20 minutes. Remove from skillet; permit or stand 5 min. Then, add broth to skillet; cook over medium warmth, stirring to loosen browned bits from pan. Bring to a boil. Reduce warmth; add strawberry. Then heat it.

Place green vegetables on a serving platter; sprinkle with cheese. Slice pork; set up over veggies. Top with strawberry mixture.

Nutrition
291 calories, 16g fat (5g saturated fat), 81mg cholesterol, 444mg sodium, 12g carbohydrate (7g sugars, 3g fibre), 26g protein.

Peppered Tuna Kabobs

Ingredients
- 1/2 cup frozen corn, thawed
- Four green onions, chopped
- One jalapeno pepper, seeded and chopped
- Two tablespoons coarsely chopped fresh parsley
- Two tablespoons lime juice
- 1 pound tuna steaks, cut into 1-inch cubes
- One teaspoon coarsely ground pepper
- Two large sweet red peppers, cut into 2x1-inch pieces
- One medium mango, peeled and cut into 1-inch cubes

For salsa, in a small bowl, combine the first five ingredients; set aside.

Rub tuna with pepper. On 4metal or soaked wooden skewers, alternately thread red peppers, tuna and mango.

Place skewers on greased grill rack. Cook, covered, over medium heat, occasionally turning, until tuna is slightly pink in centre (medium-rare) and peppers are tender 10-12 minutes. Serve with salsa.

Nutrition
205 calories, 2g fat (0 saturated fat), 51mg cholesterol, 50mg sodium, 20g carbohydrate (12g sugars, 4g fibre), 29g protein.

Weeknight Chicken Chop Suey

Ingredients
- Four teaspoons of olive oil
- 1 pound of boneless chicken breast side, cut into 1-inch cubes
- 1/2 teaspoon dried tarragon
- 1/2 teaspoon dried basil
- 1/2 teaspoon dried marjoram
- 1/2 teaspoon grated lemon zest
- 1-1/2 cups chopped carrots
- 1 cup unsweetened pineapple tidbits, drained (reserve juice)
- One can (8 ounces) sliced water chestnuts, drained
- One medium tart apple, chopped
- 1/2 cup chopped onion
- 1 cup cold water, divided
- Three tablespoons unsweetened pineapple juice
- Three tablespoons reduced-sodium teriyaki sauce
- Two tablespoons cornstarch
- 3 cups hot cooked brown rice

In a massive solid iron or some other heavy skillet, heat oil at medium temperature. Add chicken, herbs and lemon zest; leave it until lightly browned. Add the next five ingredients. Stir in 3/four cup water, pineapple juice and teriyaki sauce; bring to a boil. Reduce warmness; simmer covered till chicken is no longer purple, and the carrots are gentle 10-15 minutes.

Combine cornstarch and remaining water. Gradually stir into hen mixture. Leave for boiling; cook and stir till thickened, about 2 minutes. Serve with rice.

Nutrition
330 calories, 6g fat, 42mg cholesterol, 227mg sodium, 50g carbohydrate (14g sugars, 5g fibre), 20g protein

Thai Chicken Pasta Skillet

Ingredients
- 6 ounces uncooked whole-wheat spaghetti
- Two teaspoons canola oil
- One package (10 ounces) fresh sugar snap peas, trimmed and cut diagonally into thin strips
- 2 cups julienned carrots (about 8 ounces)
- 2 cups shredded cooked chicken
- 1 cup Thai peanut sauce
- One medium cucumber, halved lengthwise, seeded and sliced diagonally
- Chopped fresh cilantro, optional

Cook spaghetti according to package directions; drain.

Then, in a large skillet, heat oil a medium-high heat. Add snap peas and carrots; stir-fry 6-8 minutes or until crisp-tender. Add chicken, peanut sauce and spaghetti; heat through, tossing to combine.

Transfer to a serving plate. Top with cucumber and, if desired, cilantro.

Nutrition Facts
403 calories, 15g fat (3g saturated fat), 42mg cholesterol, 432mg sodium, 43g carbohydrate (15g sugars, 6g fibre), 25g protein

Spinach-Orzo Salad With Chickpeas

Ingredients
- One 14-1/2 ounces reduced-sodium chicken broth
- 1-1/2 cups of uncooked whole wheat orzo pasta
- 4 cups of fresh baby spinach
- 2 cups of grape tomatoes, halved
- Two cans (15 ounces each) of chickpeas *or* garbanzo beans, rinsed and drained
- 3/4 cup chopped fresh parsley
- Two green onions, chopped

DRESSING:
- 1/4 cup olive oil
- Three tablespoons lemon juice
- 3/4 teaspoon salt
- 1/4 teaspoon garlic powder
- 1/4 teaspoon hot pepper sauce
- 1/4 teaspoon pepper

Take a large saucepan and bring broth to a boil. Stir in orzo; return to a boil. Reduce heat; simmer, covered, until al dente, 8-10 minutes.
Take a large pan and add spinach and warm orzo, allowing the spinach to wilt slightly. Add tomatoes, chickpeas, parsley and green onions.
Whisk together dressing ingredients. Toss with salad.

Nutrition
122 calories, 5g fat, 0 cholesterol, 259mg sodium, 16g carbohydrate (1g sugars, 4g fibre), 4g protein. Diabetic Exchanges: 1 starch, one fat.

Roasted Chicken Thighs With Peppers & Potatoes

Ingredients
- 2 pounds red potatoes (about six medium)
- Two large sweet red peppers
- Two large green peppers
- Two medium onions
- Two tablespoons olive oil, divided
- Four teaspoons minced fresh thyme or 1-1/2 teaspoons dried thyme, divided
- Three tablespoons minced fresh rosemary or one teaspoon dried rosemary, crushed, divided
- Eight boneless skinless chicken thighs (about 2 pounds)
- 1/2 teaspoon salt
- 1/4 teaspoon pepper
- Preheat oven to 450°. Cut potatoes, peppers and onions into 1-in. Pieces. Place vegetables in a roasting pan. Drizzle with one tablespoon oil; sprinkle with two teaspoons each thyme and rosemary and toss to coat. Place chicken over greens. Brush chicken with remaining oil; sprinkle with remaining thyme and rosemary. Drizzle vegetables and chicken with salt and pepper.
- Roast until a thermometer inserted in chicken reads 170° and green vegetables are tender 35-40 minutes.

Nutrition Facts
308 calories, 12g fat (3g saturated fat), 76mg cholesterol, 221mg sodium, 25g carbohydrate (5g sugars, 4g fibre), 24g protein. Diabetic Exchanges: 3 lean meat, one starch, one vegetable, 1/2 fat.

Spiced Split Pea Soup

Ingredients
- 1 cup dried green split peas
- Two medium potatoes, chopped
- Two medium carrots, halved and thinly sliced
- One medium onion, chopped
- One celery rib, thinly sliced
- Three garlic cloves, minced
- Three bay leaves
- Four teaspoons curry powder
- One teaspoon ground cumin
- 1/2 teaspoon coarsely ground pepper
- 1/2 teaspoon ground coriander
- One carton (32 ounces) reduced-sodium chicken broth
- One can (28 ounces) diced tomatoes, undrained

In a 4-qt. Slow cooker combines the first 12 ingredients. Cook, covered, on low until peas are tender, 8-10 hours.
Stir in tomatoes; heat through. Discard bay leaves.

Nutrition Facts
139 calories, 0 fat (0 saturated fat), 0 cholesterol, 347mg sodium, 27g carbohydrate (7g sugars, 8g fibre), 8g protein. Diabetic Exchanges: 1 starch, one lean meat, one vegetable.

Escarole And Bean Soup

Ingredients
Two tablespoons olive oil
Two chopped garlic cloves
1 pound of escarole, chopped
Salt
4 cups of low-salt broth chicken
1 can of cannellini beans
1 (1-ounce) piece of Parmesan
Freshly ground black pepper
Six teaspoons extra-virgin olive oil

Directions
Heat olive oil in a big heavy pot at normal heat. Add the garlic and sauté till fragrant, for 15 seconds. Add the escarole and sauté till wilted, for 2 min. Add salt. Add the chicken, beans, and then Parmesan cheese. Cover and simmer till the beans are heated through, approximately five minutes — season with salt and pepper, to taste.
Ladle the soup into six bowls. Sprinkle one teaspoon extra-virgin olive oil over each. Serve with crusty bread.

Snacks

Chili-Lime Grilled Pineapple

Ingredients
- 1 fresh pineapple
- 3 tablespoons brown sugar
- 1 tablespoon lime juice
- 1 tablespoon olive oil
- 1 tablespoon honey or agave nectar
- 1-1/2 teaspoons chili powder
- Dash salt

Peel pineapple, removing any eyes from fruit. Cut lengthwise into 6 wedges; remove core. Take a small bowl and mix other ingredients until blended. Brush pineapple with half of the glaze; reserve remaining mixture for basting.
Grill pineapple, covered, over medium heat or broil 4 in. from heat 2-4 minutes on each side or until lightly browned, basting occasionally with reserved glaze.

Nutrition
97 calories, 2g fat (0 saturated fat), 0 cholesterol, 35mg sodium, 20g carbohydrate (17g sugars, 1g fiber), 1g protein.

Spicy Almonds

Ingredients
- 1 tablespoon sugar
- 1-1/2 teaspoons kosher salt
- 1 teaspoon paprika
- 1/2 teaspoon ground cinnamon
- 1/2 teaspoon ground cumin
- 1/2 teaspoon ground coriander
- 1/4 teaspoon cayenne pepper
- 1 large egg white, room temperature
- 2-1/2 cups unbalanced almonds

· Preheat oven to 325°. Take a small bowl, mix the first 7 ingredients. In another small bowl, whisk egg white until foamy. Add almonds; toss to coat. Sprinkle with spice mixture; toss to coat. Spread in a single layer in a greased 15x10x1-in. baking pan. Bake for 30 minutes, stirring every 10 minutes. Spread on waxed paper to cool completely. Store in an airtight container.

Nutrition
1/4 cup: 230 calories, 20g fat (2g saturated fat), 0 cholesterol, 293mg sodium, 9g carbohydrate (3g sugars, 4g fiber), 8g protein.

Italian Sausage-Stuffed Zucchini

Ingredients
- 6 medium sized zucchini (about 8 ounces each)
- 1 pound of Italian turkey sausage links, casings removed
- 2 medium sized tomatoes, seeded and chopped
- 1 cup of panko (Japanese) bread crumbs
- 1/3 cup of grated Parmesan cheese
- 1/3 cup of minced fresh parsley
- 2 tbsp of minced fresh oregano or 2 teaspoons dried oregano
- 2 tablespoons of minced fresh basil or 2 teaspoons dried basil
- 1/4 teaspoon of pepper
- 3/4 cup of shredded part-skim mozzarella cheese
- Additional minced fresh parsley, optional

Set oven at 350°. Cut each zucchini lengthwise in half direction. Tout the pulp, and leave a 1/4-in. Put zucchini shells in a large microwave-safe dish. In batches, microwave, covered, on excessive 2-3 minutes or till crisp-tender.
In a massive skillet, cook dinner sausage and zucchini pulp over medium warmness 6-8 mins or till sausage is not pink, break sausage into crumbles; drain. Mix in tomatoes, bread crumbs, Parmesan cheese, herbs and pepper. Spoon into zucchini shells.
Place in 2 ungreased 13x9-in. Baking dishes. Bake, covered, 15-20 mins or till zucchini is tender. Drizzle with cheese. Bake and uncovered for 5-8 minutes longer or until cheese is melted. If desired, sprinkle with extra minced parsley.

Nutrition
206 calories, 9g fat, 39mg is cholesterol, 485mg sodium, 16g carbohydrate (5g sugars, 3g fiber), 17g protein.

Mimi's Lentil Medley

Ingredients
- 1 cup dried lentils, rinsed
- 2 cups water
- 2 cups sliced fresh mushrooms
- 1 medium cucumber, cubed
- 1 medium zucchini, cubed
- 1 small red onion, chopped
- 1/2 cup chopped soft sun-dried tomato halves (not packed in oil)
- 1/2 cup rice vinegar
- 1/4 cup minced fresh mint
- 3 tablespoons olive oil
- 2 teaspoons honey
- 1 teaspoon dried basil
- 1 teaspoon dried oregano
- 4 cups fresh baby spinach, chopped
- 1 cup (4 ounces) crumbled feta cheese
- 4 bacon strips, cooked and crumbled, optional

Place lentils in a small saucepan. Add water; boil it. Dheat; simmer, covered, 20-25 minutes or until tender. Drain and rinse in cold water.
Transfer to a large bowl. Add mushrooms, cucumber, zucchini, onion and tomatoes. In a small bowl, whisk vinegar, mint, oil, honey, basil and oregano. Drizzle over lentil mixture; toss to coat. Add spinach, cheese and, if desired, bacon; toss to combine.

Nutrition
225 calories, 8g fat (2g saturated fat), 8mg cholesterol, 404mg sodium, 29g carbohydrate (11g sugars, 5g fiber), 10g protein.

Tomato Green Bean Soup

Ingredients
- 1 cup chopped onion
- 1 cup chopped carrots
- 2 teaspoons butter
- 6 cups reduced-sodium chicken or vegetable broth
- 1 pound of fresh green beans, cut into 1-inch pieces
- 1 garlic clove, minced
- 3 cups diced fresh tomatoes
- 1/4 cup minced fresh basil or 1 tablespoon dried basil
- 1/2 teaspoon salt
- 1/4 teaspoon pepper

In a large saucepan, saute onion and carrots in butter for 5 minutes. Stir in the broth, beans and garlic; boil it. Decrease temp; cover and simmer for 20 minutes or until vegetables are tender.
Stir in the tomatoes, basil, salt and pepper. Cover and simmer 5 minutes longer.

Nutrition
1 cup: 58 calories, 1g fat (1g saturated fat), 2mg cholesterol, 535mg sodium, 10g carbohydrate (5g sugars, 3g fiber), 4g protein. **Diabetic Exchanges:** 2 vegetable.

Shrimp Orzo With Feta
Ingredients
- 1-1/4 cups of uncooked whole wheat orzo pasta
- 2 tablespoons olive oil
- 2 garlic cloves, minced
- 2 medium tomatoes, chopped
- 2 tablespoons lemon juice
- 1-1/4 pounds uncooked shrimp (26-30 per pound), peeled and deveined
- 2 tablespoons minced fresh cilantro
- 1/4 teaspoon pepper
- 1/2 cup crumbled feta cheese

Cook orzo according to package directions. A in a large skillet, heat oil over medium heat. Add garlic; cook and stir 1 minute. Add tomatoes and lemon juice. Bring to a boil. Stir in shrimp. Reduce heat; simmer, uncovered, until shrimp turn pink, 4-5 minutes.
Drain orzo. Add orzo, cilantro and pepper to shrimp mixture; heat through. Sprinkle with feta cheese.

Nutrition
406 calories, 12g fat (3g saturated fat), 180mg cholesterol, 307mg sodium, 40g carbohydrate (2g sugars, 9g fiber), 33g protein. **Diabetic Exchanges:** 4 lean meat, 2 starch, 1 fat.

Garden Vegetable Beef Soup
Ingredients
- 1-1/2 of pounds lean ground beef (90% lean)
- 1 medium sized onion, chopped
- 2 garlic cloves, minced
- 1 package of jcarrots
- 2 celery ribs, chopped
- 1/4 cup of tomato paste
- 1 can of diced tomatoes, undrained
- 1-1/2 cups of shredded cabbage
- 1 medium sized zucchini, coarsely chopped
- 1 medium sized red potato (about 5 ounces), finely chopped
- 1/2 cup of fresh or frozen cut green beans
- 1 teaspoon of dried basil
- 1/2 teaspoon of dried oregano
- 1/4 teaspoon of salt
- 1/4 teaspoon of pepper
- 4 cans of reduced-sodium beef broth
- Grated Parmesan cheese, optional

In a 6-qt. sized stockpot, cook beef, onion and garlic over medium heat 6-8 minutes or until beef is no longer pink, breaking up beef into crumbles; drain. Add carrots and celery; cook and stir 6-8 minutes or until tender. Stir in tomato paste; cook 1 minute longer.
Add tomatoes, cabbage, zucchini, potato, green beans, seasonings and broth; bring to a boil. Reduce heat; simmer, covered, 35-45 minutes or until vegetables are tender. If desired, top each serving with cheese.

Nutrition
207 calories, 7g fat (3g saturated fat), 57mg cholesterol, 621mg sodium, 14g carbohydrate (7g sugars, 3g fiber), 21g protein.

Layered Hummus Dip
Ingredients
- 1 carton (10 ounces) hummus
- 1/4 cup finely chopped red onion
- 1/2 cup Greek olives, chopped
- 2 medium tomatoes, seeded and chopped
- 1 large English cucumber, chopped
- 1 cup crumbled feta cheese
- Baked pita chips

Spread hummus into a shallow 10-in. dish. Make layers with onion, olives, tomatoes, cucumber and cheese. Refrigerate until serving. Serve with chips.

Nutrition
88 calories, 5g is fat (2g saturated fat), 5mg is cholesterol, 275mg sodium, 6g is carbohydrate (1g sugars, 2g fiber), 4g protein.

Mango Rice Pudding
Ingredients
- 2 cups water
- 1/4 teaspoon salt
- 1 cup uncooked long grain brown rice
- 1 medium ripe mango
- 1 cupvanillasoymilk
- 2 tablespoons sugar
- 1/2 teaspoon ground cinnamon
- 1 teaspoon vanilla extract
- Chopped peeled mango, optional

In a large heavy saucepan, bring water and salt to a boil; stir in rice. Reduce heat; simmer, covered, 35-40 minutes or until water is absorbed and rice is tender. Meanwhile, peel, seed and slice mango. Mash mango with a potato masher or fork.

Stir milk, sugar, cinnamon and mashed mango into rice. Cook, uncovered, on low 10-15 minutes longer or until liquid is almost absorbed, stirring occasionally.

Remove from heat; stir in vanilla. Serve warm or cold, with chopped mango if desired.

Nutrition
1 cup (calculated without chopped mango): 275 calories, 3g fat (0 saturated fat), 0 cholesterol, 176mg sodium, 58g carbohydrate (20g sugars, 3g fiber), 6g protein.

Fruit & Almond Bites

Ingredients
- 3-3/4 cups sliced almonds, divided
- 1/4 teaspoon almond extract
- 1/4 cup honey
- 2 cups finely chopped dried apricots
- 1 cup finely chopped dried cherries or cranberries
- 1 cup finely chopped pistachios, toasted

Place 1-1/4 cups almonds in a food processor; pulse until finely chopped. Remove almonds to a shallow bowl; reserve for coating.

Add remaining 2-1/2 cups almonds to food processor; pulse until finely chopped. Add extract. While processing, gradually add honey. Remove to a large bowl; stir in apricots and cherries. Divide mixture into 6 portions; shape each into a 1/2-in.-thick roll. Wrap in plastic; refrigerate until firm, about 1 hour.

Unwrap and cut rolls into 1-1/2-in. pieces. Roll half of the pieces in reserved almonds, pressing gently to adhere. Roll remaining half in pistachios. If desired, wrap individually in waxed paper, twisting ends to close. Store in airtight containers, layered between waxed paper if unwrapped.

Nutrition
86 calories, 5g fat 0 cholesterol, 15mg sodium, 10g carbohydrate (7g sugars, 2g fiber), 2g protein. **Diabetic Exchanges:** 1 fat, 1/2 starch.

Peppered Tuna Kabobs

Ingredients
- 1/2 cup of frozen corn, thawed
- 4 green onions, chopped
- 1 jalapeno pepper, seeded and chopped
- 2 tablespoons of coarsely chopped fresh parsley
- 2 tablespoons of lime juice
- 1 pound of tuna steaks, cut into 1-inch cubes
- 1 teaspoon of coarsely ground pepper
- 2 large sized sweet red peppers, cut into 2x1-inch pieces
- 1 medium size mango, peel it and cut into 1-inch cubes

· For making salsa, in a small bowl, combine the first five ingredients; set aside.

· Rub tuna along with pepper. On four metal or soaked wooden skewers, alternately thread red peppers, tuna and mango.

· Place skewers on greased grill rack. Cook, covered, over medium heat, turning occasionally, until tuna is slightly pink in center (medium-rare) and peppers are tender, 10-12 minutes. Serve with salsa.

Nutrition
205 calories, 2g fat (0 saturated fat), 51mg cholesterol, 50mg sodium, 20g carbohydrate (12g sugars, 4g fiber), 29g protein. **Diabetic Exchanges:** 3 lean meat, 1 starch.

Asparagus With Horseradish Dip

Ingredients
- 32 fresh asparagus spears (about 2 pounds), trimmed
- 1 cup reduced-fat mayonnaise
- 1/4 cup grated Parmesan cheese
- 1 tablespoon prepared horseradish
- 1/2 teaspoon Worcestershire sauce

· Place asparagus in a steamer basket and then place in a large saucepan over 1 in. of water. Bring to a boil; cover and steam until crisp-tender, 2-4 minutes. Drain and immediately place in ice water. Drain and pat dry.

· In a small bowl, mix the remaining ingredients. Serve with asparagus.

Nutrition
2 asparagus spears with 1 tablespoon dip: 63 calories, 5g fat (1g saturated fat), 6mg cholesterol, 146mg sodium, 3g carbohydrate (1g sugars, 0 fiber), 1g protein. **Diabetic Exchanges:** 1 fat.

California Quinoa

Ingredients
- 1 tablespoon olive oil
- 1 cup quinoa, rinsed and well drained
- 2 garlic cloves, minced
- 1 medium zucchini, chopped
- 2 cups water
- 3/4 cup of canned garbanzo beans or chickpeas, rinsed and drained
- 1 medium sized tomato, finely chopped
- 1/2 cup crumbled feta cheese
- 1/4 cup finely chopped Greek olives
- 2 tablespoons minced fresh basil
- 1/4 teaspoon pepper

· In a large saucepan, heat oil over medium-high heat. Add quinoa and garlic; cook and stir 2-3 minutes or until quinoa is lightly browned. Stir in zucchini and water; bring to a boil. Reduce heat; simmer, covered, until liquid is absorbed, 12-15 minutes. Stir in remaining ingredients; heat through.

Nutrition
310 calories, 11g fat (3g saturated fat), 8mg cholesterol, 353mg sodium, 42g carbohydrate (3g sugars, 6g fiber), 11g protein. **Diabetic Exchanges:** 2 starch, 1-1/2 fat, 1 lean meat, 1 vegetable.

Raspberry Peach Puff Pancake

Ingredients
- 2 medium peaches, peeled and sliced
- 1/2 teaspoon sugar
- 1/2 cup fresh raspberries

- 1 tablespoon butter
- 3 large eggs, lightly beaten
- 1/2 cup fat-free milk
- 1/8 teaspoon salt
- 1/2 cup all-purpose flour
- 1/4 cup vanilla yogurt

· Preheat oven to 400°. ta small bowl, toss peaches with sugar; gently stir in raspberries.
· Place butter in a 9-in. pie plate; heat in oven until butter is melted, 2-3 minutes. Meanwhile, in a small bowl, whisk eggs, milk and salt until blended; gradually whisk in flour. Remove pie plate from oven; tilt carefully to coat bottom and sides with butter. Immediately pour in egg mixture.
· Bake until pancake is puffed and browned, 18-22 minutes. Remove from oven; serve immediately with fruit and yogurt.

Nutrition
199 calories, 7g fat (3g saturated fat), 149mg cholesterol, 173mg sodium, 25g carbohydrate (11g sugars, 3g fiber), 9g protein. **Diabetic Exchanges:** 1 medium-fat meat, 1 fruit, 1/2 starch, 1/2 fat.

Turkey Medallions With Tomato Salad

Ingredients
- 2 tablespoons olive oil
- 1 tablespoon red wine vinegar
- 1/2 teaspoon sugar
- 1/4 teaspoon dried oregano
- 1/4 teaspoon salt
- 1 medium green pepper, coarsely chopped
- 1 celery rib, coarsely chopped
- 1/4 cup chopped red onion
- 1 tablespoon thinly sliced fresh basil
- 3 medium tomatoes

TURKEY:
- 1 large egg
- 2 tablespoons lemon juice
- 1 cup panko (Japanese) bread crumbs
- 1/2 cup grated Parmesan cheese
- 1/2 cup finely chopped walnuts
- 1 teaspoon lemon-pepper seasoning
- 1 package (20 ounces) turkey breast tenderloins
- 1/4 teaspoon salt
- 1/4 teaspoon pepper
- 3 tablespoons olive oil
- Additional fresh basil

· Whisk together first five ingredients. Stir in green pepper, celery, onion and basil. Cut tomatoes into wedges; cut wedges in half. Stir into pepper mixture.
· Take a shallow bowl, whisk together egg and lemon juice. In another shallow bowl, toss bread crumbs with cheese, walnuts and lemon pepper.
· Cut tenderloins crosswise into 1-in. slices; flatten slices with a meat mallet to 1/2-in. thickness. Sprinkle with salt and pepper. Dip in egg mixture, then in crumb mixture, patting to adhere.
· Take a large skillet, heat 1 tablespoon oil over medium-high heat. Add a third of the turkey; cook until golden brown, 2-3 minutes per side. Repeat twice with remaining oil and turkey. Serve with tomato mixture; sprinkle with basil.

Nutrition
351 calories, 21g fat (3g saturated fat), 68mg cholesterol, 458mg sodium, 13g carbohydrate (4g sugars, 2g fiber), 29g protein.

Skinny Quinoa Veggie Dip

Ingredients
- 2 cans (15 ounces) black beans, rinsed and drained
- 1-1/2 teaspoons ground cumin
- 1-1/2 teaspoons paprika
- 1/2 teaspoon cayenne pepper
- 1-2/3 cups water, divided
- Salt and pepper to taste
- 2/3 cup quinoa, rinsed
- 5 tablespoons lime juice, divided
- 2 medium ripe avocados, peeled and coarsely chopped
- 2 tablespoons plus 3/4 cup sour cream, divided
- 1/4 cup minced fresh cilantro
- 3 plum tomatoes, chopped
- 3/4 cup peeled, seeded and finely chopped cucumber
- 3/4 cup finely chopped zucchini
- 1/4 cup finely chopped red onion
- Cucumber slices

· Pulse beans, cumin, paprika, cayenne and 1/3 cup water in food processor until smooth. Add salt and pepper to taste.
· In a small saucepan, cook quinoa with remaining 1-1/3 cups water according to package directions. Fluff with fork; sprinkle with 2 tablespoons lime juice. Set aside. Meanwhile, mash together avocados, 2 tablespoons sour cream, cilantro and remaining lime juice.
· In a 2-1/2-qt. dish, layer bean mixture, quinoa, avocado mixture, remaining sour cream, tomatoes, chopped cucumber, zucchini and onion. Serve immediately with cucumber slices for dipping, or refrigerate.

Nutrition
65 calories, 3g fat (1g saturated fat), 4mg cholesterol, 54mg sodium, 8g carbohydrate (1g sugars, 2g fiber), 2g protein.

Simple Asparagus Soup

Ingredients
- 1 tablespoon butter
- 1 tablespoon olive oil
- 2 pounds of fresh asparagus and trim it and cut into 1-inch pieces
- 1 medium onion, chopped
- 1 medium carrot, thinly sliced
- 1/2 teaspoon salt
- 1/4 teaspoon pepper
- 1/4 teaspoon dried thyme
- 2/3 cup uncooked long grain brown rice
- 6 cups reduced-sodium chicken broth
- Reduced-fat sour cream, optional

- Salad croutons, optional
· In a 6-qt. pan, melt butter and oil at medium tempreature. Stir in vegetables and seasonings; cook until vegetables are tender, 8-10 minutes, stirring occasionally.
· Stir in rice and broth; bring to a boil. Reduce heat; simmer, covered, until rice is tender, 40-45 minutes, stirring occasionally.
· Puree soup using an immersion blender, or cool slightly and puree soup in batches in a blender. Return to pot and heat through. If desired, serve with sour cream and croutons.
· **Freeze option:** Freeze cooled soup in freezer containers. To use, partially thaw in refrigerator overnight (soup may separate). In a saucepan, reheat to boiling, whisking until blended.
Nutrition
79 calories, 3g fat (1g saturated fat), 3mg cholesterol, 401mg sodium, 11g carbohydrate (2g sugars, 2g fiber), 4g protein.

Brunch Banana Splits
Ingredients
- 4 small bananas, peeled and halved lengthwise
- 2 cups fat-free vanilla Greek yogurt
- 2 small peaches, sliced
- 1 cup fresh raspberries
- 1/2 cup granola without raisins
- 2 tablespoons sliced almonds, toasted
- 2 tablespoons sunflower kernels
- 2 tablespoons honey

· Divide bananas among four shallow dishes. Top with remaining ingredients.
Nutrition
340 calories, 6g fat (1g saturated fat), 0 cholesterol, 88mg sodium, 61g carbohydrate (38g sugars, 9g fiber), 17g protein.

Citrus-Herb Pork Roast
Ingredients
- 3 to 4 pounds boneless pork sirloin roast
- 1 teaspoon of dried oregano
- 1/2 teaspoon of ground ginger
- 1/2 teaspoon of pepper
- 2 medium size onions, cut into thin wedges
- 1 cup and 3 tablespoons of orange juice, divided
- 1 tablespoon of sugar
- 1 tablespoon of white grapefruit juice
- 1 tablespoon of steak sauce
- 1 tablespoon of reduced-sodium soy sauce
- 1 teaspoon of grated orange zest
- 1/2 teaspoon of salt
- 3 tablespoons of cornstarch
- Hot cooked egg noodles
- Minced fresh oregano, optional

· Cut roast in half. In a small bowl, **integrate** the oregano, ginger and pepper; rub over **pork**. In a **massive** nonstick skillet **covered** with cooking spray, brown roast on all sides. Transfer to a 4-qt. gradual cooker; add onions.

· Take a small bowl, combine 1 cup orange juice, sugar, grapefruit juice, steak sauce and soy sauce; pour over top. Cover and cook dinner on low for 4-five hours or till meat is tender. Remove meat and onions to a serving platter; keep warm.
· Skim fats from cooking juices; switch to a small saucepan. Add orange zest and salt. Bring to a boil. Combine cornstarch and the last orange juice until smooth. Gradually stir into the pan. Bring to a boil; cook dinner and stir for 2 minutes or till thickened. Serve with pork and noodles; if desired, sprinkle with clean oregano.
Nutrition
289 calories, 10g fat (4g saturated fat), 102mg cholesterol, 326mg sodium, 13g carbohydrate (8g sugars, 1g fiber), 35g protein. Diabetic Exchanges: 5 lean meat, 1 starch.
QUICK RECIPES

Macaroni And Cheese
Ingredients:
- ½ cup elbow macaroni
- ½ cup water
- 3 tablespoons milk
- salt, to taste
- pepper, to taste
- ¼ cup shredded cheddar cheese
- fresh chive, to decorate

Directions
1. Mix the ingredients macaroni, water and salt in a microwaveable mug.
2. Microwave the mug for 2-3 minutes, and then stir.
3. Add the milk, cheese, salt and pepper, and then mix.
4. Microwave for more 30 sec, stir and garnish with a sprinkle of chives.

Bacon In The Microwave
Ingredients
- Bacon

Preparation:
Lay sheets of kitchen towel on a microwave secure pan.
Lay slices of bacon, don't overlap them!
Top with some other two sheets of kitchen towel.
Cook for 4-6 mins on excessive heat. Check every 30 seconds or so to maintain an eye fixed on it. Cook longer for crispier bacon!

Strawberry Microwave Breakfast Bowl
Ingredients:
- 1/4 cup oat bran
- 2 Tbsp oat flour
- 2 Tbsp buckwheat groats
- 1 Tbsp ground flaxseed
- 1/2 tsp baking powder
- pinch salt
- 1/4 tsp cinnamon
- 1/2 tsp vanilla
- 2 Tbsp unsweetened applesauce
- 1/4 cup almond milk

- 1/2 cup fresh strawberries

Preparation:
1. Mix the oat bran, oat flour, buckwheat grouts, flaxseed, baking powder, salt, and cinnamon.
2. Stir inside the vanilla, applesauce, and almond milk until all of the dry elements are incorporated. Gently fold in the diced strawberries.
3. Spray a microwave ramekin, and pour batter into dish.
4. Heat for 1 min and 30 seconds, or till the pinnacle is set.
5. Let cool for 2-three minutes.

Microwavecinnamonmaple Breakfast Quinoa

Ingredients
- 1/2 cupquinoa
- 1 cup cold water
- 1/2 teaspoon cinnamon + more for garnish
- 2 teaspoons butter
- milk or cream to taste
- maple syrup to taste
- banana slices

Instructions
1. Place quinoa in water and rinse well.
2. Drain quinoa, and then stir in 1 cup cold water, 1/2 teaspoon cinnamon and 1 teaspoon butter.
3. Microwave on high for 4 minutes. Stir and microwave 3 more minutes. Remove from microwave.
4. Cover with foil and sit 2 minutes. Fluff quinoa and stir in remaining butter. Divide between 2 bowls
5. Top with milk, cinnamon, maple syrup and banana slices to taste.

Mug Banana Bread

Ingredients
- 3 T. and 1 t. flour (all-purpose)
- 1 packet of stevia
- 2 tablespoon of brown sugar
- 1/8 tsp. of salt
- 1/8 tsp. of baking powder
- 1/8 tsp. of baking soda
- 1 egg
- 1/4 t. of vanilla extract
- 1 T. of vegetable oil
- 1 T. of low fat milk
- Half a banana, mashed
- Cinnamon, for sprinkling (optional)

Preparation
- In a big microwaveable mug lightly misted with non-stick spray, mixture flour, sugars, salt, baking powder & baking soda. Add egg & mix until all of the dry elements are incorporated. Stir in vanilla, oil & milk, then mashed banana. Microwave 1-half minutes to three minutes, depending in your microwave.
- You can prevent it & peek within the door at ninety seconds to test if it's done - it'll probably upward thrust over the pinnacle of the mug as it's heating, & if it's nonetheless runny it's no longer executed yet. But be careful not to overcook! I even have a pretty awful microwave, and mine took about 2 1/2 minutes

Second English Muffin

Ingredients
- 1/4 cup almond meal
- 1/2 tablespoon melted butter
- 1 egg
- 1/8 teaspoon baking powder
- A pinch of salt

Preparation
Mix all ingredients in a small bowl and spray cooking on the sides of the bowl and then microwave it for 90 seconds. Then take out bowl from the oven and scoop out the muffin. Leave it for cooling about 1 min and then cut it into pieces. Then you can top it, stuff it, eat it plain do whatever your little heart desires.

Chocolate Chip Pecan Mug Cake

Ingredients
- 1/3 cup whole wheat flour
- 1/4 tsp baking soda
- 1/4 tsp salt
- 1 egg
- 3 tbsp maple syrup
- 1/4 tsp vanilla extract
- 2 tbsp pecans
- 1 tbsp chocolate chips

Instructions
- Mix the ingredients flour, baking soda and salt in a microwave-safe mug; stir.
- Add egg, syrup and vanilla extract and mix with a fork.
- Stir in pecans and chocolate chips--stir everything together REALLY well.
- Microwave for approximately 1 minute and 20 seconds***
- Drizzle with extra maple syrup and enjoy!

Spiced Pumpkin Molten Mug Cake

Ingredients
- 4 tbsp of flour
- 1 1/2 tbsp of sugar
- 1/3 tsp of baking powder
- 1/2 tsp of mixed spice or pumpkin spice
- 1/4 tsp of cinnamon
- 1/2 tbsp of oil
- 2 tbsp of canned pumpkin/cooked pureed pumpkin
- 2 tbsp of milk
- 1 tbsp of Bis coff spread
- whipping cream

Directions
Mix all dry ingredients in a medium sized mug with a fork.
Then, add pumpkin, oil and milk and mix till properly combined.
Drop a tablespoon of Biscoff spread right within the middle.

Microwave on high for 70 seconds.
Top with a dollop of whipped cream.

Minute Microwave Cheesecake
Ingredients
- 2 ounces of cream cheese, softened
- 2 Tbsp of sour cream
- 1 egg
- ½ tsp of lemon juice
- ¼ tsp of vanilla
- 2-4 Tbsp of sugar replacement sub (taste as you go)

Preparation
Mix all ingredients thoroughly in a bowl. Cook on excessive heat for 90 seconds, stirring each 30 seconds incorporating all ingredients. Refrigerate until serving.
Optional: Top with clean fruit, whipped cream and nut meal.

Granola Cereal Bars
Ingredients
- 1/2 cup packed brown sugar
- 1/2 cup creamy peanut butter
- 1/4 cup light corn syrup
- 1 teaspoon vanilla extract
- 2 cups old-fashioned oats
- 1-1/2 cups crisp rice cereal
- 1/4 cup miniature chocolate chips

Preparation
In a microwave-safe bowl, combine the brown sugar, peanut butter and corn syrup; cover and microwave on high for 2 minutes or until mixture comes to a boil, stirring once. Stir in the vanilla; add oats and cereal. Fold in chocolate chips. Press into a 9-in. square pan coated with cooking spray. Cool and cut into bars.

Bart's Black Bean Soup For Two
Ingredients
- 3/4 cup of canned black beans, rinsed and drained
- 3/4 cup chicken broth
- 1/3 cup salsa
- 1/4 cup whole kernel corn
- Dash hot pepper sauce
- 1 teaspoon lime juice
- 1/2 cup Kerry gold shredded cheddar cheese
- 1 tablespoon green onion

Preparation
In a microwave-safe bowl, combine the first five ingredients. Cover and microwave on high for 2 min or until heated through. Pour into two serving bowls; drizzle each with lime juice. Sprinkle with cheese and green onions.

Microwave Egg Sandwich
Ingredients
- 1 piece Canadian bacon
- 1/4 cup egg substitute
- 1 tablespoon salsa
- 1 tablespoon shredded reduced-fat cheddar cheese
- 1 whole wheat English muffin, split, toasted
- 3 spinach leaves

Preparation
Place Canadian bacon on backside of a 6-ounces. Custard cup coated with cooking spray. Pour egg replacement over top. Microwave, uncovered, on excessive for 30 seconds; stir. Microwave 15-30 seconds or till egg is almost set. Top with salsa; sprinkle with cheese. Microwave just till cheese is melted, approximately 10 seconds.
Line bottom of English muffin with spinach. Place egg and Canadian bacon over spinach; update English muffin top.

Microwave Parmesan Chicken
Ingredients
- 2 boneless skinless chicken breast halves (4 ounces each)
- 4 teaspoons reduced-sodium soy sauce
- 1/4 teaspoon garlic powder
- 1/8 teaspoon pepper
- 1/4 cup grated Parmesan cheese
- 1 teaspoon butter

Preparation
Place chicken in a microwave-safe dish. Top with soy sauce, garlic powder and pepper. Sprinkle with cheese and dot with butter. Cover and cook on high tempreature for 4-5 minutes or until a thermometer reads 170°.

Salmon With Tarragon Sauce
Ingredients
- 4 salmon fillets (6 ounces each)
- 1/4 teaspoon salt
- 1/4 teaspoon white pepper
- 2 tablespoons white wine or chicken broth
- 1 tablespoon butter
- 1 green onion, finely chopped
- 1 tablespoon all-purpose flour
- 1 teaspoon Dijon mustard
- 1/2 teaspoon dried tarragon
- 2/3 cup 2% milk

Preparation
- Place salmon in a greased 2-qt. microwave-safe dish; sprinkle with salt and pepper. Pour wine over top. Cover and microwave on high tempreature for 4-6 minutes or until fish flakes easily with a fork. Remove salmon and keep warm.
- Add butter and onion to the pan juices; cover and microwave on high for 1 minute. Stir in the flour, mustard and tarragon until blended; gradually stir in milk. Cook, uncovered for 1-2 minutes or until thickened; stirring every 30 seconds. Serve with salmon.

Coconut Acorn Squash
Ingredients
- 2 small acorn squash
- 1/4 cup mango chutney
- 1/4 cup sweetened shredded coconut
- 3 tablespoons butter, melted

- 1/4 teaspoon salt
- 1/8 teaspoon pepper

Preparation
- Cut each squash in half; then remove and discard seeds. Place squash in a dish, cut side down. Microwave, and covered, on high tempreature for 10-12 minutes or until tender.
- Turn squash cut side up. Mix chutney, coconut and melted butter; spoon into centers of squash. Sprinkle with salt and pepper. Microwave and covered, on high tempreature for 2-3 minutes or until heated through.

Microwave Peanut Butter And Jam Brownies

Ingredients
- 75g of butter, and a little extra for greasing
- 50g of peanut butter
- Only 1 egg
- 25g of cocoa powder
- 50g of plain flour
- 100g of sugar
- Few tsp of jam

Preparation
- Add the butter and peanut butter to a microwave-secure bowl and cook on High for 30 secs to soften. Remove from the microwave and stir thoroughly. Allow to chill slightly then add the egg and stir to combine. Grease with butter and line a 2d microwaveable round dish (about 15cm wide) with dangle film. Tip the peanut butter blend into the covered dish then sieve within the cocoa powder and flour and tip within the sugar. Mix lightly to shape a thick, sticky paste. Smooth the top of the combination with the lower back of a massive spoon.
- Using a teaspoon, make crater-holes inside the pinnacle of the brownie combination and fill every generously with jam as it will soften and bubble down whilst cooked. Pop in the microwave for 3-four minutes on High. Remove and depart to cool for 15 minutes (it will keep on cooking because it cools) then enjoy!

Sweet & Spicy Popcorn

Ingredients
- 100g bag salted microwave popcorn
- ¼ tsp chili powder
- ½ tsp cinnamon
- 1 tbsp agave syrup

Preparation
Cook the microwave popcorn according to the packet instructions. Tip into a large bowl. Sprinkle over the spices, and then pour over the agave syrup. Stir and serve warm or pour into a bag and take to work as an afternoon snack.

Fastest Ever Lemon Pudding

Ingredients
- 100g caster sugar
- 100g softened butter
- 100g self-raising flour
- 2 eggs
- Zest of 1 lemon
- 1 tsp essence (vanilla)
- 4 tbsp of lemon curd
- Crème fraîche or ice cream, to serve

Preparation
- Mix the sugar, butter, flour, eggs, lemon zest and vanilla together until creamy, then spoon right into a medium microwave-proof baking dish. Microwave on High for 3 mins, turning halfway via cooking, till risen and set all the way via. Leave to stand for 1 min.
- Meanwhile, warmness the lemon curd for 30 secs within the microwave and stir till smooth. Pour throughout the pinnacle of the pudding and serve with a dollop of crème fraîche or scoops of ice cream

DESSERT RECIPES

Almond And Apricot Biscotti

Ingredients
- 3/4 cup of whole-wheat (whole-meal) flour
- 3/4 cup of all-purpose (plain) flour
- 1/4 cup of firmly packed brown sugar
- 1 teaspoon of baking powder
- 2 eggs and beat them
- 2 tablespoons of 1% low-fat milk
- 2 tablespoons of canola oil
- 2 tablespoons of dark honey
- 1/2 teaspoon of almond extract
- 2/3 cup of chopped dried apricots
- 1/4 cup of coarsely almonds and chop them

Directions
Heat the oven to 350 F.
In a big bowl, integrate the ingredients flours, brown sugar and baking powder. Whisk to blend. Then, add the eggs, canola oil, milk, almond and honey extract. Mix with the help of wooden spoon till the dough just starts offevolved to come back together. And then, add the chopped almonds and apricots. With floured hands, stir till the dough is mixed.
Then, place the dough on a long sheet of plastic wrap and shape through hand into a flattened log 12 inches long, three inches wide and approximately 1 in high. Lift up the plastic wrap to invert the dough onto a nonstick baking sheet. Bake till lightly browned, 25 to 30 minutes. Transfer to any other baking sheet to cool for 10 minutes. Leave the oven set at 350 F.
Place the cooled go browsing a slicing board. With a serrated knife, reduce crosswise on the diagonal into 24 slices half inch huge. Arrange the slices, cut-facet down, at the baking sheet. Back to the oven and bake till crisp, 15 to twenty minutes. Transfer to a cord rack and permit cool completely. Store in an airtight container.

Nutrition
Calories75 Total fat2 g Cholesterol15 mg Sodium17 mg Total carbohydrate12 g Dietary fiber1 g Total sugars6 g Added sugars2 g Protein2 g

Ambrosia With Coconut And Toasted Almonds

Ingredients
- 1/2 cup of slivered almonds
- 1/2 cup of unsweetened shredded coconut
- 1 small of pineapple, cubed (about 3 cups)
- 5 oranges
- 2 red apples
- 1 banana, and halved it lengthwise, peeled and sliced crosswise
- 2 tablespoons of cream sherry
- Fresh mint leaves for garnishing

Instructions
Set the oven at 325 F. Spread the almonds on a baking sheet and bake, stirring occasionally, till golden and fragrant, approximately 10 minutes. Transfer at once to a plate to cool. Add the coconut to the sheet and bake, stirring often, till lightly browned, about 10 minutes. Transfer immediately to a plate to cool.
In a large bowl, integrate the pineapple, oranges, apples, banana and sherry. Toss gently to combine well. Divide the fruit combination lightly among character bowls. Sprinkle calmly with the toasted almonds and coconut and garnish with the mint. Serve at once.

Nutrition
Calories177 Cholesterol0 mg Sodium2 mg Dietary fiber6 g Total sugars21 g Added sugars0 g Protein3 g

Apple-Berry Cobbler

Ingredients
- 1 cup of fresh raspberries
- 1 cup of fresh blueberries
- 2 cups of chopped apples
- 2 tablespoons of turbinado or brown sugar
- 1/2 teaspoon of ground cinnamon
- 1 teaspoon of lemon zest
- 2 teaspoons of lemon juice
- 1 1/2 tablespoons of corn-starch

For the topping:
- Take Egg white portion from 1 large egg
- 1/4 cup of soy milk
- 1/4 teaspoon of salt
- 1/2 teaspoon of vanilla
- 1 1/2 tablespoons of brown sugar
- 3/4 cup of wholewheat pastry flour

Instructions
Set the oven at 350 F. Lightly coat 6 man or woman ovenproof ramekins with cooking spray.
In a medium bowl, upload the raspberries, blueberries, apples, sugar, cinnamon, lemon zest and lemon juice. Stir to combine evenly. Add the corn-starch and stir until the cornstarch dissolves. Set aside.
In a separate bowl upload the egg white and whisk till lightly mixed. Then, add the soy milk, salt, vanilla, sugar and pastry flour. Stir to mix well.
Divide the berry mixture evenly amongst the prepared dishes. Pour the topping over each. Arrange the ramekins on a large baking pan and area in oven. Bake until the berries are tender and the topping is golden brown, approximately 30 minutes. Serve warm.

Nutrition
Calories136 Cholesterol0 mg Sodium111 mg Total carbohydrate31 g Dietary fiber4 g Added sugars7 g Protein3 g

Apple-Blueberry Cobbler

Ingredients
- 2 large apples, peel them, sliced them
- 1 tablespoon of lemon juice
- 2 tablespoons of sugar
- 2 tablespoons of cornstarch
- 1 teaspoon of ground cinnamon
- 12 ounces of fresh blue-berries

For the topping
- 3/4 cup of all-purpose flour
- 3/4 cup of whole-wheat flour
- 2 tablespoons of sugar
- 1 1/2 teaspoons of baking powder
- 1/4 teaspoon of salt
- 4 tablespoons of cold trans-free margarine, cut into pieces
- 1/2 cup of fat-free milk
- 1 teaspoon of vanilla

Instructions
Set the oven at 400 F. Coat a 9-in square baking dish with cooking spray.
In a large bowl, add the apple slices. Sprinkle with lemon juice. In a small bowl, integrate the sugar, cornstarch and cinnamon. Add the aggregate to the apples and toss gently to mix. Stir within the blueberries. Spread the apple-blueberry combination evenly within the organized baking dish. Set aside.
In another large bowl, integrate the flours, sugar, baking powder and salt. Using a fork, cut the bloodless margarine into the dry ingredients till the combination resembles coarse crumbs. Then, add the milk and vanilla. Mix just until a moist dough forms. With floured hands, knead gently 6 to eight times till the dough is clean and manageable. Usea rolling pin, and roll the dough into a rectangle 1/2-inch thick. Use a cookie cutter to reduce out shapes. Cut near collectively for at the least scraps. Together the scraps and roll out to make extra cuts.
Place the dough pieces on the apple-blueberry mixture till the top is covered. Bake till the apples are soft and the topping is golden, approximately 30 minutes. Serve warm.

Nutrition
Calories222 Total fat6 g Sodium202 mg Total carbohydrate38 g Dietary fiber4 g Added sugars6 g Protein4 g

Baked Apples With Cherries And Almonds

Ingredients

- 1/3 cup of dried cherries, chopped
- 3 tablespoons of chopped almonds
- 1 tablespoon of wheat germ
- 1 tablespoon of firmly packed brown sugar
- 1/2 teaspoon of ground cinnamon
- 1/8 teaspoon of nutmeg
- 6 small Golden apples, about 1 and 3/4 pounds of total weight
- 1/2 cup of apple juice
- 1/4 cup of water
- 2 tablespoons of dark honey
- 2 teaspoons of walnut oil

Directions

Set the oven at 350 F temperatures.
Take a small bowl; toss the cherries, almonds, wheat germ, brown sugar, cinnamon and nutmeg until all of the substances are distributed evenly. Set them aside. The apples can be left unpeeled, if you like. To peel the apples in a decorative fashion, with a vegetable peeler or a pointy knife, put off the peel from every apple in a circular motion, skipping every different row in order that rows of peel alternate with rows of apple flesh. Working from the stem end, core every apple, stopping 3/4 inch from the bottom.
Divide the cherry aggregate frivolously a number of the apples, pressing the aggregate lightly into each hole. Arrange the apples upright in a heavy ovenproof frying pan or small baking dish just huge sufficient to hold them. Pour down the apple juice and water into the pan. Drizzle the honey and oil frivolously over the apples, and cowl the pan snugly with aluminum foil. Bake till the apples are tender while pierced with a knife, 50 to 60 minutes.
Transfer the apples to man or woman plates and drizzle with the pan juices. Serve heat or at room temperature.

Nutrition

Calories200 Total fat4 g Cholesterol0 mg Sodium7 mg Total carbohydrate39 g Dietary fiber5 g Total sugars31 g Added sugars8 g Protein2 g

Grilled Angel Food Cake

Ingredients
- 1 1/2 cup of strawberries, chopped
- 3/4 cup of chopped rhubarb
- 1/2 cup of sugar
- 6 tablespoons of water
- 1 3/4 teaspoons of vanilla
- 1/8 teaspoon of cinnamon
- 1 prepared angel food cake and cut it into 6 pieces
- 3/4 cup of reduced-fat whipped for topping

Instructions

Set a hot fire in a charcoal grill or warmness a gasoline grill or broiler. Away from the heat source, coat the grill rack or broiler pan with cooking spray. Position the cooking rack four to 6 inches from the warmth source.
To make the sauce, in a saucepan, integrate the strawberries, rhubarb, sugar, water, vanilla and cinnamon. Cook on medium warmth until the aggregate simply starts offevolved to boil, approximately five minutes. Remove the saucepan from the warmth and set aside.
Place the angel meals cake closer to the edge of the grill rack where there is much less warmth or on the broiler pan. Grill or broil till each facet turns brown, about 1 to a few minutes.
Place the angel meals cake on individual serving plates. Top each piece with 1/four cup of the strawberry-rhubarb sauce and 2 tablespoons of the whipped topping. Serve immediately.

Nutrition

Cholesterol0 mgCalories180 Sodium214 mg Total fat1 g Dietary fiber1 g Added sugars17 g Protein2 g

Grilled Fruit With Balsamic Vinegar Syrup

Ingredients
- 1 small sized pineapple, peeled, cored and cut into 4 wedges
- 2 large sized mangoes, cored and cut in half
- 2 large sized peaches, cored and cut in half
- cooking spray butter-flavored
- 2 tablespoons of brown sugar
- 1/2 cup of balsamic vinegar
- Mint leaves for garnishing

Directions

In a big bowl, integrate the pineapple, mangoes and peaches. Spray generously with cooking spray. Toss and spray again to make sure the fruit is well-coated. Sprinkle with brown sugar. Toss to coat evenly. Set aside.
In a small saucepan, heat the balsamic vinegar over low warmth. Simmer until the liquid is decreased in half, stirring occasionally. Remove from the warmth. Prepare a hot hearth in a charcoal grill or warmness a gas grill or broiler. Away from the warmth source, gently coat the grill rack with cooking spray. Place the cooking rack 4 to 6 in. from the heat source. Place the fruit on the grill rack. Grill over medium warmth till the sugar caramelizes, about 3 to five minutes.
Remove the fruit from the grill and arrange onto individual serving plates. Drizzle with balsamic vinegar and garnish it with mint or basil. Serve immediately.

Nutrition

Calories208 Protein1 g Cholesterol0 mg Total carbohydrate50 g Dietary fiber4 g Sodium9 mg Added sugars12 g

Grilled Pineapple

Ingredients
For marinating
- 2 tablespoons of dark honey
- 1 tablespoon of olive oil
- 1 tablespoon of fresh lime juice
- 1 teaspoon of ground cinnamon
- 1/4 teaspoon of ground cloves
- 1 ripeed pineapple

- 8 wooden skewers, and soak them in water for 30 min, or metal skewers
- 1 tablespoon dark rum
- 1 tablespoon of lime zest

Instructions

Set hot fire in a charcoal grill or broiler (grill). Away from the warmth source, gently coat the grill rack or broiler pan with cooking spray. Position the cooking rack four to six inches from the warmth source.
For marination, in a small bowl, mix the lime juice, honey, olive oil, cinnamon and cloves and mix to mix. Set them apart.
Cut off the leaves and the bottom of the pine-apple. place the pineapple upright and, using a large, sharp knife, pare off the skin, cutting downward just under the floor in lengthy, vertical strips and leaving the small brown "eyes" on the fruit. Lay the pineapple on its facet. Align the knife blade with the diagonal rows of eyes, cut a shallow furrow, following a spiral pattern across the pineapple, to eliminate all of the eyes. place the peeled pineapple upright and cut it in half of lengthwise. Place each pineapple 1/2 cut-facet down and cut it lengthwise into 4 lengthy wedges; slice away the core. Cut every wedge crosswise into 3 portions. Thread the 3 pineapple portions onto every skewer.
Lightly brush the pineapple with the marinade. Grill or broil, turning once and basting a few times with the closing marinade, until gentle and golden, about five mins on each aspect.
Remove the pineapple from the skewers and vicinity on a platter or individual serving plates. Brush with the rum, if the usage of, and sprinkle with the lime zest. Serve hot or warm.

Nutrition
Carbohydrate13 g Dietary fiber1 g Sodium1 mg Total fat2 g Cholesterol0 mg Protein<1 gCalories70

Mixed Berry Whole-Grain Coffeecake

Ingredients
- 1/2 cup of skim milk
- 1 tablespoon of vinegar
- 2 tablespoons of canola oil
- 1 teaspoon of vanilla
- Only 1 egg
- 1/3 cup of packed brown sugar
- 1 cup of whole-wheat pastry flour
- 1/2 of teaspoon baking soda
- 1/2 of teaspoon ground cinnamon
- 1/8 of teaspoon salt
- 1 cup of frozen mixed berries, such as blueberries, raspberries and blackberries (do not thaw)
- 1/4 cup of low-fat granola and crush them

Directions

Heat oven to 350 F. Spray an 8-inch round cake pan with cooking spray and coat with flour.
In a big bowl, mix the milk, vinegar, oil, vanilla, egg and brown sugar till smooth. Stir in flour, baking soda, cinnamon and salt just until moistened. Fold half of the berries into the mixture. Spoon into the prepared pan. Sprinkle with remaining berries and top with the granola.
Bake 25 to half-hour or until golden brown and top springs returned when touched in center. Cool in pan on cooling rack for 10 minutes. Serve warm.

Nutrition
Cholesterol23 mgCalories144 Sodium139 mg Total fat4 g Total carbohydrate23 g Dietary fiber3 gadded sugars7 g Protein4 g

Orange Dream Smoothie

Ingredients
- 1 1/2 cups of orange juice
- 1 cup of light vanilla soy milk
- 1/3 cup of silken or tofu
- 1 tablespoon of dark honey
- 1 teaspoon of grated orange zest
- 1/2 teaspoon of vanilla extract
- 5 ice cubes
- 4 peeled orange segments

Instructions

In a blender, mix the ingredients orange juice, soy milk, tofu, honey, orange zest, vanilla and ice cubes. Blend until smooth and frothy, about 30 sec.
Pour into chilled glasses and garnish each glass with an orange segment.

Nutrition
Total carbohydrate20 g Sodium40 mg Total fat1 g Cholesterol0 mg Protein3 gCalories101 Total sugars14 g

Orange Slices With Citrus Syrup

Ingredients
- 4 medium sized oranges
- Zest of 1 orange and cut it into thin strips 4 inches long and 1/8 inch wide

For syrup:
- 1 1/2 cups of fresh orange juice, strained
- 2 tablespoons of dark honey

For garnish:
- 2 tablespoons of orange liqueur, such as Grand Marnier or Cointreau
- 4 fresh mint sprigs

Directions

Working with 1 orange at a time, reduce a skinny slice off the pinnacle and the bottom, exposing the flesh. Stand the orange upright and, the usage of a pointy knife, cut off the peel, following the contour of the fruit and removing all the white pith and membrane. Cut the orange crosswise into slices half of in thick. Transfer to a shallow bowl or dish. Repeat with the closing oranges. Set them apart.
Take a small saucepan on medium-high tempreature, combine the strips of zest with water to cover. Boil itl and boil for 1 minute. Drain and straight away plunge the zest into a bowl of bloodless water. Set aside.
To make the syrup, integrate the orange juice and honey in a big saucepan on medium-high tempreature. Boil it, stirr to mix the honey. Lessen the tempreature to medium-low and simmer,

uncovered, till the mixture thickens to a mild syrup, about 5 minutes. Drain the orange zest and upload to the syrup. Cook till the zest is translucent, three to 5 minutes.
Pour the aggregate over the oranges. Cover and refrigerate till chilled, or for 3 hours time.
For serving, divide the orange slices and syrup in person plates. Drizzle each serving with 1 half teaspoons of the orange liqueur, if the usage of. Garnish with the mint and serve right now.
Nutrition
Total carbohydrate39 g Dietary fiber4 g Sodium3 mg Saturated fat0 g Cholesterol0 mg Protein2 gCalories183 Total sugars33 g

Peach Crumble

Ingredients
- 8 ripe peaches,peel them, and pitted and sliced
- Juice from 1 lemon(3tbsp)
- 1/3 teaspoon of ground cinnamon
- 1/4 teaspoon of ground nutmeg
- 1/2 cup of whole-wheat flour
- 1/4 cupof packed dark brown sugar
- 2 tablespoons of trans-free margarine, cut into thin slices
- 1/4 cup of quick-cooking oats

Instructions
Set the oven at 375 F. Lightly coat a 9-inch pie pan with cooking spray.
Arrange peach slices inside the organized pie plate. Drizzle with lemon juice, cinnamon and nutmeg.
In a small bowl, whisk together flour and brown sugar. With your fingers, collapse the margarine into the flour-sugar mixture. And then add the uncooked oats and stir to mix evenly. Sprinkle the flour mixture on pinnacle of the peaches.
Bake until peaches are tender and the topping is browned, about 30 minutes. Cut into eight even slices and serve warm.
Nutrition
Total fat4 gCalories152 Protein3 g Cholesterol0 mg Total carbohydrate26 g Dietary fiber3 g Sodium41 mg

Pumpkin-Hazelnut Tea Cake

Ingredients
- 3 tablespoons canola oil
- 3/4 cup homemade or unsweetened canned pumpkin puree
- 1/2 cup honey
- 3 tablespoons firmly packed brown sugar
- 2 eggs, lightly beaten
- 1 cup whole-wheat (whole-meal) flour
- 1/2 cup all-purpose (plain) flour
- 2 tablespoons flaxseed
- 1/2 teaspoon baking powder
- 1/2 teaspoon ground allspice
- 1/2 teaspoon ground cinnamon
- 1/2 teaspoon ground nutmeg
- 1/4 teaspoon ground cloves
- 1/4 teaspoon salt
- 2 tablespoons chopped hazelnuts (filberts)

Instructions
Set the oven at 350 F. Lightly coat an 8-by-4-inch loaf pan with cooking spray.
Take a large bowl, using an electric mixer on low speed, beat together the canola oil, pumpkin puree, honey, brown sugar and eggs until well blended.
In a small bowl, whisk together the flours, flaxseed, baking powder, allspice, cinnamon, nutmeg, cloves and salt. Add the flour mixture to the pumpkin and, using the electric mixer on medium speed, beat until well blended.
Pour the batter into the prepared pan. Sprinkle the hazelnuts evenly over the top and press down gently to lodge the nuts into the batter. Bake until a toothpick inserted into the center of the loaf comes out clean, about 50 to 55 min. Let cool it in the pan on a wire rack for 10 minutes. Turn the loaf out of the pan onto the rack and let cool completely. Cut into 12 slices to serve.
Nutrition
Calories166 Total fat6 g Saturated fat1 g Cholesterol31 mg Sodium73 mg Total carbohydrate28 g Dietary fiber2.5 g Total sugars15 Protein4 g

Rainbow Ice Pops

Ingredients
- 1 1/2 cups of diced strawberries, cantaloupe and watermelon
- 1/2 cup of blueberries
- 2 cups of 100% apple juice
- 6 paper cups
- 6 craft sticks

Directions
Mix the fruit collectively and divide evenly into the paper cups. Pour 1/three cup of juice into every paper cup.
Place the cups on a level surface within the freezer. Freeze till partially frozen, approximately 1 hour. Insert a stick into center of each cup. Freeze until firm.
Nutrition
Total carbohydrate14 g Dietary fiber1 g Sodium6 mg Cholesterol0 mg Protein0.5 gCalories60 Total sugars11 g

Sautéed Bananas

Ingredients
Sauce
- 1 tablespoon of butter
- 1 tablespoon of walnut oil
- 1 tablespoon of honey
- 2 tablespoons of firmly packed brown sugar
- 3 tablespoons of 1 percent low-fat milk
- 1 tablespoon of dark raisins or golden raisins (sultanas)

saute
- 4 bananas, about 1 pound total weight

- 1/2 tsp of canola oil
- 2 tablespoons of dark rum

Directions

Start by making the sauce. In a small saucepan soften the butter over medium heat. Whisk within the walnut oil, brown sugar and honey. Stirring it continuously, cook until the sugar is dissolved, approximately 3 min. Add the milk 1 tbsp at a time, and then cook, stirring continuously until the sauce thickens slightly, about three minutes. Remove from the warmth and stir inside the raisins. Set apart and keep warm.

Peel the bananas, after which cut every crosswise into 3 sections. Cut every phase in half of lengthwise. Lightly coat a massive nonstick frying pan with the canola oil and region on medium-high tempreature. Add the bananas and saute until they start brown, three to 4 minutes. Transfer to a plate and hold warm. Add the rum to the pan, carry to a boil and deglaze the pan, stirring with a timber spoon to scrape up any browned bits from the bottom of the pan. Cook till reduced by way of half, about 30 to forty five sec. Back to the bananas to the pan to rewarm.

To serve, divide the bananas among character bowls or plates. Drizzle with the nice and cozy sauce and serve immediately.

Nutrition

Total carbohydrate27 g Dietary fiber2 g Sodium21 mg Total fat5 g Cholesterol5 mg Protein1 gCalories145 Total sugars18 g

Summer Fruit Gratin

Ingredients

Filling
- 1 pound of cherries, halved them
- 4 cups peeled, pitted and sliced mixed summer stone fruits, such as nectarines, peaches and apricots
- 1 tablespoon of whole-wheat flour
- 1 tablespoon of turbinado sugar or firmly packed light brown sugar

For the topping:
- 1/2 cup of old-fashioned rolled oats
- 1/4 cup of sliced (flaked) almonds
- 3 tablespoons of whole-wheat flour
- 2 tablespoons of turbinado sugar or firmly packed light brown sugar
- 1/4 teaspoon of ground cinnamon
- 1/8 teaspoon of ground nutmeg
- 1/8 teaspoon of salt
- 2 tablespoons of walnut oil or canola oil
- 1 tablespoon of dark honey

Directions

Heat the oven to 350 F. Lightly coat a 9-inch (23-cm) rectangular baking dish with cooking spray. In a bowl, integrate the cherries and stone fruits. Sprinkle with the flour and turbinado sugar and toss gently to mix. To make the topping, in some other bowl, integrate the oats, almonds, flour, turbinado sugar, cinnamon, nutmeg and salt. Whisk to blend. Stir within the oil and honey and mix until well-blended.

Spread the fruit mixture evenly in the organized baking dish. Sprinkle the oat-almond combination frivolously over the fruit. Bake until the fruit is effervescent and the topping is lightly browned, forty five to fifty five minutes. Serve warm or at room temperature.

Nutrition

Total carbohydrate39 g Dietary fiber5 g Sodium56 mg Total fat7 g Cholesterol0 mg Protein4 gCalories235 Total sugars25 g

Warm Chocolate Souffles

Ingredients
- 1/2 cup of unsweetened cocoa powder
- 6 tablespoons of hot water
- 1 tablespoon of unsalted butter
- 1 tablespoon of canola oil
- 3 tablespoons of all-purpose (plain) flour
- 1 tablespoon of ground hazelnuts (filberts) or almonds
- 1/4 teaspoon of ground cinnamon
- 3 tbsp of firmly packed dark brown sugar
- 2 tablespoons of honey
- 1/8 teaspoon of salt
- 3/4 cup of 1 percent low-fat milk
- 4 egg whites
- 3 tablespoons of granulated sugar
- 1 teaspoon of powdered (confectioner's) sugar
- 1 cup of rasp-berries

Directions

Set the oven at 375 F. Coat six 1-cup each souffle dishes or ramekins with cooking spray.

Take a small bowl, combine the cocoa and hot water, stirr it until smooth. Set apart.

Take a small, heavy saucepan on medium tempreature, melt the butter. Add the canola oil and stir to mix. Add the flour, hazelnuts and cinnamon and cook dinner for 1 minute, stirring constantly with a whisk. Stir within the brown sugar, honey and salt. Gradually add the milk and prepare dinner, stirring constantly, till thickened, about three minutes. Remove from the warmth and stir into the cocoa aggregate. Let cool slightly.

In a big, thoroughly cleaned bowl, using an electric mixer on excessive speed, stirr the egg whites until foamy apprence. Add the sugar 1 tbsp at a time and beat till stiff peaks form. Using a rubber spatula, gently fold 1/three of the egg whites into the cocoa aggregate to lighten it. Then fold the ultimate egg whites into the cocoa combination, mixing lightly only till no white streaks remain.

Gently scoop the cocoa egg white combination into the prepared dishes. Bake till the souffle rises above the rim and is set in the center, 15 to 20 minutes for character souffles or forty to forty five mins for the big souffle.

Cool down the souffles on a wire rack for 15 mins. Using a fine-mesh sieve, dust the pinnacle with the powdered sugar. Garnish with raspberries and serve immediately.

Nutrition
Calories203 Total fat7 g Cholesterol7 mg Sodium106 mg Total carbohydrate29 g Dietary fiber4 g Total sugars22 g Protein6 g

Watermelon-Cranberry Agua Fresca

Ingredients
- 2 and 1/2 pounds of seedless watermelon, rind removed and diced (about 7 cups)
- 1 cup of fruit-sweetened cranberry juice (sometimes called cranberry nectar)
- 1/4 cup of fresh lime juice
- 1 lime, cut into 6 slices

Directions
Place the melon in a blender. Process till smooth. Pass the puree via a fine-mesh sieve located over a bowl to take away the pulp and make clear the juice. Pour the juice into a massive pitcher Add the cranberry and lime juices and mix to combine. Refrigerate till very cold. Pour it into tall chilled glasses and garnish each with a slice of lime.

Nutrition
Total carbohydrate20 g Dietary fiber1 g Sodium9 mg Saturated fat0 g Total fat0 g Cholesterol0 mg Protein1 gCalories84 Total sugars16 g

Skillet Apple-Ginger Crisp

Ingredients
3/4 cup of all-purpose flour (about 3 1/4 ounces)
1/4 cup of packed light brown sugar
1 tablespoon of granulated sugar
1/2 teaspoon of ground cinnamon
1/2 teaspoon of kosher salt
1/4 teaspoon of ground ginger
1/4 teaspoon of baking powder
5 tbsp of cold unsalted butter, cut into pieces
1/3 cup of uncooked old-fashioned regular rolled oats
FILLING
2 tablespoons of unsalted butter
1/2 cup of sugar
2 and 1/4 pounds Granny Smith apples (about 6 medium apples), peeled and sliced (about 7 cups)
1 tablespoon of fresh lemon juice
Pinch of kosher salt
2 tablespoons of all-purpose flour
1 tablespoon of apple brandy (such as Calvados) or cognac
1/4 cup of thinly sliced crystallized ginger candy (such as Gin Gins)

Directions
Make the toppings
Set oven at 375°F. Pulse flour, brown sugar, granulated sugar, cinnamon, salt, ginger, and baking powder in a meals processor until combined, about 2 times. Add butter, and process until flour mixture is going beyond the crumbly stage and begins to clump collectively and appearance moist, about 30 sec. Add oats, and pulse to mix, nabout 3 times. Transfer to a bowl, break up any large clumps, and chill, covered, till prepared to use.
Make the filling
Heat a 9-inch cast-iron skillet over medium-high. Add butter, and melt till sizzling. Stir in sugar to moisten in spots. Cook, stirring occasionally, till sugar is a deep amber color, about 5 mins. Then, add apples (cook down slowly), lemon juice, and salt. Cooking, stirring often, until apples have softened and liquid is barely reduced, 5 to 6 min. heStir in flour and apple brandy until combined. Scatter oat topping frivolously over apple mixture, and pinnacle evenly with ginger candy. Bake in preheated oven till oat topping is golden brown, 30 to 35 minutes. Let cool slightly, about 10 minutes. Spoon into bowls,serve with vanilla ice cream or whipped cream.

Cast-Iron Cornmeal Cake With Buttermilk Cream

Ingredients
3 large-sized eggs

Directions
Place a 10-inch solid iron skillet in oven; preheat oven to 425°F. Let skillet preheat in oven 15 minutes. Whisk together eggs and buttermilk in a massive bowl until frothy, approximately 1 minute. Whisk in brown sugar and cane syrup. Set buttermilk combination aside.
Mix baking powder, cornmeal, flour, salt, and baking soda in a separate bowl collectively.
Add cornmeal aggregate to buttermilk aggregate; stir the use of a timber spoon till combined.
Carefully do away with preheated skillet from oven. Add butter to skillet; swirl skillet to soften butter, frivolously coating backside, and facets of the skillet. Pour melted butter into cornmeal batter in a bowl; quickly stir to incorporate. Pour mixture into greased warm skillet; right now, switch to the preheat the oven.
Reduce and set oven temperature at 375°F; bake cake until pinnacle is flippantly browned and sides are darkish golden and turn away from skillet, 30 to 35 minutes. Immediately invert cake onto a wire rack. Let cool 15 minutes. Serve warm with Buttermilk Cream.

Recipes by type of food
Vegan and vegetarian recipes

Quick And Easy Vegetarian Biryani Recipe
Ingredients
- 2 tablespoons of olive oil
- 1 large-sized onion, thinly sliced
- 1 –2 cups of chopped or thinly sliced veggies (bell pepper, zucchini, or carrots)
- 3 garlic cloves, chopped
- 1 tablespoon of ginger, chopped
- 1 tablespoon of cumin
- 1 tablespoon of *coriander*
- 1 teaspoon of chili powder
- 1 teaspoon of *cinnamon*
- 1/2 teaspoon of *cardamom*
- 1/2 teaspoon of turmeric
- 1 bay leaf
- 4 cups of veggie stock
- 2 cups *basmati rice*, rinsed
- 3/4 teaspoon of salt
- 1 can of chickpeas
- 1/2 cup of raisins
- 1/4 cup of cashews and chopped parsley or cilantro

Directions
- in a huge skillet, or shallow Dutch oven, warmness oil over medium-excessive warmness. Add the onion and sauté, often stirring, till tender and golden, five mins. Turn heat to medium, add your preference of veggies and garlic and ginger, and cook 4-5 minutes. Remove one cup of the aggregate and set aside.
- Add spices and bay leaf, and stir one minute, toasting the spices. Add basmati rice, and saute one-minute stirring. Add stock and salt.
- Top with chickpeas, raisins, and the cup of veggies you place aside. Bring to a simmer over high heat, then decrease temperature to low. Cover the pot with a skinny dish towel, vicinity the lid over the top of the towel, and bring the four corners of the towel up and over the lid. This will tighten the seal and continues the steam in, permitting the rice to cook extra speedy and evenly.
- Simmer on low 2030 mins or until the rice has soaked up the liquid. See notes.
- While it's far simmering make the Cilantro Mint Chutney
- Uncover the Vegetarian Biryani and fluff up with a fork. Top with the toasted cashew and cilantro. Serve with optional Chutney.

Nutrition
Calories 385 Fat 6.8 cholesterol 0 sodium 416.2 protein 8.6

Whole Roasted Cauliflower With Tahini Sauce
Ingredients
1 whole cauliflower
2 tablespoons olive oil, divided
½ teaspoon salt
1 tablespoon *zaatar* spice
1 cup of water
Garnish with fresh herbs and parsley, dill and or mint, sprinkle

Instructions
Preheat oven to 425F.
Trim the cauliflower – cutting off the stem (more natural) or leaving it intact, trimming and slicing the bottom, so it stands up straight.
Place it in an ovenproof skillet. Drizzle 1 tablespoon oil everywhere in the cauliflower, sprinkle with salt, and Zaatar spice. Pour one cup of water into the lowest of the pan.
Cover tightly with foil and bake for forty five-fifty five minutes. Smaller cauliflower's heads will take 45 minutes. Use your nice judgment.
Take the foil off, minding the new steam (it's going to burn!). Drizzle with a little greater olive oil, region back within the oven for 30 minutes, perhaps rotating halfway through. At this point, it have to be deeply golden, however if not, preserve roasting until it is another 10-15 minutes.
Remove from the oven and sprinkle with sparkling herbs, optional Aleppo chili flakes, and either drizzle the tahini sauce over the whole thing right inside the pan, or cut it up, like a cake, into wedges and serve the tahini sauce at the side.

Nutrition
Calories 127 Fat 8 protein 5

Vegan Ramen With Miso Shiitake Broth
Ingredients
Flavorful Vegan Ramen Broth:
- 1 large sized onion-diced
- 2 smashed garlic cloves
- 1–2 tbsp of olive oil
- 4 cups of veggie stock
- 4 cups of water
- 1/2 cup of *dried Shiitake* Mushrooms, broken into small pieces
- 1 sheet of *Kombu* seaweed (available at *Asian markets*) –*optional,* but edible!
- 1/8 cup of mirin
- 1–2 tablespoons of white *miso paste*
- Add pepper to taste
- For more spicy, add *sriracha* to taste

RAMEN:
6– 8 ounces *Ramen Noodles*
8 ounces Cubed *Crispy Tofu*
Steamed or sauteedbok choy, sparkling spinach, shredded carrots or cabbage, roasted winter squash, roasted cauliflower, roasted carrots, roasted sweet potato, sauteed mushrooms, smoked mushrooms, infant corn, Bamboo shoots, Enoki mushrooms, Kimchi, Soft, boiled eggs (obviously no longer vegan) daikon radish, pickled radish, fresh herbs.

Garnishes: scallions, *sesame seeds*, *sriracha*, and *sesame oil*

Instructions

Make the BROTH: Over medium-high heat, saute the onion in 1 tablespoon oil until tender about 3 minutes. Turn heat to medium, add the smashed garlic cloves and continue cook onions until they are deeply golden brown. Add the veggie stock, water, dried shiitakes, a sheet of *kombu* (rinsed), and mirin. Bring to a Simmer.

Simmer for 25-30 min uncovered on med heat, *and then remove the Kombu*. Add miso and pepper to your taste. Keep heated. If this decreases too much it may become salty and then simply add a little water to taste.

Cook the *ramen noodles*.

Prep other veggies and toppings.

Assemble Ramen Bowls:

Fill the bowls with cooked noodles, *crispy tofu*, and any other veggies you want. Pour the flavorful Shiitake broth over the top of dish. Garnishing with a little drizzle of *sesame oil* and *sriracha*. Top with scallions and *sesame seeds*.

Serve immediately.

Nutrition

Calories 408 Fat 13.8g Protein 13.9g

Chipotle Portobello Tacos (Vegan!)

Ingredients
- 2 extra-large portobello mushrooms
- 1 red bell pepper
- ½ an onion – optional

Chipotle Marinade
- 1 tablespoon of oil
- 2 tbsp of *canned Chipotle* in *Adobo sauce* (SAUCE ONLY)
- 1 minced garlic clove
- ½ teaspoon of cumin
- ½ teaspoon of *coriander*
- salt to your taste

4 tortillas, warmed
1 can refry black beans
cilantro, *pickled onions*, *Vegan Cilantro Crema*, or guacamole or sliced avocado.

Directions

Set oven at 425F.

Slice the Portobello's into ½ inch thick wedges and sliced bell pepper into ½ adhesive strips. Add onion, and cut into ½ inch thick rings or half-moons. Place all on a sheet-pan lined sheet pan & Mix marinade ingredients together in a small bowl. Brush both facets of mushrooms liberally with the marinade, then closing purple bell pepper and onion lightly. Sprinkle Portobellos with salt. Roast 20 mins or until portobellos are fork-tender.

While that is roasting, heat the beans any prep any extra garnishes. Pickled onions and Vegan cilantro Crema both take about 10 minutes to make. Or actually use avocado slices.

When equipped to serve, heat the tortillas (over a gasoline flame on the stove or in a toaster oven) and spread generously with the refried black beans. Divide chipotle Portobello's and peppers (and onions if used) many of the tortillas. Top with Cilantro Crema or avocado, sparkling cilantro, and non-obligatory pickled onions.

Nutrition

Calories 307 Fat 1.5g Protein 9.4g

Chinese Eggplant With Spicy Szechuan Sauce

Ingredients
- 1 1/2 lbs of Japanese Eggplant
- 2 teaspoons of salt
- A bowl of water
- 2 tablespoons of cornstarch
- 2-4 tablespoons of *peanut oil*
- 4 cloves garlic, chopped
- 2 teaspoons of ginger, finely minced
- 5-10 dried red chilies

Szechuan Sauce:
- 1 teaspoon of *Szechuan peppercorns*
- 1/4 cup of soy sauce
- 1 tablespoon of garlic chili paste (or sub 1 teaspoon chili flakes)
- 1 tablespoon of *sesame oil*
- 1 tablespoon of *rice vinegar*
- 1 tablespoon of *Chinese cooking wine* (or mirin)
- 3 tablespoons of sugar, brown sugar, *coconut sugar*, *maple syrup* or alternative
- 1/2 teaspoon of *five-spice*

Then garnish with scallions and *roasted peanuts*.

Instructions

Cut eggplant into half inch thick half of-moons or bite-sized pieces. Place in a large bowl covered with water and stir in 2 teaspoons salt. Cover with a plate and permit stand 15 minutes.

At the sametime, chop the garlic and ginger and make the Szechuan Sauce.

To make the Szechuan Sauce: Toast the Szechuan peppercorns in a dry skillet at medium temp for 1-2 min. Crush. Place these along with the last ingredients (soy, chili paste, sesame oil, rice vinegar, Chinese cooking wine, sugar, and five spices) in a small bowl and whisk. Set with the aid of the stove.

Drain the eggplant and dry with a towel. Mix with the corn starch.

Working in 2 batches, heat 1 -2 tbsp oil in an extra-large skillet over medium warmness. Add half the eggplant is spreading them out. You need to get both sides great and golden, and the insides cooked through -so take your time right here and don't rush this step. Let one facet brown then turn them over the usage of tongs. This will take approximately 10 mins for each batch. Set the eggplant aside.

Add 1 extra tablespoon oil to the skillet, and over medium warmness, upload the garlic and ginger, stirring for 2 minutes. Turn the fan on, upload the dried chilies and mix one min. Pour the Szechuan

sauce into the pan and convey to a simmer for 20 seconds. Add the eggplant returned into the skillet, tossing lightly for about 1 minute. If it appears dry, add a tablespoon of water to loosen.
Place in a serving plate and top with scallions and optional peanuts.
Nutrition
Calories 323 Fat 21.8 Protein 5.9g

Crispy Vegan Quinoa Cakes With Tomato-Chickpea Relish

Ingredients
Quinoa Cakes
- 2 cups of water
- 1 cup *rinsed, white* quinoa
- Two teaspoons olive oil
- 1 tsp cumin
- One teaspoon of *granulated garlic* powder
- 1/2 tsp of *kosher salt*
- 1/2 tsp of herbs de Provence (or Italian dried herbs)
- zest from one small lemon (optional)
- 1/4 cup of chopped Italian parsley (optional)

Fresh Tomato Chickpea Relish
- 2 cups of cherry or grape tomatoes, sliced in half
- 1 cup of cucumber, diced
- 1/4 cup of fresh basil (or flat-leaf parsley, dill, or mint, or a combo!) chopped
- 1/4 cup of chopped scallions (or finely sliced red onion)
- 1 ½ cup of cooked chickpeas (1 can be drained and rinsed)
- 3 Tbs of olive oil
- 3 Tbs of *balsamic vinegar*
- 1/4 tsp of salt
- One small minced garlic clove (optional)

Instructions
In a medium pot, over high warmth, upload rinsed quinoa, salt, garlic powder, cumin, dried herbs, olive oil, and stir. Brint to a roiling boil. Cover, decrease warmness to low, and simmer lightly for 20 min. Set the time.
When the quinoa is cooking, you can make the Tomato Chickpea relish, stirring all ingredients collectively in a medium bowl.
Check quinoa- making sure all of the water is gone. If no longer, hold cooking covered, five greater minutes, and until steam, holes appear (this typically takes me a complete of 25 minutes), and quinoa has soaked up all the water and looks fantastically dry.) quinoa must be dry-ish and no longer watery.
Mix the quinoa with a fork, repeatedly, for a minute, till you start to see the man or woman grains start to interrupt apart. This may seem strange, but preserve stirring. Eventually, after a complete minute of stirring, the grains will spoil apart and begin to clump. Remove from stove, permit cool down inside the pot to wherein it's cool enough to address with your palms, about 15 minutes. Stir inside the lemon zest and clean parsley if you want.

Using wet fingers form into four balls, the size of a tennis ball. Place on a plate or sheet pan. Using moist arms press into a 1 – 1 1/2 inch thick cake (about 3-four inches wide), smoothing any cracks at the edges, and making them exceptional and tidy. Wet fingers are key. Place within the refrigerator for 15 minutes, or overnight. (These will hold 3-4 days if made ahead.) As the cakes cool they will come to be even sturdier.
Pan the Quinoa Cakes in a well-oiled skillet at medium warmness. You can pan-sear them with none coating, or for an additional crispy crust, dredge in rice flour or GF Panko. I regularly do these without any coating at all. Just make sure to no longer mess around with. Them- permitting them to expand a great crust earlier than flipping. As then develop the crust, they'll clearly release themselves from the pan. You also can bake these in a toaster oven (right at the rack) or in a 400F oven (on a parchment-covered pan) till warmed through, approximately 20 minutes.
Divide amongst plates and top with the sparkling tomato chickpea relish. Spoon any closing dressing over top and around the desserts.
Garnish with crumbled goat cheese if you want or a balsamic glaze.
Nutrition
Calories 388 Fat 17.6g Protein 12.3g

Spicy Mexicanoaxacan Bowl

Ingredients
Spicy Rub
- 2 teaspoons of cumin
- 1 teaspoon of ground chipotle
- ½ teaspoon of *kosher salt*

Sheet Pan **Ingredients**
- ½ a red onion, cut in ½ in wedges
- 1 medium sized yam or sweet potato- diced into ¾ inch cubes (leave skin on)
- 8 baby sized bell peppers, cut in half
- ½ cup of pecans
- 2 teaspoons of *maple syrup*
- 1 15-16 ounce can of Seasoned Black Beans

For garnishing: Avocado, cilantro, scallions, Cabbage Slaw, *Mexican Secret Sauce* or *Vegan Avocado Sauce*
Quick Cabbage Slaw
- ¼ of a a red cabbage, shredded
- 1 tablespoon olive oil
- ¼ cup chopped cilantro or scallions or both
- 1 teaspoon *coriander*
- 1/8 teaspoon *kosher salt*
- 1 tablespoon lime juice

Instructions
Preheat oven to 425F
Mix cumin, chipotle and salt collectively in a small bowl.
Place onion, candy potato and peppers on a parchment lined sheet pan. Drizzle onion and potato with a bit olive oil and sprinkle generously with spice mix, tossing to coat all sides well. Use approximately ½ or ⅔ of the spice.

Place within the oven for 20-30 minutes, tossing halfway through.

On some other smaller parchment-covered pan, toss the pecans with 2 teaspoons maple syrup and 1 teaspoon of the spice mix. Place within the oven for 10-12 minutes, until gently browned. When you pull it out, provide nuts a short toss to loosen them up and "fluffen" them, so when they cool, they're smooth to remove.

Heat the beans in a pot on the stove and make the slaw. Finely chop or shred the cabbage and place in a medium bowl with the rest of the ingredients, toss. Taste, regulate lime and salt.

Slice the avocado.

When the greens are fork tender, assemble the bowls. Divide the beans amongst 2-three bowls. Divide all the vegetables, placing them over the beans, and top with slaw and upload the avocado.

Serve with the Mexican Secret Sauce in case you like, or sour cream and warm sauce– it's first-rate without although too.

Nutrition
Calories 489 Fat 18.4g Protein 16.6g

Instant Pot Mujadara

Ingredients
- 1 cup brown lentils (do not *split lentil*)
- 1 1/2 tablespoons of olive oil
- 2-3 fat shallots, thinly sliced
- 4 cloves garlic, chopped
- 2 teaspoons of cumin
- 1 teaspoons of *coriander*
- 1 teaspoon of *allspice*
- ½ teaspoon of *cinnamon*
- ½ teaspoon of turmeri
- ¼ teaspoon of ground ginger
- 1 ½ teaspoons of *kosher salt*
- 1 teaspoon of dried mint or parsley
- lemon zest from one small lemon
- 3 ½ cups of water (be accurate)
- 1 cup brown of *basmati rice*

Directions
Place lentils in a bowl and cover with hot tap water (or boiling water), permitting them to soak until time to feature to the immediate pot.

Set Instant Pot to Saute function. Saute shallots in the oil, 4-five minutes, stirring constantly, until soft and aromatic and slightly caramelized. Remove half, saving for the topping. Add the garlic and saute till fragrant, approximately 1-2 minutes. Add all of the spices, salt, lemon zest and water. Stir. Drain the lentils and upload them together with the rinsed rice to the immediate pot. Give an amazing stir.

Cover the on the spot pot and set to Normal Pressure, High for 14 minutes. Let clearly release for as a minimum 10 min.

In the mean time, prepare any garnishes you like.
To serve, gently fluff Mujadara with a fork. Divide among bowls, drizzle with olive oil, add tomatoes, avocado, caramelized shallots, sprouts, a spoonful of yogurt or zhoug yogurt, or tahini sauce – and sparkling parsley or mint. Feel loose to serve with other seasonal veggies (roasted root veggies, shredded cabbage or carrots, etc).

Nutrition
Calories 429 Fat 14.8g Protein 14.4g

Black Pepper Tofu With Bok Choy

Ingredients
- 8-12 ounces of firm tofu, cut into 1 inch cubes
- corn starch for dredging
- 2 tablespoons of wok oil (high heat oil like peanut, coconut or vegetable)
- 5 finger pinch of salt
- 1 teaspoon of fresh cracked *peppercorns*
- 1 fat shallot, sliced
- 4 cloves garlic, rough chopped
- 6 ounces of baby bok choy (about 4) quartered lengthwise (or if very thick, in half again)

Black Pepper Sauce:
- 2 tablespoons of soy sauce (or Gluten-free Liquid Aminos)
- 2 tablespoons of Chinese Cooking Wine (Shaoxing Rice Wine) or sub dry white wine, pale sherry, or rice wine.
- 2 tablespoons of water
- 1 teaspoon of brown sugar (or sub palm sugar, coconut sugar or agave)
- ½ teaspoon of fresh cracked peppercorns
- 1 teaspoon of chili paste (optional)

Instructions
Cut the tofu into cubes and blot dry with paper towels, pressing down gently.

Make the wok sauce, stirring ingredients collectively in a small until most of the sugar dissolves. Place it with the aid of the stove.

Prep the shallots, garlic and bok choy.
Dredge the tofu in a mild coating of cornstarch (cornstarch is optional, but gives a crispier texture). Heat oil in a wok or large solid iron skillet over medium-high heat and upload the salt and overwhelmed peppercorns to the oil, swirling it around until fragrant, approximately one minute. Add the tofu to the oil, and sear on all sides until golden and crispy, turning the warmth down if want be. Be affected person and take your time, it will take about 5-6 minutes.

Set the crispy tofu apart on a paper towel-lined plate, and wipe the pan out.

Heat every other teaspoon or two of oil over medium warmth, and upload shallots, garlic and bok choy. Stir continuously till bok choy starts to wilt and shallots turn out to be golden, approximately 3-four minutes. It will smell superb. Add the wok sauce to the pan, get all of the sugar which could have settled inside the bowl.

Simmer for multiple minutes, or until bok choy is just tender.

At the last, toss the tofu back into the pan with the bok choy and sauce. Cooking any further will do

away with the first rate crispiness! Taste for salt and warmness, adjusting on your preference.
Serve immediately, diving between two bowls.
Nutrition
Calories 463Fat 24.4g Protein 24.8g

Spicy Miso Portobello Mushroom Burger (Vegan)

Ingredients
- 2 large sized portobello mushrooms
- 1 Tablespoon of Miso (any color)
- 1 tablespoon of toasted *sesame oil*
- 1 tablespoon of *sriracha*
- pinch of salt and pepper

Cucumber Ribbon Salad
- 2 turkish cucumbers, cut it length-wise into ribbons
- 1 scallion, sliced
- 1/4 teaspoon of salt
- ¼ teaspoon of sugar
- 2 teaspoons *of vinegar*
- ½ teaspoon of toasted *sesame seeds*

Carrot Slaw
- 1 1/2 cups of matchstick carrots (or grated)
- 1 scallion
- 1/4 teaspoon of salt
- ¼ teaspoon of sugar
- 2 teaspoons of *rice vinegar*
- ½ teaspoon of toasted *sesame seeds*

Asian Guacamole
- 1 extra large sized avocado, cubed
- 1 teaspoon of finely chopped ginger (or use *ginger paste*)
- 1 teaspoon of rice wine vinegar
- 1 teaspoon of *sesame oil*
- ¼ teaspoon of salt and pepper
- pinch chili flakes and *sesame seeds*

2 whole wheat buns, grilled

Instructions
Preheat the grill. Using a fork or mini whisk, blend the miso, siracha and sesame oil …. & pinch salat and pepper together in a small bowl to make a paste. Brush liberally onto each aspects of the portobello mushrooms.
Using a mandolin or veggie peeler, reduce the cucumber into lengthy thin ribbons. Place them in a bowl with scallions and upload the dressing components and lightly toss.
Make the carrot slaw the identical way. Place in a bowl, toss with dressing ingredients. To save time you could integrate the each the carrots and cucumber (and double the dressing) and serve them together in one bowl
Make the Asian Guacamole, with the aid of placing the whole thing in a small bowl, mashing and stirring a bit until creamy and combined. It doesn't must be smooth. Sprinkle with sesame and chili flakes.
Grill the portobellos, top facets down first, for 4-5 mins over medium heat, until juicy and tender. Flip, grill a few greater minutes. Grill the Buns.

Assemble the burgers….spread buns with generous quantity of Asian Guac, location the portobello- gills side up (to catch all of the flavorful juices) then mound with cucumber ribbon and carrot salad, a little squeeze of sriacha, non-obligatory pickled ginger. Use the remaining Asian Guac at the bun tops, and pinnacle the burgers.
Eat immediately.
Nutrition
Calories 415 Fat 21.2g Protein 6g

Simple Baked Sheet-Pan Ratatouille!

Ingredients
- 3 Japanese eggplant
- 1 red or yellow color bell pepper
- 2 medium sized tomatoes
- 2 zucchini or summer squash
- 1 medium onion
- 12–14 garlic cloves, peeled
- 2–3 tablespoon of fresh herbs – thyme or rosemary or combination of both
- olive oil for sprinkling
- salt and pepper to taste
- splash *balsamic vinegar*

Serve with pasta, soft polenta, whole grains, or feel free to add beans, sausage, chicken.

Easy Creamy Polenta
- 1 cup *corn meal*
- 4 ½ cups water or stock
- 1 tablespoon olive oil or butter
- ½ cupgratedcheese(cheddar, Parmesan, mozzarella, *goatcheese*)
- salt and pepper to taste

Directions
Set the oven at 400 F and place a piece of parchment on 1-2 huge sheet pans.
Using a vegetable peeler, peel eggplant in case you want – or simply remove some of the skin in lengthy stripes. Or in case you prefer, go away the pores and skin on. Cut into ½ inch thick bite-sized pieces. Slice the bell pepper into ½ inch extensive strips. Cut the tomatoes into 3/four inch wedges. Slice the zucchini the lengthy way and then slice into ½ inch thick 1/2 moons. dice the onion into ¼-½ inch thick half moons.
Spread out the vegetables on the sheet pan in a unmarried laye (this is why you maximum likely want sheet pans). Add complete garlic cloves (peeled) and herbs.
Sprinkle with olive oil and toss, using enough oil to coat. Sprinkle with a generous quantity of salt and pepper. Toss well.
Roast within the hot oven for 20 minutes, mix, roast 20 more minutes, mix again. Turn warmness right down to 300 and roast 10-20 more minutes, or until tender and edges start to caramelize.
Taste, alter salt, and drizzle with a bit splash of balsamic.
Use right away or cool and refrigerate (or freeze) till geared up to use.

Nutrition
Calories 147 Fat 9.7g Protein 2.5g

Blackened Tempeh With Avocado, Kale, Vegan Cajun Ranch

Ingredients
Cajun Vegan Ranch Dressing
- ⅓ cup of *vegan ranch dressing* (or sub your favorite store-bought ranch)
- ½ –1 teaspoon of cajun spice blend

Blackened Tempeh:
- 1 block of tempeh
- 2–3 tablespoons of Cajun Spice like Black Magic
- 2 tablespoons of olive-oil
- 4–5 leaves of lacinato kale, tough stems removed
- 1 tsp of oil, pinch salt, lemon zest from ½ a lemon
- 4 radishes, sliced
- 1 scallion, sliced
- 1 avocado, sliced
- ¼ cup *pickled onions*

Instructions
Stir the cajun spice into the dressing, beginning conservatively. Taste, and add extra to taste. You need it bold!
Add the tempeh, entire to a sauté pan of generously salted water, just sufficient to cover it. Let simmer lightly 8-10 mins to help soften and reduce bitterness. Slice it into ½ inch extensive slices and generously coat each side with Cajun Spices.
Pan-sear the tempeh in oil, until crispy and heated through. Set aside.
Stack the kale (getting rid of any thick stems) and reduce in to skinny ribbons. Place in a bowl and then add a teaspoon or of olive oil (just enough to slightly coat) a pinch salt and lemon zest. Massage with your fingers till tender. To the kale upload the radishes, scallion, pickled onion and avocado. Toss with a number of the Vegan Ranch dressing, sufficient to coat. (You can also preserve the whole thing separate, specially if making grain bowls)
Either divide the salad among bowls or region it in warm, entire wheat tortillas, topped with the blackened tempeh and sprouts.
The salad is hearty that it will flavor exact the following day.

Nutrition
Calories 281 Fat 18.1g Protein 16.9g

Veggie Lo Mien

Ingredients
4-5 ounces of dry *lo mein noodles*
Lo Mein Sauce:
- 3 tablespoons of soy sauce (or GF Braggs)
- 2 tablespoons of *Chinese cooking wine*
- 1 tablespoon of *oyster sauce*
- 2 teaspoons of *sesame oil*
- 1 teaspoon of *maple syrup*, sugar or *honey*
- 1/4 teaspoon of *liquid smoke*
- 1/8 teaspoon of *white pepper*
- 1/2– 1 teaspoon of *sriracha* (or chili paste)

Lo Mein Stir Fry:
- 2 tablespoons of *wok oil, peanut oil* or *coconut oil*
- 1/2 an onion, sliced
- 2 cups of sliced mushrooms
- 3 garlic cloves, chopped
- 1 teaspoon of ginger, minced
- 1/2 red bell pepper, sliced
- 1 cup of matchstick carrots
- 1 cup of shredded cabbage
- 1 cup of snow peas

Garnish: scallions, sliced

Instructions
1. Set water to boil and cook dinner the noodles according to directions at the package.
2. Stir together the Lo mein Sauce components in a small bowl.
3. Prep any and all veggies and set close to the stove.
4. In a wok or huge skillet, warmness oil over medium-excessive warmth. Add the onions and mushrooms and saute 3-four minutes, stirring continuously. Turn heat to medium, add the garlic and ginger and saute 2 minutes. Add the bell pepper, carrots, cabbage and snow peas and stir often, just permitting them to get tender, however still crisp, 3-four minutes.
5. Add the noodles and give an excellent stir and toss a few times to incorporate.
6. Add the Lo Mein Sauce and stir and toss constantly 2 minutes. If it receives too dry add a little splash of water to loosen.
7. Serve in bowls, garnish with scallions.

Nutrition
Calories 464 Fat 16.6g Protein 13.8g

Szechuan Tofu And Veggies

Ingredients
- 8 ounces of tofu, patted dry and cubed
- 2 tablespoons of olive or high heat oil
- Small pinch of salt and pepper
- ½ cup of thinly sliced onion
- 4 ounces of sliced mushrooms
- 2 cups of shredded cabbage
- 1 cup of shredded carrots or matchstick
- ½ red bell pepper sliced in fine pieces
- 1 cup of asparagus, snap peas
- 6- 8 small dried red Chinese
- For garnishing use scallions, *sesame seeds*, chili flakes

Serve this on its own, over rice or over *soba noodles* or zucchini noodles.
¼ cup *Szechuan Sauce* and more to taste!

Instructions
• Heat oil in a skillet. Season oil generously with salt and pepper. With tofu, use ½ teaspoon kosher salt **in** keeping with ½ pound of tofu. Swirl the pro-oil around till unfold out uniformly. Add tofu and sear on **as a** minimum side, till crispy and golden. Be affected person here. Set aside.
• To the same pan, add a little higher oil if needed, onion, and mushrooms and sauté over

medium-high warmth – continually stirring, until smooth, about three minutes. Add the remaining veggies, upload **the** dried chilies **if** you like -and lower heat to medium, and sauté, tossing & stirring for **3-5** minutes till just gentle or al dente. Tender, however colorful and still slightly crisp!

- Add the Szechuan Sauce, starting with ¼ cup and adding **more** to taste and Cook the sauce 2 minutes, letting it thicken a bit. **Toss** inside the crispy tofu (or shrimp or chicken) proper on end, simply **to** heat it.
- Divide **among** bowls. Sprinkle with sesame seeds and scallions. Add chili flakes for more exceptional warmth.
- Serve this just because it is, or over rice, or noodles and remember, do not devour the dried chilies!

Nutrition
Calories307%Fat 20.3g31%SaturatedFat2.9g Cholesterol 0mg0% Sodium 368.4mg15%Total Carbohydrate 23.9g8%Dietary Fiber 7g28%Sugars 11.9g Protein 14.2g28%

How To Make Tlayudas

Ingredients
- 4 whole grain tortillas 8-10 inches wide

Cabbage Slaw:
- ½ head of cabbage, shredded
- 1 cup of shredded carrots
- 4 radishes -sliced
- ¼ cup of thinly sliced red onion – or sub *pickled onions* or pickled shallots
- 3/4 teaspoon of salt, plus more taste
- ½ an english cucumber- sliced
- 1 tablespoon of jalapeno- finely chopped- optional
- ¼-½ cup of scallions sliced
- ¼-½ cup of cilantro- chopped
- 2 tablespoons of olive oil
- 3 tablespoons of fresh lime juice, plus a little zest

Toppings:
- 1 can of refried beans
- *Chicken carnitas* or *Turkey Chorizo*
- Crumbled Queso Freso Cheese
- *Chipotle Mayo* or Avocado Cilantro Sauce
- Garnish with avocado, cilantro, lime wedges, scallions, fresh summer tomatoes, *hot sauce*, or sour cream.

Avocado Cilantro Sauce:
- 1 medium avocado (perfectly ripe)
- 4-6 jalapeno slices
- 1 garlic clove
- handful cilantro- ¼ -½ cup
- 2 tablespoons of olive oil
- 2 tablespoons of lime juice
- 4 tablespoons of water
- ½ teaspoon of salt

Instructions
1. Pre-warmth oven to 275 F
2. Toast tortillas dry, at once at the oven racks (no sheet pan) till crisp, about 20 minutes. This is key- they want to be very crispy and dry, no longer bendy. You can make these in advance.
3. Mix the cabbage, carrots, radish, onion, and toss in a huge bowl with the salt.
4. Then, add the cucumber, jalapeño, scallions and cilantro, Toss well, then add olive oil and lime juice and a bit zest. Let it rest on the kitchen counter – or make this in advance and refrigerate.
5. If you want to make the avocado sauce- make this now- placing the whole lot in a meals processor and blending until smooth. Taste, adjust salt and spice degree including more jalapeño if needed. Place in a bowl.
6. When ready to assemble, heat the refried beans, adding ¼-½ cup water (to loosen them) and using a fork, whip in a pinch of salt, cumin and coriander to season to taste.
7. If the usage of hen or chorizo, warmth them up now and if using cheese, switch on the broiler.
8. To assemble, cautiously lather up a few beans at the tortilla (like you pizza sauce on a pizza). At this point you can add chicken and cheese (and melt) or go away off and preserve it vegan. Top with the warmed base with a generous mound of cool slaw. Spoon over avocado sauce.
9. garnishing with cilantro sprigs, hot sauce, lime wedge, pickled onions.

Serve immediately while the beans are warm and the tortillas are still crisp.

Nutrition
Calories 406 Fat 22.5g Protein 10.3g

Middle Eastern Salad Tacos

Ingredients
Middle Eastern Spiced Chickpeas
- 2 teaspoons of olive oil
- 1 can of chick peas, rinsed and drained
- 1 teaspoon of *sumac*
- 1 teaspoon of cumin
- ¼-½ teaspoon of salt
- 1 teaspoon of *sesame seeds*

½ cup of Hummus
6 x 6 inch of tortillas, warmed or lightly toasted
Salad
- giant handful arugula
- 1 medium sized tomato
- 2 Turkish cucumbers, diced
- 1–2 tablespoon of olive oil
- 1–2 tablespoon of lemon juice
- 1 teaspoon of ground *coriander*
- ¼ teaspoon of salt, more to taste

Instructions
Heat oil in a skillet at mediumtempreature. Then, add chickpeas and other spices and salt. Warm through, mixing. During the last min add the *sesame seeds*. Turn heat off.
Mix the salad in a bowl. Toast the tortillas until warm and pliable.

Together. Spread hummus onto the warm tortilla. Top with warm chickpeas and a heaping mound of the salad. Sprinkle with herbs and scallions.
Nutrition
Calories405%TotalFat 15.9g24%SaturatedFa:2.1g Cholesterol 0mg0% Sodium 539.9mg22%TotalCarbohydrate 56.7g19%Dietary Fiber 11.9g48%Sugars 5.5g Protein 13.6g27%

Roasted Chiles Rellenos With Black Beans

Ingredients
- 4–6 poblano peppers leave
- 6 ripe, medium tomatoes,
- 6 fat garlic cloves
- one medium-large sized onion, sliced into ½ inch wedges or slices
- 2 small sized jalapeños
- 1–2 tablespoon of olive oil
- 1 can of black beans
- 4–6 ounces of grated jack cheese or Mexican queso fresco
- ½ cup of stock (veggie) or sub water
- 1 teaspoon of cumin
- 1 teaspoon of *coriander*
- 1 teaspoon of chili powder
- 1 teaspoon of dried oregano
- 1 teaspoon of salt
- 2 tablespoons of tomato paste
- ¼ cup of fresh cilantro plus more for garnishing

You can Serve with rice, sour cream, toasted *pumpkin seeds*, cilantro

Directions
Set oven at 450 F
Cut the tomatoes in half and set up them at the sheet pan. Add the onions to sheet pan, along side the complete garlic cloves, halved jalapeños and entire poblano peppers, making sure they're no longer overcrowded. You may need to use sheet pans.
Sprinkle with olive oil, sprinkle with salt and pepper and place within the oven and test after 15 mins. If the peppers are tender cast off them (pasilla peppers will cook much faster than poblanos- please see notes) and take a look at the garlic. Otherwise hold roasting with the tomatoes and onions another 15-20 minutes, till peppers and onions are gentle and tomatoes are juicy.
In the interim make the filling. together the beans (drained) with the cheese. If vegan, mix the beans with 1 cup of vegan herbed tofu ricotta. Season the mixture with salt and pepper.
When the poblanos are just gentle, take the sheet pan out of the oven (depart the oven on) and allow it cool. Add ⅓ of the onions, reducing them up, into the filling mixture and stir.
Blend up the Roasted Ranchos Sauce. Place the alternative half of of the onions right into a blender at the side of the tomatoes, pan juices, jalapeño, garlic, ½ cup stock, cumin, coriander, chili powder, oregano, salt, tomato paste and sparkling cilantro – and blend until smooth. Set aside.
Cut a slit inside the poblano peppers from stem to pointy stop and the use of your fingers, gently eliminate seeds whilst rinsing them under cold walking water. If the thin skins slip off, allow them, however don't worry about actively peeling them, in particular poblanos – their skins are pretty thin - Leaving some of the skin on is perfectly fine. Pasillo peppers have thick pores and skin and have to be peeled.
In a big baking dish (or oven proof skillet) pour a touch of the roasted tomato ranchero sauce to coat the bottom. Place the peppers over-top of the sauce, slit facet up, then spoon the filling into every one. Pour the relaxation of the flavorful ranchero sauce over the top. At this point you may add more shredded cheese to the top, or leave it off.
Cover with foil and bake 20-25 mins in a 425F oven- or till the filling is warm and melty, uncover and bake 5 greater min.
Garnishing with cilantro leaves, toasted pumpkin seeds and bitter cream if you like.

Nutrition
Calories 302 Fat 4.8g Protein 16.6g

Roasted Portobello Mushrooms With Walnut Coffee Sauce

Ingredients
- 4 extra large sized portobello mushrooms
- 2 tablespoons of olive oil
- 1 tablespoon of *balsamic vinegar*
- generous pinch salt and pepper

Walnut Coffee Sauce:
- 3 tablespoons of olive oil
- 2 extra large shallots, diced
- 4 garlic cloves, chopped
- 1 cup of walnuts
- 1 ¼ cup of black coffee (cold is ok)
- ½ teaspoon of salt
- ½ teaspoon of pepper
- 1 teaspoon of miso
- 1 teaspoon of balsamic

Instructions
Set he oven at 400 F
Mix oil and vinegar in a bowl and brush the portobellos on each facets with this. Sprinkle with salt and pepper and region gills facet down, on a parchment lined sheet pan. Bake for 20 -25 minutes till tender. Wrap in foil till equipped to utilize.
When the portobellos are roasting you can prepare the sauce.
Heat oil in a sauce pan, at medium heat. Saute the shallots and garlic till aromatic and tender, about 4-five min, mixing often. Then, add the walnuts and mix for 2 min. Then add the coffee, scraping up any brown bits. Pour all right into a blender, add the salt, pepper, miso paste, balsamic and mix for sometime, till become smooth. Place the sauce back into the pan and heat up gently proper before serving.
When the portobellos are prepared, either slice them and place over the Coffee Walnut sauce in a serving

dish, or personally serve them with roasted garlic mashed potatoes.
Topping with a sprig of thyme and pomegranate seeds for color! Season with clean cracked pepper.
Nutrition
Calories408%TotalFat 37.5g58%SaturatedFat4.4g Cholesterol 0mg0% Sodium 307.1mg13%Total Carbohydrate 16.7g6%Dietary Fiber 4.6g19%Sugars 6.9g Protein 7.9g16%

Roasted Spaghetti Squash w/ Eggplant Puttanesca

Ingredients
- 3 lb of Spaghetti Squash- (or sub pasta noodles)
- 4 tablespoon of olive oil- divided
- 1 medium sized eggplant – cut into a small dice (4 cups)
- 1 red onion- diced
- 4–6 cloves garlic- rough chopped
- 1 red bell pepper- diced
- 14 ounce can of crushed tomatoes
- 1 tablespoon of dry Italian herbs
- 1 teaspoon of *kosher salt*
- ¼ teaspoon of red chili flakes, more to taste
- Splash red wine
- 2 tablespoons of *capers*, more to taste, plus a splash of the brine
- 3 tablespoons of slice olives
- Garnish with fresh Italian parsley, grated Romano or Parmesan cheese, or a drizzle olive oil

Instructions
1. Pre heat oven to 425F
2. Cut squash in half size, and scrape out seeds with a spoon and location open side down, on a parchment-covered baking sheet in the oven and roast for 30- 40 mins or till tender. (You ought to this the night earlier than after which refrigerate and reheat.)
3. When the squash is cooking, roasting, you can make the Eggplant Puttanesca sauce.
4. In a massive heavy bottom skillet or dutch oven, heat three tablespoons oil over med-excessive warmness.
5. Add finely diced onion and eggplant, and saute, stirring frequently for 4-5 mins. Add garlic and red bell pepper, turn warmness down to medium and maintain cooking till eggplant is tender, approximately 10-12 more minutes, stirring occasionally.
6. Add beaten tomatoes, a generous splash of wine, chili flakes, salt, pepper, Italian herbs, and simmer on low warmth 5-10 greater minutes. Add capers and olives.
7. Taste, alter salt, spice level and add more capers or olives to taste. Sometimes add a little splash of the caper or olive brine, to bump up the flavor.
8. When spaghetti squash is tender, scoop it out right into a strainer, allow it drain for a few mins, then vicinity a platter or bowl, and fluff and toss properly with salt, pepper and 1 tablespoon olive oil.
9. Divide among bowls and pinnacle with the eggplant puttanesca. Sprinkle with sparkling Italian parsley and grated cheese (optional) or a drizzle olive oil. Alternatively you can serve this proper out of the spaghetti squash shell (making sure to season the squash, mixing with a fork earlier than topping with the putttanesca.

Nutrition
Calories427%TotalFat 22.8g35%SaturatedFat3.5g Cholesterol 0mg0% Sodium 1246.2mg52%TotalCarbohydrate 58.5g19%Dietary Fiber 14.3g57%Sugars 26.1g Protein 6.9g14%

Bali Bowls With Peanut Tofu

Ingredients
- 14 ounces of tofu
- 1 large sized sweet potato, cut into ¾ inch cubes
- drizzle of olive oil
- 3/4 cup of uncooked *black rice*

Peanut Sauce Ingredients:
- 3 thin slices of ginger- cut across the grain, about the size of a quarter.
- 1 fat clove garlic
- 1/4 cup of *peanut butter* (or sub almond butter!)
- ¼ cup of fresh orange juice (roughly ½ an orange)
- 2 tablespoons of soy sauce or GF Braggs Liquid Amino Acids
- 3 tablespoons of *maple syrup, honey*, agave
- 3 tablespoons of toasted *sesame oil*
- ½ –1 teaspoon of cayenne pepper
- 3/4 teaspoon of salt

Bowl Veggie Options:
- 1–2 cups of shredded cabbage
- 1–2 cups of shredded carrots
- 1–2 cups of shredded beets
- 1 cup of sliced snap peas
- ½ cup of thinly sliced radishes
- 1 medium sized avocado
- fresh sunflower sprouts

Instructions
Set oven at 425 F
Blot dry, and then cut the tofu into 2 inch squares or 2-3 inch lengthy strips (which might be ¾ inch thick). Place on a parchment-lined sheet pan. Sprinkle lightly with salt.
Cut the yam into ¾ inch cubes and area at the other side of the sheet pan. Sprinkle with olive oil and sprinkle with salt. Toss and unfold out.
Make the peanut sauce, placing everything in a blender, and blend till smooth. Reserve ½ of the peanut sauce for the bowl. Use the remaining to coat the tofu. Pour over tofu and brush tops and facets and lather them up. I want to leave a very generous amount at the pinnacle of every piece. Place within the hot oven for 25-30 minutes.
Cook the rice like you'll pasta – the use of this basmati rice method.
Prep all your veggies. And FYI, these are just alternatives for you, feel free to use what you like, adding or subtracting from the list.

When the tofu is caramelized and the candy potatoes are fork tender, assemble your bowls.
Drizzle with the closing peanut sauce. Or place the peanut sauce in a bit dish on each bowl.
Nutrition
Calories 496 Fat 14.8g Protein 14.4g

Jade Noodles

Ingredients
- 8 ounces of dry noodles- *soba noodles*, *linguini*, *rice noodles*
- 1 small bunch of asparagus -8 ounces
- 4 ounces of snow peas
- 1 small bunch of broccolini – or sub broccoli or green beans -8 ounces
- 8–16 onces of edamame (shelled)
- 8 ounces of *baked tofu* (or seared tofu, pressed tofu, or sub chicken breast)
- 3-4 generous handfuls baby spinach- 4 ounces
- 3 scallions- sliced
- garnishes -toasted *sesame seeds*, avocado, cilantro, sprouts

Sesame Ginger Dressing
- ⅓ cup of olive oil
- 2 tablespoons of *sesame oil*
- ⅓ cup of soy sauce or gluten free Bragg's liquid amino acids
- ¼ cup of rice wine vinegar
- 3 tablespoons of brown sugar
- 1 tablespoon of chili sauce
- 2 tablespoons of finely chopped ginger
- 3 fat cloves garlic- minced

Instructions
Bring a massive pot of salted water to boil for the pasta and cook pasta according to directions
Make the Sesame Ginger dressing by way of stirring the ingredients collectively in a medium bowl.
During the ultimate couple mins of cooking the pasta, upload any veggies that want a brief blanching immediately into the boiling pasta water (broccolini, asparagus, snow peas, edamame) for 1-2 mins, until they turn brilliant green. Drain and rinse with cold walking water till chilled. Drain well and region in a massive bowl.
Pour dressing over top and upload tofu (or chicken) and child spinach, a handful at a time, tossing the whole thing together well. Toss in the scallions. Taste, adjust salt and heat (add more chili paste if you want).
Serve in bowls with optionally available garnishes.
Nutrition
Calories 422 Fat 20.6g Protein 12.3g

Vegan Mushroom Pasta With Roasted Sun Chokes

Ingredients
- 8 ounces of dry pasta- tagliatelle, fettuccine, linguine, spaghetti
- 8 ounces of sunchokes
- 2 teaspoons of olive oil
- salt and pepper
- 8 ounces of sliced mushrooms- cremini, shittake, porto's, chanterelles
- 2 tsp of olive oil

Artichoke Sauce:
- 1 jar of artichoke hearts (about 1 ½ cups)
- ½ cup of water
- ¼ cup of olive oil
- 10 fresh sage leaves
- 2 garlic cloves
- ½ teaspoon of salt
- ½ teaspoon of cracked pepper
- lemon to taste
- Garnishes- grated *Pecorino*, *truffle oil*

Instructions
Preheat oven to 400.
Wash and pat dry sunchokes. Don't trouble peeling. Quarter them and mix in a bowl with olive oil, salt and pepper. Place on a parchment linked baking sheet within the oven and roast for 20 mins or until tender.
Bring pot of generously salted water to a boil (for the pasta). Cook the pasta to al dente.
While water is boiling, in a huge skillet, saute the mushrooms over medium heat in a bit olive oil. Season with salt and pepper, set aside.
Make the Sauce: drain the artichoke hearts and region them in a blender. Add the water, olive oil, sage, garlic, salt and pepper. Blend till creamy and really very smooth. If sauce seems "stringy" from the aritchokes, you want to preserve mixing on high speed. Taste. If the usage of frozen artichoke hearts or artichokes packed in water, add a little squeeze of lemon to taste. (The marinated artichokes in oil commonly have a piece of vinegar or acid already.)
Add the cooked, drained pasta (do not rinse) to the cooked mushrooms inside the saute pan. Toss with the artichoke sauce and warmth up, lightly stirring. Taste for salt, adding extra if necessary. Add the roasted sunchokes and toss well.
To garnish, you may drizzle a bit truffle oil over top and dust some finely grated Parmesan.—or hold it vegan, as much as you. Chili flakes are excellent too.
Nutrition
Calories436%TotalFat 17.7g27%SaturatedFat2.5g Cholesterol 0mg0% Sodium 324.1mg14%TotalCarbohydrate 60.9g20%Dietary Fiber 6.9g28%Sugars 8g Protein 10.9g22%

Roasted Eggplant With Zaatar

Ingredients
- 1 eggplant (about 1– 1 ⅛ lb)
- 1 ½ tablespoons of olive oil
- 1 tablespoon of zataar spice mix- or see notes
- ¼ teaspoon of salt, more to taste
- 1 fat garlic clove

Served with:
- 2 cups of cooked rice or grains (freaked, *faro*, *quinoa*)

- 1–2 cups of fresh chopped veggies- tomato, cucumber, radish, grated carrot or beets
- plain yogurt, or tzatziki
- Italian parsley, kalamata olives, *aleppo* chili flakes, feta or *goat cheese* crumbles

Instructions
Preheat oven to 400F
Slice Eggplant in half, then slice deeply at a diagonal at one inch intervals -"crosshatching"(see photographs above) careful no longer to cut through skin.
Season each side with ⅛ teaspoon kosher salt, sprinkling it into the slices if possible.
Mix oil, spices, garlic collectively in a bowl to make a paste. Brush or spoon the whole contents over the eggplant and area on a sheet pan in the oven and bake for 1 hour rotating halfway via. After an hour, pierce with a fork and if they're very tender and juicy, they are are done. Bigger eggplants can also take longer.
In the suggest time, prepare dinner the grain and chop or prep some other vegetables.
When the eggplant is done, collect the plates, topping the warm rice or grain with the roasted eggplant, then surround with fresh veggies and drizzle with tahini sauce, yogurt or tzatziki- or you can surely season the clean veggies and rice with salt, lemon and olive oil. Add olives or cheese in case you wish. Sprinkle with sparkling Italian parsley. Enjoy!

Nutrition
Calories 343 Fat 16.1g Protein 9.5g

Fresh Spring Rolls With Peanut Sauce

Ingredients
- 8–10 Rice paper wrappers (10 inches in diameter)
- 1 head green leaf lettuce
- 1 red or yellow color bell pepper, cut into thin strips
- 1 1/2 cups of *shredded* purple cabbage
- 1 ½ cups of shredded carrots
- ½ of an English cucumber, cut into thin long strips
- ¼ cup of fresh Thai basil leaves, torn (or regular basil)
- ¼ cup of fresh mint leaves, torn (or cilantro, but mint is best!)
- Garnishing: daikon radish strips, avocado, grated radishes, grated turnips, grated beets, spicy greens like watercress or arugula, sprouts

Instructions
If using the Baked Tofu, make this first, see observe for cutting into strips.
Prep all your filling ingredients. Cut the vegetables, gather the herbs. Gather all of the fillings close to you. I like to region those all on a cutting board close to my spring roll rolling area. Miser en vicinity.
Fill a large bowl (big enough to dip rice paper) with lukewarm water and area it behind your rolling area. Wet the counter in the front of you. (Or drench a thin kitchen towel with water, wring it out and lay it on the counter, rolling the spring rolls on pinnacle of the towel.
Do a "tester" roll. Dip the rice paper within the water. If using "thin" rice paper (package must say) just a brief dip is all you need. Otherwise, dip for 5-15 seconds. Pull when barely pliable (no longer too soft) and location it at the wet counter or towel. If rice paper still feels overly stiff, dip your hand in the water bowl and moist the rice paper a little, it'll soften up.
Place a 1/four leaf of lettuce down first in the front center of the rice paper (to save you shredded veggies from poking out of rice paper) leaving 2- three inches of area on the sides.
Top the leaf with shredded greens, tofu and torn herbs. Then firmly wrap up, tucking within the facets as you go. Place seam facet down on a wet cutting board, cover with a moist paper towel

Nutrition
Calories116%TotalFat 4.5g7%SaturatedFat0.6g Cholesterol 0mg0% Sodium 254.1mg11%Total Carbohydrate 5.2g2%Dietary Fiber 1.6g6%Sugars 2.2g Protein 3.9g8%

Bucatini Pasta With Arugula Pesto & Heirloom Tomatoes

Ingredients
- 16 ounces of Bucatini Pasta
- ½ cup of smoked salted almonds
- 4 cloves garlic
- 2 cups of basil leaves
- 2 cups of arugula
- 1 cup of olive oil
- 1 teaspoon of salt
- ½ teaspoon of fresh cracked pepper
- 1 tablespoon of plus 1 teaspoon juice

For garnishing: mini heirloom tomatoes (sliced in half), grated Romano cheese lemon zest

Instructions
Cook pasta in line with guidelines on package.
Make the pesto.
In a meals processor, place garlic, and almonds. Pulse 4-5 times.
Add basil, arugula and pulse a few greater times.
Add oil, lemon, salt and pepper.
Process till combined, but now not too smooth, a bit grain is good.
Toss with drained pasta.
Garnishing with: mini heirloom tomatoes (sliced in half), grated romano cheese and a touch lemon zest, fresh arugula leaves.

Nutrition
Calories 475 Fat 31.7g Protein 10.4g

Middle Eastern Eggplant Wrap

Ingredients
- 1 small sized eggplant (1 pound)
- olive oil, salt and pepper for taste

Kale Slaw

- 6–7 lacinato kale leaves – 2 cups of shredded (packed)
- 1 bunch of italian parsley
- handful mint leaves
- ¼ cup of finely diced onion
- 2 tablespoons of olive oil
- 2 tablespoons of lemon juice
- ¼ teaspoon of salt
- sliced tomato, radishes, cucumber, feta, yogurt for garnishing

Quick *tahini sauce*
- 2 tbsp of *tahini paste*
- 3 tablespoons of hot tap water
- 1 tablespoon of lemon juice
- ⅛ tablespoon of salt
- 1 minced garlic clove
- 2– 4 wraps or tortillas about 8-10 inch

Instructions
Preheat oven to 425F
Slice eggplant into ¼ inch thick disks.
Brush the sides with olive oil and season with salt and pepper. Place on a parchment coated sheet pan and roast the oven for 25-30 minutes, flipping over after 20 minutes. While they're baking, make the slaw filling and sauce.
Slice the kale into thin ribbons, and then stack them. Then, place in a pot. Finally chop the parsley and mint, thin stems are ok. Add to the bowl along side the onion. Mix with oil, lemon juice, salt, pepper. You want this to be quite "juicy", so if wanted upload a little greater oil and lemon juice in same portions. You can upload radishes and/ or tomatoes here in case you want or sprinkle them over pinnacle of the wrap.
Whisk collectively the tahini sauce substances in a small bowl.
Lightly heat or toast the tortilla or wrap. Spread the inner with tahini sauce. Top with warm eggplant and a large mound of the dressed greens. Topping with tomatoes, radishes and feta if you like.
This recipe make 2 full-size wraps or 4 smaller ones. Or 3 medium ones.
For even more flavor, grill the eggplant for the duration of the nice and cozy months. Both the eggplant and the kale slaw may be made ahead and refrigerated.

Chili Garlic Tofu With Sesame Broccolini
Ingredients
- 8 –12 ounces of extra firm tofu
- 2 Tablespoons of *peanut oil*
- ½ teaspoon of salt
- ½ teaspoon of fresh cracked *peppercorns*
- 4 smashed garlic cloves
- 8 ounces of broccolini
- 1 Tablespoon of Chili Garlic Sauce
- 2 Tablespoons of *Honey*
- 1 1/2 teaspoons of Soy Sauce
- Garnishing – 2 small sheets roasted seaweed, sliced into thin strips
- 1 Tablespoon of toast *sesame seeds*

Directions
Drain the tofu with paper towels and reduce into half of inch thick pieces. Blot again.
Heat oil in a skillet at medium temp.
Then, add salt and pepper and smashed garlic, directly in the skillet. Swirl and cook dinner for 1-2 minutes till the garlic is being fragrant.
Sear tofu till it is golden brown, over medium heat, about 5 mins on each side
Meantime, fill a medium pot with ¾ in of water, and set at the stove. Place a steam basket internal and layer up the broccolini. Cover with a lid and convey to a boil. Steam for 5 mins or desired doneness – much less for inexperienced beans.
Together the chili sauce, honey and soy sauce in a small bowl. Set aside.
Cut the seaweed strips.
When the tofu is done, divide amongst serving plates. With tongs, move the garlic from the skillet, transfer the broccolini to the skillet and deliver it a terrific mix for coating.
Add the toasted sesame seeds, and mix for one min at medium tempreature. Divide many of the serving dishes.
Sprinkle the tofu with the chili sauce and topping with the seaweed strands.

Nutrition
Calories 435 Fat 26.6g Protein 33g

Crispy Sheet Pan Jackfruit Tacos
Ingredients
8 x six-inch taco shells (corn or flour)
1 can of vegan refried beans (pinto or black beans)
Shredded cabbage
1 avocado or sour cream
Tomatillo Salsa
pickled onions
cilantro for garnishing

Directions
Set oven at 400 F
On a parchment-lined sheet pan, lay out the tortillas. Spread with a few tbsp of refried beans. Topping with cheese if you like or maintain this vegan.
Divide the jackfruit carnitas the various tortillas and region them inside the oven. Bake till heated via and the rims of the tortillas are crispy about 12-15 min.
Topping with cabbage slaw and avocado, pickled onions and salsa or hot sauce. Serve with non-compulsory sour cream or vegan-adaptable chipotle Mayo.
Fold up into tacos and consume immediately!

Nutrition
Calories 459 Fat 18.4g Protein 12.3g

Lentil Dal With Sweet Potatoes
Ingredients
- 1 cup of *red lentils* (*split lentils*)
- 1–2 tablespoon of *coconut oil*, *ghee*, or olive oil
- 1 yellow onion

- 1 tablespoon of grated fresh ginger
- 4 cloves garlic
- 1 teaspoon of *cumin seeds* (or substitute ground cumin)
- 1 tablespoon of *Garam Masala* Spice
- 1 teaspoon of *fenugreek leaves* (optional)
- ¾ teaspoon of salt
- 1 teaspoon of *honey* or maple
- 2 bay leaves
- 1 serrano chili pepper, slit down the side vertically
- 1 medium sized sweet potato, diced into ¾ inch cubes
- 3 cups of water
- 2 medium sized tomatoes, diced
- chopped scallions for garnishing
- Flaked coconut

Tempering oil -Optional highly recommended!!!
- 2–3 tablespoons of *coconut oil*
- 1 teaspoon of *cumin seeds*
- 1 teaspoon of *fennel seeds*
- 1 teaspoon of *black mustard seeds*
- 8 *curry leaves*

Directions

Rinse lentils and soak lentils in a bowl of water.
Take a pot or Dutch over, warmness oil over medium excessive warmth.
Saute onion for 2-3 minutes, stirring, then upload ginger. Saute two greater minutes, then add garlic and turn heat to medium. Add spices, salt, bay leaves and chili. Stir for any other minute letting spices toast, then add honey, and candy potato.
Strain lentils and then add to the pot, along side water and tomatoes. Give a stir, convey to boil, cover, and turn heat down, and let gently simmer, approximately 15 min. After 15 min, uncover and take a look at consistency, If watery, retain to simmer uncovered until it reduces and becomes thicker. Adjust salt, adding extra in your taste, retaining in mind you need this to be salty if serving it over rice in dish.
Make oil to drizzle over top: heat oil or ghee over medium high tempreature, upload seeds and curry leaves and swirl or stir till you pay attention popping, about 30- forty five seconds. Turn warmth off.
Drizzle it onthe dal, after dishing it up.
Serve it with toasted naan bread, and garnishing with cilantro and flaked coconut.

Nutrition
Calories 355 Fat 14.8g Protein 14.4g

Zaatar Roasted Cauliflower Steaks With Sauce

Ingredients
- 1 whole cauliflower- leaves- sliced into ½ inch thick steaks
- 1 tablespoon of olive oil
- 3-4 teaspoons of *zaatar* spice
- salt and pepper to your taste

Green Tahini Sauce
- 3/4 cup of water
- 3 tablespoons of lemon juice
- 2 tablespoons of olive oil
- 2 fat garlic cloves
- 1 small bunch cilantro
- 2-3 slices jalapeno (
- 1/4 teaspoon of salt
- ½ cup of *tahini paste*

Directions

Set oven at 425 F
Trim the leaves of cauliflower leaving the long stem in tact. Slice the very cease off the stem. Slice the Cauliflower into 5-6 slices.
Brush the sides with olive oil and sprinkle with salt and pepper. Sprinkle generously with zaatar spice and area on a parchment coated sheet pan within the oven, to roast till fork tender approximately 20-25 minutes.
While it's roasting make the inexperienced tahini sauce.
Place all of the ingredients except the tahini paste in the blender, and mix until combined (however no longer smooth). Add paste and mix again until favored smoothness. Sprinkle salt according to your taste.
Dish up the Zaatar Cauliflower Steaks and Drizzle with Green Tahini Sauce! Serve along the Everyday Kale Salad!

Nutrition
Calories308%TotalFat 27.1g42%SaturatedFat3.9g Cholesterol 0mg0% Sodium 224mg9%Total Carbohydrate 14.6g5%Dietary Fiber 5.7g23%Sugars 3.1g Protein 7.9g16%

Tofu Stir-Fry With Broccoli And Mushrooms

Ingredients
- 8 ounces of broccolini
- 1–2 tablespoons of *coconut oil* or *peanut oil.*
- 8–10 ounces of tofu- patted dry, cubed
- 1 shallot- diced
- 5 garlic cloves- rough chopped
- 8 ounces of shiitake mushrooms, stems removed, sliced
- 4-5 red chilies
- 2 tablespoons of chopped peanuts or cashews
- 2 tablespoons of sweetened *black vinegar*
- 2 tablespoons of soy sauce
- 2 tablespoons of water
- Garnishing- *crispy shallots*, scallions, *sesame seeds*

Instructions

Place broccolini in a steamer basket, interior a medium pot with 1 inch water. Bring to a boil. Cover, turn warmth down and simmer five minutes. Turn tempreature off. Uncover it.
Meantime, chop the shallots, garlic and slice the mushrooms.
Mix the rest of the ingredients together via the stove.
In a wok or cast iron skillet, warmth the coconut oil over medium high warmth. When it becomes hot, season the oil with a generous 5 finger pinch of salt

and fresh cracked pepper. Add tofu (or bird or shrimp) and browning all aspects flipping and turning till maximum facets aspects are golden and crispy, about five-6 min. If it is sticking, make sure that pan is nicely oiled, and permit it increase a touch golden crust earlier than flipping. (When it receives this "crust" it'll clearly release itself from the pan- if its sticking, you will be flipping it prematurely) Set the tofu (or chook or shrimp) aside.
Add a little extra coconut oil to the wok and heat. When it becomes hot, add shallot and garlic, stirring constantly till golden and fragrant, about 2 minutes. Add sliced shiitake mushrooms. Continue cooking turning warmness to medium, stirring often till tender. Add dried chilies and elective nuts. Saute 1 min.
Then, add vinegar, soy and water. Mix it. Using tongs, add the steamed broccolini and toss to coat. Add tofu, supply a few stirs, coating all. Taste for salt, add greater if necessary. Divide amongst 2 bowls. Garnishing with crispy shallots, scallions or toasted sesame seeds. Serve immediately.
Nutrition
Calories359% Daily Value*Total Fat 21.2g33%Saturated Fat 12.3g Cholesterol 0mg0% Sodium 489.6mg20%Total Carbohydrate 28.3g9%Dietary Fiber 8.1g32%Sugars 7.4g Protein 20.6g41%

Sesame Brussel Sprouts, Mushrooms & Tofu

Ingredients
- 8–10 ounces of tofu (firm or pressed), blotted dry and cut into flat-ish cubes
- 1 tablespoon of olive or *coconut oil*
- salt and pepper
- 1 shallot or ½ onions diced
- 10 ounces of shredded Brussels sprouts, cabbage slaw or broccoli slaw
- 4 ounces of sliced mushrooms
- 1 teaspoon of soy sauce
- Garnishing: toasted *sesame seeds*, toasted *sesame oil* sliced scallions, nuts, sprouts

Instructions
Heat oil in a large skillet (or wok) over medium excessive warmth.
Season oil with a generous pinch salt and clean cracked pepper
Add tofu and sear all sides, turning warmness all the way down to medium if necessary.
When golden, set tofu aside. Blot.
In the equal pan add a bit greater oil if necessary. Sauté shallot (or onion) over medium high heat, stirring till smooth 2-three minutes.
Add mushrooms. Cook until tender, 3-four minutes, turning warmth down if want be.
Add shredded Brussels sprouts and cook, usually stirring until gentle and bright green, about three minutes. If pan feels dry add a splash of water or cooking wine.

Keep the Brussels slightly crisp, yet soft.
Stir in soy sauce.Taste for salt.
Divide veggies amongst two bowls. Top with seared tofu. Drizzle with a touch sesame oil, sprinkle with toasted sesame seeds(or Gomasio), nuts if you want and scallions. Add Sriracha in case you like.
Serve immediately.

Make Life Simple Instant Pot Lentil Soup

Ingredients
- 1 onion, diced
- 6 –8 cloves garlic, chopped
- 2 tablespoons of olive oil
- 4 cups diced veggies
- 1 and 1/2 teaspoons of salt, more to taste.
- 1 tablespoon of cumin
- 2 teaspoons of *coriander*
- 2 teaspoons of curry powder
- 1 teaspoon of turmeric
- 1/2 teaspoon of *allspice*
- 1 teaspoon of Italian herbs
- 2 tablespoons of tomato paste
- 2 medium sized tomatoes, diced
- 4 flavorful cups chicken or veggie stock
- 2 cups of water
- 1 and ¼ cup of small Black *Caviar lentils* or French Green Lentils
- Finishing with olive oil, lemon juice, chopped Italian parsley, diced tomatoes and optional chili flakes and toasted pita.

Instructions
Saute onion and garlic within the Instant Pot in 2 tablespoons oil until fragrant and tender, approximately 2-three minutes. (Or prepare dinner in a dutch oven on the range, over medium-excessive heat)
Add the veggies, spices and salt. Saute 4-5 extra min. Then, add the tomato paste and brown it a bit on heat. Add the tomatoes and their juices, inventory and water, scraping up any browned bits. Add the lentils, stir and cover, placing the Instant pot to Pressure Cook on Normal for 12 minutes. (Alternately if cooking on the stove top, carry to a simmer and cover, simmering on low for 20-25 min)
Let the stress launch both manually or naturally. Divide amongst bowls and drizzle with olive oil, a squeeze of lemon, chili flakes, sparkling parsley and sparkling diced tomato

Nutrition
Calories287%TotalFat 3.2g5%SaturatedFat0.8g Cholesterol 5.8mg2% Sodium 316.7mg13%Total Carbohydrate 43.1g16%Dietary Fiber 8.2g33%Sugars 7.5g Protein 18g36%

Vegan Stuffed Poblanos With Avocado Crema

Ingredients
- 6 whole sized poblano peppers
- 1 sweet medium sized potato- 2 Cups,
- 1 corn on the cob, kernels cut

- 1 tablespoon of olive oil
- 1 C thinely diced onion
- 4 garlic cloves- chopped
- 1 14 ounce can of black beans
- 1 T Cumin
- 2 tsp of *coriander*
- ½ tsp of chile powder
- ½ tsp of *kosher salt*
- ⅓ Cup of chopped cilantro
- ¼ C -½ C of crumbled queso fresco cheese, mozzarella, jack, *goat cheese*

Avocado Crema (Vegan)
- ⅔ C of Avocado (one small avocado)
- ⅓ C of cilantro
- 2/3 C of water- plus more as needed
- ½ teaspoon of *kosher salt*
- 1 tsp of *coriander*
- ⅛ C of lime juice
- 2 garlic cloves
- cracked pepper to taste

Instructions

Preheat oven to 400F. Dice the candy potatoes, into 1/2 in cubes. The smaller the dice, the better it is. Toss with a drizzle of olive oil, region on a parchment-covered baking sheet, in conjunction with the 6 poblano peppers and roast till golden and tender, about 20 minutes, turning peppers over, midway.

While that is baking Make the Avocado Crema, placing all of the ingredients in the blender, and blend till smooth, adding a bit more water if needed to get the blade going. Set aside.

Then cut the kernels off. Set aside. Dice the onion. Take out peppers and sweet potatoes from the oven. when tender. Enclose the poblano peppers in foil for 5-10 minutes so that they steam, to make removing the skins easier. Hold the peppers underneath cool, slow strolling water and gently get rid of skins trying to maintain the peppers intact. It's OK, if all of the skins don't release, just peel off what wants to come off naturally. Carefully, with a pointy knife, slice the top off of the peppers (wherein stuffing will go) and rinse the seeds out with running water. Keep the stems and set aside.

In skillet warmness olive oil over med-high warmness, upload onions and sauté for 2-3 minutes. Turn warmness to down medium, add garlic and hold stirring until fragrant and golden, approximately 3-4 greater minutes. Add corn. Saute more than one minutes, then fold within the black beans, roasted candy potatoes, spices, salt and pepper, sautéing till warmed through. Fold in cilantro. Taste and alter salt on your liking. Turned warmth off. Stir in cheese if using.

Stuff the peppers: Spoon inside the filling into the peppers then region stuffed peppers on a greased or parchment sheet pan or in a baking dish in 375 F oven for 10-15 minutes — or longer to soften the cheese in the filling.

Serve the stuffed peppers over a generous mattress of Avocado Cream sauce. Top with cilantro sprigs, crumbled queso fresco.

Nutrition
Calories280%TotalFat 6.6g10%SaturatedFat1g Cholesterol 0mg0% Sodium 62mg3%Total Carbohydrate 50.9g17%Dietary Fiber 12.7g51%Sugars 11.8g Protein 11.1g22%

Vegan Lentil Cakes With Zhoug Sauce

Ingredients
- 2 cups of cooked lentils
- 1 tablespoon of olive oil
- ½ red onion, diced
- 4–6 garlic cloves, chopped
- 8 ounces of mushrooms, sliced
- ½ cup of rolled oats
- ½ cup of walnuts
- 1 teaspoon of cumin
- 1 teaspoon of *coriander*
- ¾ teaspoon of *kosher salt*
- 1 tablespoon of ground flax
- 3 tablespoons of water
- 1 tablespoon of Braggs Liquid Amino's (or 2 teaspoons soy sauce)
- ¼ cup of chopped parsley or cilantro

Zhoug Yogurt
- ½ –1 cup of plain yogurt (feel free to use vegan yogurt)
- 1–2 tablespoons of *zhoug* – a spicy Israeli condiment available at Trader joes and upscale markets
- salt and lemon to your taste

Instructions

Cook ⅔ -¾ cup dry lentils in simmering water until gentle. Drain. You will need 2 cups cooked.

In the suggest time, sauté the onion, garlic and mushrooms in olive oil over medium warmth for five minutes. Add a bit water if it receives too dry. Turn warmth right down to low and cook till very gentle and cooked through. Set aside.

In a food processor, combination the oats right into a direction flour. Add walnuts, pulse 10 times. Add 1/2 of the lentils, half of the mushroom mixture, salt, spices, flax, water, (or egg) and pulse repeatedly till it's well blended and bureaucracy a thick dough. It doesn't need to be smooth…a bit texture is good. Scrap right into a medium bowl and stir in the final complete lentils and fresh herbs.

Using moist hands form into 8-10 little desserts or 4- five burger patties.

Sear in a skillet, in a little oil, over medium heat, taking care to let them brown and form a crust, before flipping. (FYI This will make sure they don't stick to the skillet. As they form a crust, they release from the pan almost naturally.)

Serve with the closing mushrooms and optional Zhoug Yogurt (vegan adaptable).

To make zhoug yogurt sincerely stir a 1-2 tablespoons zhoug into to the yogurt to taste. Add salt and lemon if you like.
Nutrition
Calories 252% TotalFat 11.3g17%SaturatedFat1.3g Cholesterol 0mg0% Sodium 447.8mg19%Total Carbohydrate 28g9%Dietary Fiber 9g36%Sugars 3.6g Protein 12.4g25%

Vegan Tikka Masala With Cauliflower
Ingredients
- 1–2 tablespoons of *coconut oil*, olive oil or *ghee*
- 1 shallot – chopped roughly
- 1 tablespoon of chopped ginger
- 4 fat garlic cloves, rough chopped
- 1 teaspoon of cumin
- 1 teaspoon of *coriander*
- 1 teaspoon of turmeric
- ½ teaspoon of paprika
- 1 teaspoon of curry powder
- 1 teaspoon of *mustard seeds*
- 1 teaspoon of *fennel seeds*
- 1 teaspoon of *fenugreek leaves*
- 1 teaspoon of salt
- 1 can of diced tomatoes
- 1 can of *coconut milk*
- 1 red bell pepper
- 1 head of cauliflower – sliced
- squeeze of lemon
- cilantro for garnish

Serve with *pita bread*, or rice.
Instructions
Heat oil in a massive heavy bottom pot or Dutch oven over medium excessive heat. (see notes for Instant Pot)
Add shallot, ginger and garlic, and decrease warmness to medium to save you burning, stirring often about three minutes till fragrant and golden.
Add spices, seeds and salt and gently toast, even as stirring 1-2 minutes, which will beautify their flavor.
Add diced tomato, cook 2 extra mins, then upload the coconut milk and stir to incorporate, bringing to a simmer. Add cauliflower and crimson bell pepper, supply a stir, cowl and let simmer 10-12 mins on medium low heat. Check the cauliflower - it need to be simply tender, and maintain cooking uncovered until preferred tenderness (the smaller you chop the portions the faster this may prepare dinner). Taste, add a squeeze of lemon juice. Add greater salt if you want.
Serve in bowls over rice or with naan or pita bread. Garnish with cilantro.
Nutrition
Calories 210 Fat 16g Protein 14.4g

Smoky Chipotle Black Bean Burger Recipe
Ingredients
- 2 cans of black beans, rinsed, drained well (3 cups cooked)
- 1 teaspoon of salt
- 2 teaspoons of cumin
- 2 teaspoon of *smoked paprika*
- 1 teaspoon of *coriander*
- ¼ teaspoon of *chipotle powder*, more to taste
- 2 tablespoon of olive oil
- zest from one small lime, 1 tablespoon
- 1 tablespoon f lime juice
- 1 egg
- ¼ cup of chopped cilantro
- ½ cup of bread crumbs

Instructions
Rinse well and drain 2 cans of black beans and vicinity in a medium sized pot.
Drizzle with salt and all the other spices. Then, add olive oil, lime zest and lime juice. Mash with a potato masher, until mainly mashed, leaving a little texture, then mix until combined. (You can also pulse in a meals processor). Taste, alter warmness level.
At this point you can upload ¼-⅓ cup floor flax seed in case you need this vegan. Otherwise, upload the egg, cilantro and the bread crumbs and blend well till mixed well. Let stand 10-15 mins o the breadcrumbs or/flax have a threat to soak up moisture.
Using easy damp hands, form into 4 big patties.
Warm 1 tbsp of oil in a pan, at medium tempreature. Sear every aspect five-7 minutes, or till golden and heated all the way through. Place in a warm oven till equipped to serve – and experience free to feature any melty cheese.
Refrigerate the seared black bean burgers for later use (let them cool, then wrap it tightly in plastic wrap).
To reheat, warm in an oven, toaster oven or at the grill.
Serve it on toasted buns, with chipotle mayo, Mexican slaw or Curtido and avocado in case you like, or over a mattress of dressed veggies and/ and grains with fresh veggies!
Nutrition
Calories290%TotalFat 9.1g14%SaturatedFat1.5g Cholesterol 35.3mg12% Sodium 1150.7mg48%Total Carbohydrate 39.5g13%Dietary Fiber 15.4g61%Sugars 1.1g Protein 14.9g30%

Hemp Crusted Tofu With Celeriac Puree
Ingredients
Hemp Crusted Tofu (or sub sunflower seeds)
- 8-12 ounce of block of tofu, patted dry and sliced into ¾-1 inch filets
- 1 tablespoon of warm water
- 1 tablespoon of miso
- 1 tablespoon of olive oil
- 1 garlic clove minced
- ¼ teaspoon of salt
- 2 –3 tablespoons of *hemp seeds*
- 1 extra large sized celeriac, peeled and diced (about 2 heaping cups)
- 1 tablespoon of olive oil
- 1 fat shallot- diced
- 2 garlic cloves-chopped

- 1 cup of water
- ¼ teaspoon of salt
- pepper to taste

Serve with *Gremolata* and *Everyday Kale Slaw.*
Instructions
Preheat oven to 400 F
Take a small bowl, whisk water, miso, olive oil, garlic and salt. Brush all facets of the tofu with the marinade and liberally coat the pinnacle -region on a parchment coated sheet pan. Spoon any final marinade over the top. Drizzle each filet liberally with hemp seeds, pressing them down lightly. Place inside the oven for half-hour or until golden.
When the tofu is baking you can make the Celeriac Puree.
Peel the celeriac the usage of a pointy paring knife and dice. Heat oil at medium tempreature in a big skillet and saute the shallot and garlic until golden and fragrant, about 2-3 min. Add the celeriac and water. Bring to a simmer, cover it and simmer it gently for 10 min or until fork tender.
When tender, upload the celeriac and any last liquid into a meals processor. Blend until smooth, upload salt, pepper and more water to get a silky clean consistency. Think of this almost as a "sauce", as opposed to a "mash". For greater richness you may add another tablespoon of olive oil, or maybe butter or ghee.
Divide the Celeriac Puree among bowls, pinnacle with the Hemp Tofu and spoon a touch Gremolata over pinnacle. Serve with the Everyday Kale Slaw or a easy aspect salad.
Nutrition
Calories308%TotalFat 24.5g38%SaturatedFat3.3g Cholesterol 0mg0% Sodium 678.3mg28%Total Carbohydrate 13.7g5%Dietary Fiber 3.3g13%Sugars 6.2g Protein 13.9g28%

Vegan Collard Green Wraps
Ingredients
- 4 extra large sized collard green leaves
- 1 cup of Hummus
- 1 cup of *crispy tofu* cubes
- ½ cup of grated carrots
- ½ cup of grated beets
- 1 cup of greens(watercress, arugula spinach) or micro greens
- fresh herbs (cilantro, parsley, basil, mint)

Drizzle with Everyday *Tahini Sauce!*
Instructions
Take a large bowl of water to a boil. Turn warmness to low, stack and area four collard vegetables inside the water, stem facets first and blanch for 30-60 seconds, or till stems are tender. Using tongs, turn so all components of the leaves are blanched and pliable enough to roll.
Pull them off form the water with the tongs, shake them within the sink and location at the counter.
When the water is heating, you can grate your carrots and beets, slice the avocado into pieces and make the tofu crispy.
In order to make the tofu crispy, pat dry an 8 ounce block of extra company tofu and cut it into ½ in cubes. Then, place in a bowl and toss with ½ teaspoon salt, and your desire of 1-2 teaspoons turmeric or garam masala spice. You also can use every other spice combination here – zaatar spice, cajun seasoning, etc., simply something to give it some flavor! Heat 2 tbsp of oil in a pan or properly seasoned solid iron skillet, and sear the tofu, on a couple facets, until crispy. Set aside.
Make the ordinary tahini sauce if using.
Assemble the collard greens wraps. Place ¼ cup hummus at the lower middle of the wrap, pinnacle with ¼ of the tofu, then the vegetables and herbs. Rolling up, tucking the sides in as you go like a burrito.
Roll up all four wraps and region seam them aspect down.
If serving right away, reduce in them in half and serve with a drizzle of the tahini sauce. Or wrap, with out cutting, in plastic wrap for later. These will preserve for 2 days inside the fridge.
Nutrition
Calories220%TotalFat 12g18%SaturatedFat1.7g Cholesterol 0mg0% Sodium 492.9mg21%Total Carbohydrate 20.5g7%Dietary Fiber 5.6g23%Sugars 3.8g Protein 10g20%

Vegan Mashed Potatoes
Ingredients
2 pounds of russet potatoes
8 cloves of garlic, peeled and smashed
1 sprig fresh rosemary
1 sprig fresh thyme
1/4 cup of olive oil
1 pinch of salt to your taste
Directions
Place the potatoes, garlic, rosemary, and thyme in a pot and cover with salted water; bring to a boil. Cook, covered until vegetables are easily pierced with a knife, about 30 minutes. Drain, reserving 1 cup of the water.
Transfer boiled potatoes and garlic to a pot; then discard rosemary and thyme. Then, add olive oil and other spices. Mash potato with a masher; add cooking water to reach desired consistency.

Poultry and Meat Recipes

Oven-Roasted Whole Chicken

Ingredients
- 2 cups of water
- 2 tablespoons of kosher salt plus 1/2 teaspoon, divided
- 2 tablespoons of granulated sugar
- 1 tablespoon of whole black peppercorns
- 1 ½ teaspoons of fennel seed
- 2 lemons, divided
- 3 cloves garlic, crushed
- 6 fresh thyme sprigs and 1 teaspoon of thyme leaves, divided
- 2 fresh bay leaves
- 6 cups of ice
- 1 (4 to 5 pound) chicken
- 2 teaspoons of extra-virgin olive oil
- 1 teaspoon of ground pepper

Directions

Mix water, 2 tablespoons salt, sugar, peppercorns, fennel seed, lemon wedges, garlic, thyme sprigs and bay leaves in a small saucepan. Bring to a boil at medium temperature and stir until the salt is dissolved, approximately 2 minutes. Remove from heat.

Place ice in a 5-quart bowl and pour the brine over it. Let cool, stirring occasionally, about 5 minutes. Add hen, making sure it is absolutely submerged inside the brine. (Add more cold water if necessary.) Refrigerate it in a single day or up to 24 hours.

To roast fowl, preheat oven to 375 levels F. Line a rimmed baking sheet with foil and area a cord rack on top. Coat the rack with cooking spray.

Remove the fowl from the brine and region it on the prepared rack. Pat it dry with a paper towel.

Zest the final lemon and juice it to get 2 tsp. Mix the zest and juice with oil, pepper and the ultimate 1 teaspoon thyme and half of teaspoon salt. Loosen and raise the pores and skin from the breast and legs together with your arms and rub the paste under and over the pores and skin. Truss the fowl with kitchen string

Roast the chook for 1 hour. Rotate the pan, and boom the heat to 400 tiers F. Cook till an instant-read thermometer registers a hundred and sixty ranges F in the thickest a part of the breast, 25 to 30 minutes more. Let the fowl rest for 10 minutes before carving.

Nutrition

263 calories; 10.7 g total fat; 118 mg is cholesterol; 361 mg is sodium. 651 mg potassium; 11.1 g is carbohydrates; 3.2 g fiber; 5 g sugar; 29.7 g protein; 18 mg vitamin c; 36 mcg folate; 62 mg calcium; 2 mg iron; 44 mg magnesium;

Cauliflower Rice Bowls With Grilled Asparagus And Chicken Sausage

Ingredients
- 2 teaspoons of olive oil
- 4 links of fully cooked sweet Italian chicken sausage, sliced
- 1 (12 ounce) of package frozen riced cauliflower
- 1 (12 ounce) of package frozen grilled asparagus spears
- 6 tablespoons of pesto

Directions

Heat oil in a pan at medium tempreature. Add sausage and cook, mixing often, until heated through and browned on each sides, about five minutes. Prepare cauliflower and asparagus in step with bundle directions (about three to 4 minutes each inside the oven). Set apart to cool it slightly before assembling bowls.

Divide pesto among four small lidded bins and refrigerate.

Divide the cauliflower among four single-serving lidded boxes. Topping each with one-fourth of the asparagus and one-fourth of the sausage. Refrigerate for up to 4 days. To reheat, vent the lid and microwave on High till steaming, 2 1/2 to three minutes. Top with pesto before serving.

Nutrition

290 calories; 19 4 g total fat; 65 mg is cholesterol; 733 mg is sodium. 193 mg is potassium; 7.5 g carbohydrates; 3.5 g fiber; 2 g sugar; 20.4 g protein; 58 mg is vitamin c; 121 mcg folate; 72 mg calcium; 2 mg iron; 19 mg magnesium;

Baked Lemon-Pepper Chicken

Ingredients
- 4 (6 ounce) of boneless, skinless chicken breasts
- ½ teaspoon of salt, and 1/8 teaspoon, divided
- 1 tablespoon of extra-virgin olive oil
- 1 medium sized lemon, thinly sliced
- 2 tablespoons of lemon juice
- 1 tablespoon of pure maple syrup
- 2 tablespoons of unsalted butter, cut into pieces
- 1 teaspoon of cracked pepper

Directions

Preheat oven to 425 levels F.

Sprinkle fowl flippantly with half tsp of salt. Heat oil in a skillet at medium-high tempreatue. Add the chicken; cook, undisturbed, till the bottom is golden brown, approximately four minutes. Flip the chook; set up lemon slices round the hen inside the pan. Transfer the skillet to the oven; bake till an instant-read thermometer inserted into the thickest part of meat registers 165 degrees F, approximately 10 minutes.

Transfer the chicken to a platter. Then add lemon juice, maple syrup to the pan. Add butter and 1 piece at a time, mixing until it melts into the sauce. Mix in pepper and the remaining 1/8 tsp of salt. Drizzle the sauce over the hen.

Nutrition

286 calories; 13.3 g total fat; 109 mg is cholesterol; 448 mg is sodium. 350 mg is potassium; 7.1 g is carbohydrates; 1.4 g fiber; 3 g sugar; 34.8 g protein; 8

mcgis folate; 43 mg calcium; 1 mg iron; 38 mg magnesium; 3 g added sugar;

Antipasto Baked Smothered Chicken
Ingredients
- 3 tablespoons of extra-virgin olive oil, divided
- ⅓ cup of chopped marinated artichoke hearts
- ⅓ cup of chopped salami
- ¼ cup of chopped pepperoncini
- 2 tablespoons of red-wine vinegar
- 1 tablespoon of chopped fresh oregano, plus more for garnish
- 1 pound of chicken cutlets
- ½ teaspoon of ground pepper
- 2 ounces of fresh mozzarella cheese, thinly sliced

Directions
Mix 2 tablespoons oil, artichoke hearts, salami, pepperoncini, vinegar and oregano in a medium bowl. Heat the final 1 tablespoon oil in a large ovenproof skillet over medium-excessive heat. Sprinkle bird with pepper and add to the pan. Cook till starting to brown, about three minutes. Turn the fowl over and pinnacle every piece with the artichoke combination and cheese. Transfer the pan to the oven and broil the fowl till the cheese is browned and an instant-read thermometer inserted inside the thickest a part of the bird registers 165 degrees F, 3 to 4 minutes more. Serve the chook with any pan drippings and oregano, if desired.

Nutrition
303 calories; 19.6 g total fat; 82 mg cholesterol; 476 mg sodium. 263 mg potassium; 2.8 g carbohydrates; 0.7 g fiber; 27.6 g protein; 5 mcg folate; 90 mg calcium; 1 mg iron; 27 mg magnesium;

Lemon & Dill Chicken
Ingredients
- 4 boneless, skinless chicken breasts, (1-1 1/4-pounds)
- Salt & freshly ground pepper, to your taste
- 3 teaspoons of extra-virgin olive oil, or canola oil, divided
- ¼ cup of finely chopped onion
- 3 cloves of garlic, minced
- 1 cup of reduced-sodium chicken broth
- 2 teaspoons of flour
- 2 tablespoons of chopped fresh dill, divided
- 1 tablespoon of lemon juice

Directions
Season chook breasts on each facets with salt, pepper. Heat 1 and 1/2 tsp of oil in a big heavy skillet over medium-excessive warmth. Add the fowl and sear till properly browned on each facets, about 3 minutes in step with side. Transfer chook to a plate and tent with foil.
Reduce warmth to medium. Add the closing 1 half of tsp oil to the pan. Then, add onion and garlic and cook, stirring, for 1 min. Whisk broth, flour, 1 tablespoon dill and lemon juice in a measuring cup and add to pan. Cook, whisking, till barely thickened, about three mins.
Back to the chicken and any accumulated juices to the pan; lessen warmth to low and simmer until the chicken is cooked through, about four minutes. Transfer the chicken to a warmed platter. Season sauce with salt and pepper and spoon over the chook. Garnish with the closing 1 tablespoon chopped sparkling dill.

Nutrition
170 calories; 6.2 g total fat; 63 mg is cholesterol; 339 mg is sodium. 272 mg potassium; 3.3 g carbohydrates; 0.3 g fiber; 1 g sugar; 24.1 g protein; 3 mg vitamin c; 12 mcg folate; 19 mg calcium; 1 mg iron

Balsamic Marinated Chicken
Ingredients
- ¼ cup of extra-virgin olive oil
- ¼ cup of balsamic vinegar
- 2 cloves of garlic, minced
- 1 tablespoon of Italian seasoning
- 1 teaspoon of salt
- ½ teaspoon of freshly ground pepper
- 1-1 1/4 pounds of boneless, skinless chicken breast (see Note)

Directions
Mix oil, vinegar, garlic, Italian seasoning, salt and pepper in a bowl until combined properly.
Place bird in a shallow dish or 1-gallon sealable plastic bag. Add the marinade and refrigerate for at the least 1 hour and as much as 12 hours. Then, remove it from the marinade and pat dry.
Heat grill to medium-high or position a rack in top third of oven and heat broiler.
To grill: Oil the grill rack. Grill the chicken, turning once, until an instant-examine thermometer inserted into the thickest part registers 165 ranges F, 4 to 8 mins in step with each side.
To broil: Line a broiler pan with foil and coat with cooking spray. Place the chook at the foil. Broil, watching cautiously and turning as a minimum once, until an instant-study thermometer inserted into the thickest element registers 165 levels F, 10 to 15 minutes total.

Nutrition
169 calories; 7.3 g total fat; 63 mg is cholesterol; 250 mg is sodium. 208 mg potassium; 1.1 g carbohydrates; 1 g sugar; 22.9 g protein; 3 mcg folate; 14 mg calcium; 1 mg iron; 22 mg magnesium;

Asian-Style Chicken Salad Bowls
Ingredients
- 1 (12 ounce) of package seasoned cooked chicken strips
- 1/2 cup of sesame dressing
- 1 (9 ounce) of package shredded coleslaw mix
- ½ cup sesame-honey-flavored almonds

Directions
Cut fowl strips into bite-size pieces; set aside.

Measure 2 tablespoons dressing into every of four small lidded containers and refrigerate.
Divide coleslaw blend among four single-serving lidded packing containers. Top each with one-fourth of the hen and 2 tablespoons almonds.
Seal the boxes and refrigerate for up to 4 days. Toss with dressing just earlier than serving.

Nutrition
330 calories; 21.6 g total fat; 55 mg cholesterol; 493 mg sodium. 47 mg potassium; 13.6 g carbohydrates; 2.3 g fiber; 9 g sugar; 22.7 g protein; 27 mg vitamin c; 101 mg calcium; 3 mg iron

Southwest Black-Bean Pasta Salad Bowls
Ingredients
- 1 (14 ounce) of package frozen Mexican-style corn
- 2 cups of black-bean rotini
- 1 (12 ounce) of package cooked chili-lime chicken
- ½ cup of mild pico de gallo
- ½ cup of cilantro salad dressing

Directions
Heat corn in line with bundle directions; set aside to cool.
Cook pasta according to package deal directions. Drain and rinse with cold water. Drain once more and toss with the corn; set apart.
Slice chicken strips into bite-length pieces; set aside.
Divide percent de gallo into 4 small lidded packing containers and refrigerate. Measure salad dressing into 4 small lidded containers and refrigerate. (Timesaving tip: You also can carry the bottle of dressing to your lunch bag--or store inside the office fridge--and dress when geared up to serve.)
Divide the corn and pasta mixture among four single-serving boxes, then top every one with one-fourth of the fowl. Seal the packing containers and refrigerate for up to 4 days. Toss with the dressing just earlier than serving and top with the p.c. de gallo.

Nutrition
436 calories; 14.4 g total fat; 64 mg cholesterol; 375 mg sodium. 46.8 g carbohydrates; 14.4 g fiber; 9 g sugar; 33.7 g protein; 6 mg vitamin c; 187 mg calcium;

Moroccan Chicken Tagine With Apricots & Olives

Ingredients
- 2 tablespoons of extra-virgin olive oil, divided
- 1 pound of boneless, skinless chicken thighs, trimmed and cut into 1-inch pieces
- ½ teaspoon of salt, divided
- 1 large sized onion, chopped
- 1 lemon, zested and juiced, divided
- 1 tablespoon of minced garlic
- 1 tablespoon of grated fresh ginger
- 1 tablespoon of tomato paste
- 2 teaspoons of ras el hanout
- 2 cups of unsalted chicken broth
- 1 (15 ounce) can of no-salt-added chickpeas, rinsed
- ½ cup of chopped dried apricots
- ½ cup of pitted green olives, halved
- ½ cup of toasted slivered almonds, divided
- Fresh cilantro for garnish

Directions
Heat 1 tablespoon oil in a big pot over medium-high warmth. Add chicken and season with 1/four teaspoon salt. Cook, stirring once in a while, till gently browned on all sides, about five minutes. Using a slotted spoon, switch the hen to a smooth plate.
Add the remaining 1 tablespoon oil and onion to the pan. Cook, stirring every so often and scraping up any browned bits, till the onion is soft and gently browned, about four minutes. Stir in lemon zest, garlic, ginger, tomato paste and ras el hanout. Cook, stirring, until fragrant, about 30 seconds. Stir in broth, chickpeas, apricots, olives, 1/four cup almonds and the bird. Bring to a simmer and cook, stirring sometimes, till the bird is cooked thru and the sauce has thickened slightly, approximately eight minutes. Remove from warmth and stir in lemon juice and the final 1/4 teaspoon salt. Serve crowned with the final 1/four cup almonds and cilantro, if desired.

Nutrition
344 calories; 16.8 g total fat; 50 mg cholesterol; 473 mg sodium. 579 mg potassium; 26.9 g carbohydrates; 5.9 g fiber; 11 g sugar; 21.5 g protein; 8 mg vitamin c 17 mcg folate; 89 mg calcium; 3 mg iron; 67 mg magnesium;

Baked Lemon-Pepper Chicken

Ingredients
- 4 (6 ounce) of boneless, skinless chicken breasts
- ½ teaspoon of salt, plus 1/8 teaspoon, divided
- 1 tablespoon of extra-virgin olive oil
- 1 medium sized lemon, thinly sliced
- 2 tablespoons of lemon juice
- 1 tablespoon of pure maple syrup
- 2 tablespoons of unsalted butter, cut into pieces
- 1 teaspoon of cracked pepper

Directions
Preheat oven to 425 ranges F.
Sprinkle chicken flippantly with 1/2 tsp of salt. Heat oil in a skillet at medium-high tempreature. Add the chook; cook, undisturbed, until the underside is golden brown, about four minutes. Flip the bird; set up lemon slices round the bird inside the pan. Transfer the skillet to the oven; bake till an instant-study thermometer inserted into the thickest part of meat registers 165 levels F, approximately 10 minutes.
Transfer the chook to a platter. Then, add lemon juice and maple syrup to the pan. Add butter and 1 piece at a time, stirring until it melts into the sauce. Stir in pepper and the final 1/8 tsp of salt. Drizzle the sauce over the bird.

Nutrition
286 calories; 13.3 g total fat;109 mg is cholesterol; 448 mg is sodium. 350 mg is potassium; 7.1 g is carbohydrates; 1.4 g fiber; 3 g sugar; 34.8 g protein;

24 mg vitamin c; 8 mcg folate; 43 mg calcium; 1 mg iron; 38 mg magnesium

Slow-Cooker Honey-Orange Chicken Drumsticks

Ingredients
- ⅓ cup of honey
- 2 teaspoons of orange zest
- 2 tablespoons of orange juice
- 3 tablespoons of reduced-sodium soy sauce or tamari
- 3 cloves of garlic, minced
- 1 ½ tablespoons of minced fresh ginger
- 1 tablespoon of rice vinegar
- ¼ teaspoon of crushed red pepper
- 12 medium sized chicken drumsticks (3-3 1/2 pounds), skin removed
- 2 tablespoons of chopped fresh cilantro
- 2 teaspoons of toasted sesame seeds

Directions
Mix honey, orange zest, orange juice, soy sauce (or tamari), garlic, ginger, vinegar and crushed crimson pepper in a small bowl.
Coat a 5- to 6-quart cooker with cooking spray. The, add drumsticks, pour within the sauce and stirr to coat. Cover and cook until an thermometer registers 165 levels F whilst inserted into the thickest a part of the meat with out touching bone, 2 to 3 hours on High heat or 4 hours on Low heat.
Transfer the drumsticks to a pot. Pour the liquid from the slow cooker right into a medium skillet. Bring to a boil over high heat. Boil till reduced and syrupy, 10 to fifteen min. Pour the sauce over the drumsticks and stir to coat. Serve sprinkled with cilantro and sesame seeds.

Nutrition
252 calories; 7.1 g total fat; 150 mg is cholesterol; 416 mg is sodium. 352 mg potassium; 17.7 g is carbohydrates; 0.4 g fiber; 16 g sugar; 28.8 g protein; 4 mg vitamin c; 8 mcg folate; 30 mg calcium; 2 mg iron; 34 mg magnesium

Buffalo-Style Bistro Lunch Box

Ingredients
- 1 (12 ounce) of package seasoned cooked chicken strips, cut into bite-size pieces
- 1 bunch of celery, trimmed and cut into sticks
- 1 pound of carrots, peeled, cut into sticks
- 1 (8 ounce) of container Buffalo-style hummus
- 2 ounces of crumbled blue cheese

Directions
Divide hen among four single-serving divided lunch packing containers with lids.
Divide celery and carrots most of the bins.
Measure 1/four cup hummus into a compartment of every container (or into every of 4 separate small lidded packing containers) and top with one-fourth of the blue cheese (approximately 2 tablespoons). Seal the packing containers and refrigerate for up to four days.

Nutrition
301 calories; 9.5 g total fat; 66 mg cholesterol; 759 mg sodium. 798 mg potassium; 25.7 g carbohydrates; 8.5 g fiber; 9 g sugar; 27.7 g protein; 9 mg vitamin c; 55 mcg folate; 144 mg calcium; 3 mg iron

Chicken Breasts With Mushroom Cream Sauce

Ingredients
- 2 5-ounce ofboneless, skinless chicken breasts, trimmed and tenders removed (see Tip)
- ½ teaspoon of freshly ground pepper
- ¼ teaspoon of salt
- 1 tablespoon of canola oil
- 1 medium-sized shallot, minced
- 1 cup of thinly sliced shiitake mushroom caps
- 2 tablespoons of dry vermouth, or dry white wine
- ¼ cup of reduced-sodium chicken broth
- 2 tablespoons of heavy cream
- 2 tablespoons of minced fresh chives, or scallion greens

Directions
Season chook with pepper and salt on both sides. Heat oil in a skillet at over medium tempreature. Add the bird and cook, turning a few times and adjusting the warmth to save you burning, until brown and an instant-study thermometer inserted into the thickest element registers 165 F, 12 to 16 min. Transfer to a plate and tent with foil to preserve warm.
Add shallot to the pan and cook it, mixing, till fragrant, about 30 sec. Add mushrooms; cooking, mixing occasionally, until tender, about 2 minutes. Pour in vermouth (or wine); simmer till nearly evaporated, scraping up any browned bits, approximately 1 minute. Pour in broth and cook till reduced by using half, 1 to 2 min. Mix in cream and chives (or scallions); return to a simmer. Return the hen to the pan, turn to coat with sauce and cook till heated through, approximately 1 minute.

Nutrition
Nutrition
274 calories; 15.4 g total fat; 4.8 g saturated fat; 83 mg is cholesterol; 425 mg sodium. 403 mg is potassium; 4.8 g carbohydrates; 0.7 g fiber; 2 g sugar; 25.2 g protein; 548 IU vitamin aiu; 4 mg vitamin c; 19 mcg folate; 33 mg calcium; 1 mg iron; 31 mg magnesium

Cauliflower Chicken Fried "Rice"

Ingredients
- 1 teaspoon of peanut oil plus 2 tablespoons, divided
- 2 large-sized eggs, beaten
- 3 scallions, thinly sliced, whites and greens separated
- 1 tablespoon of grated fresh ginger
- 1 tablespoon of minced garlic
- 1 pound of boneless, skinless chicken thighs, trimmed
- ½ cup of diced red bell pepper

- 1 cup of snow peas, trimmed and halved
- 4 cups of cauliflower rice
- 3 tablespoons of reduced-sodium tamari or soy sauce
- 1 teaspoon of sesame oil (optional)

Directions

Heat 1 teaspoon oil in a big flat-bottomed carbon-metallic wok or large heavy skillet over excessive heat. Add eggs and cook, with out stirring, till fully cooked on one side, approximately 30 seconds. Flip and cook until simply cooked through, about 15 seconds. Place it to a cutting board and cut into 1/2-inch pieces.

Add 1 tablespoon oil to the pan at the side of scallion whites, ginger and garlic; cook, stirring, till the scallions have softened, about 30 seconds. Add bird and cook, stirring, for 1 minute. Add bell pepper and snow peas; cook, stirring, till simply tender, 2 to four minutes. Transfer everything to a massive plate. Add the closing 1 tablespoon oil to the pan; upload cauliflower rice and stir until starting to soften, about 2 minutes.

Return the fowl aggregate and eggs to the pan, upload tamari (or soy sauce) and sesame oil (if using) and stir until well combined. Garnish with scallion greens.

Nutrition

304 calories; 15.5 g total fat; 200 mg is cholesterol; 591 mg is sodium. 883 mg is potassium; 12.2 g is carbohydrates; 4.2 g fiber; 5 g sugar 29.9 g protein; 108 mg vitamin c; 124 mcg folate; 75 mg calcium; 3 mg iron; 65 mg magnesium;

Chicken Club Wraps

Ingredients

- 1 pound of boneless, skinless chicken breast, trimmed
- ½ teaspoon of freshly ground pepper, divided
- 3 tablespoons of nonfat plain Greek yogurt
- 3 tablespoons of cider vinegar
- 3 tablespoons of minced onion
- 2 tablespoons of extra-virgin olive oil
- ⅛ teaspoon of salt
- 1 medium-sized tomato, chopped
- 1 avocado, chopped
- 3 strips of cooked bacon, crumbled
- 8 large-sized leaves red
- 4 10-in flour tortillas, preferably whole-wheat

Directions

Preheat grill to medium-high.

Sprinkle fowl on each aspects with 1/four teaspoon pepper. Oil the grill rack. Grill the fowl, turning as soon as or twice, until an instant-read thermometer inserted into the thickest part registers 165 levels F, 15 to 18 minutes. Transfer to a clean slicing board and let cool for about 5 minutes.

Meanwhile, mi xyogurt, vinegar, onion, oil, salt and the remaining 1/4 teaspoon pepper in a big bowl. Chop the bird into bite-size pieces and add to the bowl together with tomato, avocado and bacon; toss to combine.

To collect the wraps, place 2 lettuce leaves on each tortilla and top with bird salad (approximately 1 cup every). Roll up like a burrito. Serve cut in half, if desired.

Nutrition

526 calories; 25.6 g total fat; 70 mg is cholesterol; 901 mg is sodium. 587 mg potassium; 39 g is carbohydrates; 11 g is fiber; 4 g sugar; 33.6 g protein; 10 mg vitamin c; 52 mcg folate; 38 mg calcium; 1 mg iron; 45 mg magnesium;

Southwest Black-Bean Pasta Salad Bowls

Ingredients

- 1 (14 ounce) of package frozen Mexican-style corn
- 2 cups of black-bean rotini
- 1 (12 ounce) of package cooked chili-lime chicken
- ½ cup of mild pico de gallo
- ½ cup of cilantro salad dressing

Directions

Heat corn according to package directions; set apart to cool.

Cook pasta in keeping with bundle directions. Drain and rinse with cold water. Drain once more and toss with the corn; set aside.

Slice chook strips into bite-size pieces; set apart. Divide p.C. de gallo into four small lidded boxes and refrigerate. Measure salad dressing into 4 small lidded bins and refrigerate. (Timesaving tip: You can also bring the bottle of dressing on your lunch bag-- or store inside the workplace fridge--and get dressed when ready to serve.)

Divide the corn and pasta mixture among four single-serving packing containers, then top each with one-fourth of the chook. Seal the containers and refrigerate for up to 4 days. Toss with the dressing just earlier than serving and pinnacle with the percent de gallo.

Nutrition

436 calories; 14.4 g total fat; 64 mg is cholesterol; 375 mg sodium. 46.8 g carbohydrates; 14.4 g fiber; 9 g is sugar; 33.7 g protein; 6 mg vitamin c; 187 mg calcium; 4 mg iron;

Chicken & Shiitake Dumplings In Tangy Chile-Oil Sauce

Ingredients

Dumplings

- 8 ounces of ground chicken, thigh meat
- 4 dried shiitake mushrooms (1/2 ounce) chopped
- ½ cup of finely chopped scallions, green and white parts
- 1 ½ teaspoons of grated fresh ginger
- ⅛ teaspoon of freshly ground white or black pepper
- ½ teaspoon of kosher salt
- 1 tablespoon of Shaoxing rice wine or dry sherry
- 1 tablespoon of low-sodium soy sauce
- 1 tablespoon of canola oil or other neutral oil

- 1 ½ tablespoons of sesame oil
- 40 round dumpling wrappers
- All-purpose flour
- ¼ cup of chopped fresh cilantro, for garnish

Sauce
- 1 small clove garlic
- ¼ cup of low-sodium soy sauce
- 2 ½ tablespoons of Chinkiang vinegar
- 2-3 teaspoons of hot chile oil

Directions

To put together dumpling filling: Mix the ground chicken, chopped shiitakes, scallions, ginger, pepper, salt, Shaoxing (or sherry), soy sauce, canola oil (or other oil) and sesame oil in a medium bowl. Vigorously stir and fold with a fork or spatula to make a cohesive, thick combination with no visible big chunks of meat. Cover and let stand at room temperature for 30 min. You ought to have approximately 2 cups of filling.

At the sametime, prepare sauce: Mince garlic, then mash with the flat facet of a chef's knife. Place the garlic in a bowl; stir in soy sauce, vinegar and 2 teaspoons chile oil. Taste and add tempreature with more chile oil, if desired. Pour one-third (about 2 half of tablespoons) of the sauce onto a serving platter. Set aside near the stove with the ultimate sauce.

Half-fill a huge (5- or 6-quart) pot with water, convey to a boil, then decrease the warmth and cover to maintain hot. Line two baking sheets with parchment paper and dust generously with flour; set aside for holding the stuffed dumplings.

Lay four to six dumpling wrappers on a smooth work surface. Brush the rims of the wrappers with water. For every dumpling, preserve a wrapper in a barely cupped hand. Use a dinner knife to scoop up about 1 half of teaspoons of filling (the quantity depends at the wrapper size). Place the filling slightly off-center towards the upper 1/2 of the wrapper. Make a shape of flat mound and keep a knuckle's length (3/four inch) of wrapper clean on all sides. Bring up the wrapper facet closest to you to close, then firmly press to seal well and create a half of-moon. You can depart the dumplings like this, or, for a fancier look, form two small pleats near the center, urgent firmly to keep, or make a series of huge pleats on the rim from one stop to the different, firmly pressing into place.

Place the formed dumpling on a prepared baking sheet. Repeat, spacing the dumplings half of inch apart. Keep the finished ones included with a dry kitchen towel to hold them from drying out.

Return the water to a mild boil; add half of the dumplings, gently dropping every in; use a slotted spoon or spider to nudge them to prevent sticking. Let the dumplings cook till they waft to the floor and are translucent (the filling is fuzzily visible) and the wrapper is chewy-tender, 6 to eight minutes. If the water returns to a boil, lessen the heat. Scoop it out the cooked dumplings with a slotted spoon, letting extra water drip off. Arrange the dumplings on the organized platter and cowl with a big inverted bowl to preserve warm.

Boil the wayer and then repeat with the remaining dumplings. Drizzle the reserved sauce onto the dumplings; use huge spoons to toss. Drizzle with cilantro, if desired, and serve immediately.

Nutrition

151 calories; 6.3 g total fat; 24 mg is cholesterol; 547 mg is sodium. 192 mg is potassium; 15 g carbohydrates; 0.8 g is fiber; 1 g is sugar; 7.4 g protein; 1 mg vitamin c; 10 mcg is folate; 17 mg calcium; 1 mg iron; 14 mg magnesium;

Filipino Pancitbihon

Ingredients
- 2 tablespoons of canola oil
- 1 cup of chopped onion
- 2 tablespoons of minced garlic
- 8 ounces of pork tenderloin, thinly sliced
- 8 ounces of boneless, skinless chicken thighs, thinly sliced
- 4 cups of reduced-sodium chicken broth
- 3 cups of shredded cabbage
- 2 cups of snow peas, halved
- 1 ½ cups of halved and sliced carrots
- 1 cup of chopped leaves of celery
- 1 (8 ounce) of package pancitbihon rice noodles (see Tip)
- 2 ½ tablespoons of reduced-sodium soy sauce

Directions

Heat oil in a big pot over medium heat. Add onion and garlic; cook, stirring, till beginning to soften, 2 to three mins. Add beef and chicken; cook, stirring, until just cooked through, three to 5 mins more. Transfer to a plate.

Add the other ingredients broth, cabbage, snow peas, carrots and celery leaves to the pot. Bring to a simmer; cook till the greens are mainly tender, about 5 min. Add pancitbihon and cookig, stirring, until the liquid is absorbed, three to five mins. Stir in the red meat and chicken; cook, stirring, till heated through, 2 minutes more. Stir in soy sauce and serve.

Nutrition

341 calories; 8.2 g total fat; 61 mg is cholesterol; 379 mg is sodium. 653 mg is potassium; 45.7 g is carbohydrates; 3.4 g is fiber; 5 g sugar; 21.2 g protein; 26 mg is vitamin c; 36 mcg folate; 76 mg calcium; 3 mg iron; 41 mg magnesium; 1 mg is thiamin

Creamy Mushroom, Chicken & Asparagus Bake

Ingredients
- 1 ½ tablespoons of extra-virgin olive oil, plus 1 and 1/2 teaspoons, divided
- 2 (8 ounce) of packages sliced fresh button mushrooms
- 1 cup of chopped yellow onion
- 3 tablespoons of all-purpose flour
- 2 ½ cups of whole milk
- 2 teaspoons of chopped fresh tarragon

- ½ teaspoon of salt
- ½ cup of finely grated Parmesan cheese, divided
- 1 pound of fresh asparagus and cut into 1 inch pieces
- 1 (8.8 ounce) of pouch precooked microwaveable whole-grain brown rice
- 2 cups of chopped cooked chicken breast
- ¼ cup of whole-wheat panko breadcrumbs

Directions

Set oven at 375 degrees F. Heat 1 half of tablespoons oil in a massive cast-iron skillet over medium-high tempreature. Add mushrooms and onion; cook, stirring often, until the moisture launched from the veggies evaporates and the mushrooms are gently browned, 9 to ten minutes. Mix in flour; cook, stirring constantly, for 1 minute. Gradually upload milk; cook, stirring constantly, until the liquid thickens, approximately 2 minutes. Stir in tarragon, salt and 1/four cup Parmesan till melted. Stir in asparagus, rice and chicken. Remove from heat.
Toss panko with the ultimate 1 1/2 teaspoons oil and 1/4 cup Parmesan in a small bowl; sprinkle over the chicken aggregate. Bake until the mixture is becoming bubbly and the topping is golden, approximately 15 minutes.

Nutrition

329 calories; 12.5 g total fat; 56 mg is cholesterol; 413 mg is sodium. 745 mg potassium; 29.6 g is carbohydrates; 3.7 g fiber; 9 g sugar; 26 g protein; 9 mg vitamin c; 145 mcg is folate; 206 mg calcium; 2 mg iron; 63 mg magnesium;

Chicken Kurma

Ingredients
- 1 tablespoon of extra-virgin olive oil
- 1 small sized onion, diced
- 2 medium sized tomatoes, diced
- 3 cloves of garlic, thinly sliced
- 1 (1 inch) of piece fresh ginger, peeled and minced
- 1 serrano pepper, seeded and minced
- 1 tablespoon of tomato paste
- 1 teaspoon of ground turmeric
- 1 teaspoon of kosher salt
- ½ teaspoon of ground pepper
- 1 ½ pounds of boneless, skinless chicken breast, cut into 1-inch pieces
- ½ medium sized red bell pepper, diced
- ½ medium sized green bell pepper, diced
- Juice of 1/2 lemon
- Fresh cilantro for garnishing

Directions

Heat oil in a big saucepan over medium warmth. Add onion and cook, stirring occasionally, until soft, 2 to 3 minutes. Add tomatoes, garlic, ginger, serrano, tomato paste, turmeric, salt and pepper. Bring to a simmer. Reduce warmth to keep a simmer, cover and prepare dinner for 10 mins.
Add bird and boom heat to maintain a active simmer. Cook, stirring occasionally, till the hen is nearly cooked through, about five minutes. Add bell peppers and lemon (or lime) juice and prepare dinner, stirring occasionally, till the chicken is just cooked through, five to 10 minutes more. Garnishing with cilantro and/or mint, if desired.

Nutrition

175 calories; 5.2 g total fat; 63 mg is cholesterol; 400 mg is sodium. 436 mg potassium; 7.2 g carbohydrates; 1.8 g fiber; 3 g is sugar; 24.1 g protein; 44 mg is vitamin c; 24 mcg folate; 28 mg calcium; 1 mg iron; 35 mg magnesium;

Skillet Lemon Chicken & Potatoes With Kale

Ingredients
- 3 tablespoons of extra-virgin olive oil, divided
- 1 pound of boneless, skinless chicken thighs, trimmed
- ½ teaspoon of salt, divided
- ½ teaspoon of ground pepper, divided
- 1 pound of baby Yukon Gold potatoes, halved lengthwise
- ½ cup of low-sodium chicken broth
- 1 large sized lemon, sliced and seeds removed
- 4 cloves garlic, minced
- 1 tablespoon of chopped fresh tarragon
- 6 cups of baby kale

Directions

Preheat oven to 400 degrees F.
Heat 1 tbsp of oil in a skillet at medium-high heat. Sprinkle chicken with 1/4 teaspoon each salt and pepper. Cook, turning once, until browned on both sides, about 5 minutes total. Transfer to a plate.
Add the remaining 2 tablespoons oil, potatoes and the remaining 1/4 teaspoon each salt and pepper to the pan. Cook the potatoes, cut-side down, until browned, about 3 minutes. Stir in broth, lemon, garlic and tarragon. Return the chicken to the pan.
Transfer the pan to the oven. Roast it till the chicken is cooked through and the potatoes are tender, about 15 minutes. Stir kale into the mixture and roast until it has wilted, 3 to 4 minutes.

Nutrition

374 calories; 19.3 g total fat; 76 mg is cholesterol; 378 mg is sodium. 677 mg potassium; 25.6 g is carbohydrates; 2.9 g fiber; 2 g is sugar; 24.7 g protein; 2463 IU vitamin aiu; 41 mg vitamin c; 51 mcg folate; 65 mg calcium; 2 mg iron; 53 mg magnesium;

Crock-Pot Pineapple Chicken

Ingredients
- 1 ½ pounds of boneless, skinless chicken thighs
- 1 cup of low-sodium chicken broth
- ¼ cup of low-sodium soy sauce
- 4 teaspoons of cornstarch
- 2 teaspoons of toasted sesame oil
- 3 large sized cloves garlic, minced
- 1 tablespoon of minced fresh ginger
- ½ teaspoon of crushed red pepper
- 2 cups of cubed fresh pineapple
- 1 large sized red bell pepper, cut into 1-inch pieces

- 1 medium sized onion, cut into 1-inch pieces
- Sliced scallions for garnishing

Directions
Coat a 5- or 6-quart gradual cooker with cooking spray. Place chook in a single layer within the backside of the cooker. Whisk broth, soy sauce and cornstarch in a measuring cup till smooth. Add sesame oil, garlic, ginger and overwhelmed purple pepper; stir to combine. Pour the aggregate over the chicken, then scatter pineapple, bell pepper and onion over the top. Cover and prepare dinner on Low for four 1/2 hours or on High for two hours.
Remove the hen and veggies to a bowl. Transfer the liquid to a medium saucepan; carry to a boil over medium-high heat. Cook, stirring occasionally, till reduced to approximately 1 cup, about 10 minutes. Coarsely shred the bird; place the chicken combination in a serving bowl. Add the sauce and stir to combine. Garnish with scallions, if desired.

Nutrition
324 calories; 10 g total fat;160 mg cholesterol; 717 mg is sodium. 728 mg potassium; 21.5 g is carbohydrates; 2.7 g fiber; 11 g sugar; 36.8 g protein; 95 mg vitamin c; 46 mcg folate; 42 mg calcium; 2 mg iron; 64 mg magnesium;

Chicken Cutlets And Zucchini Noodles With Creamy Tomato Sauce

Ingredients
- 1 pound chicken cutlets
- ¼ teaspoon salt, divided
- ¼ teaspoon ground pepper, divided
- 1 tablespoon extra-virgin olive oil
- ½ cup finely chopped red onion
- ½ cup dry white wine
- ½ cup heavy cream
- 1 medium plum tomato, chopped
- 2 (10 ounce) packages zucchini noodles

Directions
Sprinkle chook with 1/8 teaspoon every salt and pepper. Heat oil in a skillet at medium-high tempreature. Add the bird and cook, turning once, until browned and cooked through, approximately 6 minutes. Transfer to a plate.
Add onion to the pan. Cook, stirring, for 1 minute. Increase heat to high and upload wine. Cookit , scraping up any browned bits, until the liquid is frequently evaporated, about 2 min. Lessen tempreature to medium and stir in cream, any gathered juices from the bird and the last 1/eight teaspoon each salt and pepper; simmer for two minutes. Stir in tomatoes, then go back the bird to the pan. Turn to coat. Divide the chicken and sauce between 4 plates.
Add zucchini noodles to the skillet over medium-excessive heat. Cook, stirring, until softened and heated through, 1 to two minutes. Serve with the chicken.

Nutrition
331 calories; 17.3 g total fat; 117 mg is cholesterol; 208 is mg sodium. 906 mg potassium; 8.1 g carbohydrates; 2.4 g fiber; 4 g is sugar; 28.6 g protein; 6 mg vitamin c; 20 mcg folate; 62 mg calcium; 1 mg iron; 42 mg magnesium;

Chicken Paillards With Blood Orange Pan Sauce

Ingredients
- 4 blood color oranges, divide them
- 1 pound of boneless, skinless chicken breast
- ¼ teaspoon of kosher salt
- ¼ teaspoon of ground white pepper
- 1 large sized egg
- ¾ cup of finely grated Parmesan cheese
- 2 tablespoons of extra-virgin olive oil
- 2 tablespoons of unsalted butter, divided
- Fresh flat-leaf parsley for garnishing

Directions
Grate half of tsp zest from 1 orange. Get juice of the orange into a pot and add the zest. Segment the ultimate three oranges. Using a sharp knife, slice each ends off and do away with the peel and white pith. Set a fine-mesh sieve on the bowl. Working over the sieve, cut the orange from their membranes. Squeeze its juice out of the membranes and peel before discarding. Reserve the orange sections and juice separately.
Cut fowl into 4 pieces. Place among sheets of plastic wrap and pound with a meat mallet or heavy skillet till approximately 1/four inch thick. Season with salt and white pepper.
Beat egg in a shallow dish. Place Parmesan on a plate. Dip the chook into the egg, then dredge lightly within the Parmesan, urgent to assist it adhere.
Warm the oil and 1 tbsp butter in a big nonstick or cast-iron skillet over medium-high heat. Add the hen and cook, flipping once, until golden and an instant-examine thermometer inserted in the thickest part registers 165 ranges F, 5 to 7 mins total. Add the stored orange juice to the pan and bring to a boil. Cook for 1 min. Add the reserved orange segments and the final 1 tablespoon butter and stir until melted. Serve the fowl with the sauce and parsley, if using.

Nutrition
392 calories; 21.9 g total fat; 157 mg cholesterol; 463 mg is sodium. 649 mg potassium; 15.6 g is carbohydrates; 2.4 g fiber; 11 g sugar; 32.3 g protein; 58 mg vitamin c; 17 mcg is folate; 175 mg calcium; 1 mg iron; 39 mg magnesium;

Creamy Lemon Chicken Parmesan

Ingredients
- ⅓ cup of all-purpose flour
- 2 large sized eggs, beaten
- ¾ cup of whole-wheat panko breadcrumbs
- ½ cup of grated Parmesan cheese, divided
- 1 teaspoon of Italian seasoning
- 1 teaspoon of garlic powder

- 4 4-ounce of chicken breast cutlets
- 3 tablespoons of extra-virgin olive oil, divided
- 2 cloves garlic, minced
- 1 cup of low-sodium chicken broth
- ¼ cup of lemon juice
- ¼ teaspoon of salt
- ½ cup of half-and-half
- ¼ cup of chopped fresh parsley

Directions

Preheat oven to 400 tiers F. Place flour in a shallow dish. Place overwhelmed eggs in every other shallow dish. Mix panko, 1/4 cup Parmesan, Italian seasoning and garlic powder in a 3rd shallow dish. Working with one at a time, coat every cutlet in flour, shaking off the excess. Transfer to the egg combination and turn to coat. Transfer to the panko aggregate and turn to coat. Reserve 1 tablespoon of the flour (it'll be cooked later) in a small bowl. Discard any ultimate flour, egg and panko mixture.

Heat 1 tablespoon oil in a big skillet at medium-high tempreature. Add 2 cutlets and cook, flipping once, until golden, 1 to 2 minutes according to side. Transfer to a huge baking sheet. Reduce warmth to medium and add any other 1 tablespoon oil to the pan. Add the closing cutlets and cook, flipping once, till golden on both sides, 1 to two minutes in step with side. Place it to the baking sheet. Bake the cutlets until cooked throughout, about 10 minutes. Meanwhile, wipe out the pan. Add the last 1 tablespoon oil and warmth over medium-high warmth. Add garlic and cooking, mixing, until fragrant, approximately 30 sec. Add broth, lemon juice and salt to the pan. Bring to a boil. Whisk half of-and-half into the reserved 1 tablespoon flour. Add to the broth combination and cook, stirring frequently, until reduced by approximately half and thickened sufficient to coat the returned of a spoon, 8 to 10 minutes. Remove from warmth.

Transfer the cutlets to a large platter. Sprinkle with the sauce and top with the ultimate 1/4 cup Parmesan and parsley.

Nutrition

378 calories; 20.8 g total fat; 130 mg is cholesterol; 466 mg is sodium. 387 mg is potassium; 15.2 g is carbohydrates; 1.4 g is fiber; 2 g sugar; 31.2 g protein; 12 mg is vitamin c; 30 mcg folate; 146 mg calcium; 2 mg iron; 34 mg magnesium;

Instant Pot Brisket

Ingredients
- 1 (3 pound) of beef brisket, cut in half crosswise
- 1 teaspoon of salt
- 1 teaspoon of ground pepper
- 1 teaspoon of paprika
- 2 teaspoons of extra-virgin olive oil
- 2 medium sized red onions, each cut into 8 wedges
- 6 cloves garlic, smashed
- 1 cup of beef broth
- ¼ cup of ketchup
- 1 tablespoon of tomato paste

Directions

Sprinkle brisket throughout with salt, pepper and paprika. Select Sauté putting on a programmable pressure multicooker (which includes Instant Pot; times, commands and settings may also vary in keeping with cooker logo or model). Select High temperature placing; upload oil to the cooker and allow to preheat for 2 to three minutes. Add 1 brisket piece; cook till well browned, about 7 minutes in step with side. Then remove from the cooker; and repeat the process with the ultimate brisket piece. Add onions and garlic to the cooker; cook them, stirring occasionally, till starting to brown, approximately 4 min. Add broth, ketchup and tomato paste, at the lowest of the cooker pot to loosen browned bits. Return the brisket to the cooker. Press Cancel. Cover the cooker and fix the lid in its place. Turn the steam release cope with to Sealing position. Select Manual/Pressure Cook placing. Select High stress for 60 minutes. (It will take 10 to 12 mins for the cooker to return up to stress before cooking begins.) When cooking is complete, permit the stress release obviously for 10 minutes. Before disposing of the lid from the cooker, carefully flip the steam release take care of to Venting function and allow the steam fully escape (the glide valve will drop; this can take 2 to a few mins).

Remove the brisket to a slicing board; allow relaxation for 10 mins. Meanwhile, blend the onion mixture within the cooker with an immersion blender till very smooth, approximately 30 seconds. Remove and discard the fats cap from the brisket. Slice the brisket towards the grain; return the slices to the sauce inside the cooker. Cover the cooker and fix the lid in its place. Turn the steam release deal with to Sealing function. Select Manual/Pressure Cook placing. Select High stress for three mins. (It will take 10 to 12 mins for the cooker to return up to strain before cooking begins.) When cooking is complete, allow the strain release obviously for 10 mins. Before taking off the lid from the cooker, carefully turn off the steam release handle to Venting function and permit the steam completely escape (the go with the flow valve will drop; this may take 2 to three mins). Place the slices on a platter; spoon the onion sauce over the brisket and serve it.

Nutrition

203 calories; 6.9 g total fat; 84 mg is cholesterol; 443 mg is sodium. 320 mg potassium; 5.1 g is carbohydrates; 0.6 g fiber; 3 g sugar; 28.8 g protein; 3 mg vitamin c; 15 mcg is folate; 26 mg calcium; 3 mg is iron; 24 mg magnesium; 1 g added sugar;

Lola Beef Kebabs

Ingredients
- 12 ounces of white potatoes, cut into 1-inch pieces
- 2 teaspoons of grapeseed or canola oil plus 2 tablespoons, divided
- 1 small sized onion, finely chopped
- 1 pound of lean ground beef

- 1 large sized egg, beaten
- 1 medium sized red bell pepper, finely chopped
- 2 cloves garlic, minced
- ¼ cup of all-purpose flour
- 2 teaspoons of garam masala
- 2 teaspoons of ground pepper
- 1 ½ teaspoons of ground coriander
- 1 teaspoon of ground ginger
- ¾ teaspoon of kosher salt
- Fresh cilantro for garnishing

Directions

Add 1 in of water to a medium saucepan outfitted with a steamer basket. Bring to a boil over high warmness. Add potatoes, cowl and steam until tender, about 20 minutes. Remove the potatoes, drain the water, then go back the potatoes to the pan. Cook, shaking, till they're dry, approximately 2 minutes. Transfer to a huge bowl and lightly mash with a potato masher. Let cool for 10 minutes.

Meanwhile, warmth 2 teaspoons oil in a large nonstick skillet over medium warmness. Add onion and cook, stirring often, till very tender, four to 6 minutes. (Reduce warmth, if necessary, to prevent burning.) Transfer to the bowl with the potatoes. Add red meat, egg, bell pepper, garlic, flour, garam masala, pepper, coriander, ginger and salt. Mix along with your arms until nicely combined.

Preheat oven to 400 tiers F. Line a baking sheet with foil.

To make every kebab, use moist arms to roll 1/four cup red meat combination into a 4-inch-lengthy log, urgent firmly so the kebab holds its shape and gently pinching the ends to form a compact torpedo. Repeat to make 15 kebabs.

Wash and dry the skillet. Heat the final 2 tablespoons oil within the skillet over medium warmth. Cook half of the kebabs, without allowing them to touch, until lightly browned and crispy, 1 to 3 minutes in step with side. Transfer to the prepared pan. Repeat with the final kebabs. Bake until an instant-read thermometer registers one hundred sixty tiers F, 8 to 10 min. Garnishing with cilantro.

Nutrition

361 calories; 17.1 g total fat; 107 mg is cholesterol; 383 mg is sodium. 639 mg is potassium; 22.7 g is carbohydrates; 2.6 g fiber; 2 g is sugar; 28.3 g protein; 37 mg vitamin c; 43 mcg folate; 36 mg calcium; 3 mg iron; 43 mg magnesium;

Instant Pot "Corned" Beef & Cabbage

Ingredients
- 2 tablespoons of pickling spice
- 1 ¼ teaspoons of salt
- 1 teaspoon of dry mustard
- 3 pounds of boneless beef roast, cut it into 1 1/2-inch pieces
- 2 tablespoons of canola oil
- 2 cups chopped of yellow onions
- 1 ½ pounds of carrots, cut into 1 1/2-inch pieces
- 12 ounces of baby red potatoes
- 4 cups of low-sodium chicken broth
- 1 small head green cabbage, cut into 8 wedges
- 2 tbsp of chopped fresh dill
- 5 tablespoons of sour cream
- 3 tablespoons of prepared horseradish

Directions

Process pickling spice in a espresso grinder or spice grinder till finely floor, approximately 10 seconds. Combine the floor pickling spice, salt and mustard in a small bowl; set aside.

Select Sauté setting on a programmable stress multicooker (together with an Instant Pot; times, instructions and settings might also vary in step with cooker brand or model). Select High temperature setting and permit to preheat for three mins. Meanwhile, sprinkle red meat frivolously with half of the pickling spice combination.

Add one-0.33 of the red meat and a couple of teaspoons oil to the cooker; cook, turning the red meat occasionally, until browned on all sides, about 6 mins total. Transfer the red meat to a bowl; repeat the process twice the usage of the last beef and oil. Add onions, carrots, potatoes, broth and the ultimate pickling spice mixture to the cooker, scraping the bottom of the cooker insert to release any browned bits. Return the red meat (and any collected juices inside the bowl) to the cooker; stir to combine. Top with cabbage wedges. Press Cancel.

Cover the cooker and lock its lid in place. Turn the steam release manage to Sealing position. Select Manual/Pressure Cook putting. Select High stress for 30 min. (It will take upto 10 to 15 min for the cooker to come back up to pressure before cooking begins.) When cooking is complete, permit the stress release evidently for five mins. Carefully flip the steam release manage to Venting function and let the steam absolutely escape (the go with the flow valve will drop; this will take 2 to a few mins). Remove the lid from the cooker.

Transfer the red meat and vegetables to a platter; sprinkle with dill. Stir together bitter cream and horseradish in small bowl; serve the sauce alongside the beef and greens

Nutrition

385 calories; 12.6 g total fat;103 mg is cholesterol; 576 mg is sodium. 1101 mg is potassium; 30.1 g carbohydrates; 8.2 g is fiber; 12 g sugar; 38.5 g protein; 75 mg vitamin c; 120 mcg folate; 137 mg calcium; 4 mg iron; 68 mg magnesium;

Shepherd's Pie With Cauliflower Topping

Ingredients
- 1 pound of lean ground beef
- 2 cups of chopped onion
- 2 tablespoons of minced garlic
- 1 (15 ounce) can of no-salt-added diced tomatoes, drained
- 1 tablespoon of reduced-sodium Worcestershire sauce
- 1 ½ teaspoons of chopped fresh rosemary

- 3 tablespoons of chopped fresh flat-leaf parsley, divided
- 1 ½ teaspoons of ground pepper, divided
- ¾ teaspoon of salt, divided
- ¼ cup of unsalted beef broth
- 1 tablespoon of all-purpose flour
- 8 cups of cauliflower florets
- 2 cups of water
- 6 tablespoons of unsalted butter
- ¼ cup of heavy cream

Directions

Set oven at 375 degrees F. Heat a 12-inch ovenproof skillet over medium-excessive warmness. Add pork, onion and garlic; cook, stirring frequently to crumble, till the red meat is browned and onion is smooth, 8 to ten minutes. Mix in drained tomatoes, Worcestershire, rosemary, 1 tablespoon parsley, 1 teaspoon pepper and 1/four tsp salt. Mix broth and flour in a small bowl; stir into the mixture in the skillet. Cook over medium-low warmness, stirring frequently, till the aggregate thickens, about 15 minutes

Meanwhile, region cauliflower and water in a huge saucepan; carry to a boil over high warmth. Cover and reduce warmness to medium-high; cook until the cauliflower is gentle when pierced with a fork, about 10 minutes. Drain. Add butter, cream and the last 1/2 teaspoon salt; mash with a fork or potato masher till smooth (you'll have about four cups mashed).

Spoon the mashed cauliflower orn the hot mixture in the skillet, spreading it over the top (do now not mix the two layers together). Sprinkle with the final half teaspoon pepper.

Bake till the top is beginning to brown and the filling is bubbly, 22 to 25 minutes. Sprinkle with the closing 2 tablespoons parsley before serving.

Nutrition

356 calories; 23.2 g total fat; 91 mg is cholesterol; 427 mg is sodium. 799 mg is potassium; 18.1 g carbohydrates; 4.6 g fiber; 8 g sugar; 20 g protein; 88 mg vitamin c; 104 mcg is folate; 85 mg calcium; 3 mg iron; 46 mg magnesium;

Instant Pot Goulash

Ingredients
- 1 and ½ pounds of beef stew meat such as chuck, cut into 1 1/2-inch pieces
- 3 tablespoons of all-purpose flour
- 1 tablespoon of canola oil
- 2 cups of thinly sliced red onions
- 1 tablespoon of chopped fresh thyme
- 5 cloves of garlic, chopped
- 1 tablespoon of no-salt-added tomato paste
- 1 tablespoon of smoked paprika
- 2 teaspoons of caraway seeds
- 3 cups of angel hair coleslaw mix or finely shredded cabbage
- 1 (14 ounce) can of stewed tomatoes, undrained
- ¾ teaspoon of salt
- ½ teaspoon of ground pepper
- 12 ounces of whole-wheat egg noodles
- ¾ cup of whole-milk plain yogurt

Directions

Toss beef and flour collectively in a medium bowl. Select Sauté putting on a programmable stress multicooker (consisting of an Instant Pot; times, instructions and settings may also vary in step with cooker logo or model). Select High temperature putting, and permit to preheat. Add oil to the cooker. Add the flour-coated pork; cook, stirring often, until browned, 7 to 8 mins. Add onions, and thyme and garlic; cook, stirring often, till the onions soften, five to 6 mins. Then add tomato paste, paprika and caraway seeds; cook, stirring constantly, for 1 minute. Stir in cabbage, tomatoes and their juice, salt and pepper. Press Cancel.

Cover the cooker and lock the lid in place. Turn the steam release deal with to Sealing position. Select Manual/Pressure Cook placing. Select High stress for 30 minutes. (It will take five to 7 mins for the cooker to return up to pressure before cooking begins.)

When cooking is complete, permit the stress release naturally (the drift valve will drop; this could take 5 to 7 mins) before doing away with the lid from the cooker.

Meanwhile, prepare noodles in line with bundle directions; drain.

Divide the noodles evenly among 6 bowls; topping with the goulash and yogurt.

Nutrition Facts

490 calories; 9.9 g total fat; 81 mg is cholesterol; 595 mg is sodium. 751 mg potassium; 57.5 g carbohydrates; 8.3 g is fiber; 11 g is sugar; 37.9 g protein; 24 mg vitamin c; 42 mcg folate; 160 mg is calcium; 4 mg iron; 47 mg magnesium;

Beef Tenderloin With Pomegranate Sauce &Farro Pilaf

Ingredients
- 1 (2 pound) of beef tenderloin, trimmed
- 1 ½ teaspoons of kosher salt, divided
- ¾ teaspoon of ground pepper, divided
- 2 tablespoons of grapeseed oil, divided
- ½ cup of finely chopped shallot, divided
- 1 clove of garlic, minced
- 1 ¼ cups of farro, rinsed
- 2 ½ cups of low-sodium beef broth, divided
- 1 teaspoon of ground cumin
- ½ cup of pomegranate juice
- ½ cup of dry red wine
- 2 tablespoons of pomegranate molasses
- 1 tablespoon of balsamic vinegar
- 2 sprigs of fresh thyme
- 1 ½ tablespoons of cold butter, cubed
- ½ cup of pomegranate arils, plus more for garnish
- ½ cup of chopped unsalted pistachios
- 1 teaspoon of lemon zest
- Fresh mint for garnishing

Directions

Preheat oven to 400 degrees F.

Sprinkle beef with half of teaspoon salt and 1/4 teaspoon pepper. Heat 1 tablespoon oil in a huge ovenproof skillet over medium-high warmness. Add the beef and cook, turning occasionally, till browned on all sides, five to 7 mins total.

Transfer the skillet to the oven. Roast, flipping the red meat once halfway, till an instant-examine thermometer inserted inside the thickest element registers 135 ranges F for medium-rare, 30 to 40 mins.

Meanwhile, warmness the closing 1 tablespoon oil in a massive saucepan over medium heat. Add 1/four cup shallot; cook, stirring, till softened, 1 to a few mins. Add garlic, farro; cook, stirring, for 1 minute. Add 2 1/4 cups broth, cumin, half of teaspoon salt and 1/4 teaspoon pepper. Bring to a boil over excessive heat. Reduce heat to preserve a simmer, cowl and cook till the liquid is absorbed, 35 to 40 minutes. Remove from heat.

Transfer the pork to a reducing board. Place the skillet at medium tempreature and add the last 1/four cup shallot. Cook, stirring, for two mins. Add the remaining 1/four cup ingredients broth, pomegranate juice, wine, pomegranate molasses, vinegar and thyme. Boil it, scraping up any browned bits. Cook till reduced to half cup, 7 to 10 mins. Strain the sauce. Stir in butter, any collected juices on the reducing board and the last 1/2 teaspoon salt and 1/four teaspoon pepper.

Stir pomegranate arils, pistachios and lemon zest into the farro. Slice the pork and serve with the sauce and farro. Garnish with mint and extra pomegranate arils, if desired.

Nutrition Facts
414 calories; 17.3 g total fat; 70 mg cholesterol; 438 mg is sodium. 507 mg is potassium; 33 g is carbohydrates; 4 g is fiber; 8 g sugar; 30.4 g protein; 3 mg vitamin c; 21 mcg folate; 54 mg calcium; 3 mg iron; 34 mg magnesium;

Slow-Cooker Ropavieja
Ingredients
- 1 medium sized red bell pepper (about 5 1/8 ounces), roughly chopped
- 1 medium sized yellow onion (about 8 ounces), roughly chopped
- 4 medium sized plum tomatoes (about 1 pound, 3 ounces), roughly chopped
- 2 garlic cloves
- 2 tablespoons of fresh oregano leaves
- 1 teaspoon of ground cumin
- ½ cup of unsalted beef stock
- 2 tablespoons of no-salt-added ketchup
- 2 pounds of flank steak, trimmed and cut crosswise into 2-inch pieces
- 2 tablespoons of extra-virgin olive oil
- ½ teaspoon of black pepper
- 1 ¾ teaspoons of kosher salt
- ⅓ cup of roughly chopped pimiento-stuffed green olives (about 3 ounces)
- 2 (15 ounce) cans of no-salt-added black beans, drained and rinsed
- 2 (8.8 ounce) packages of precooked microwavable brown rice

Directions
Place the ingredients bell pepper, onion, tomatoes, garlic, oregano, and cumin in a meals processor; pulse till finely chopped, five to six times. Transfer the bell pepper aggregate to a five- or 6-quart sluggish cooker; stir within the red meat stock and ketchup. Put the steak, oil, black pepper, and 1 tsp of the salt in a medium bowl, and toss to coat. Submerge the steak inside the bell pepper combination within the slow cooker. Cover and cook on Low tempreature until the beef could be very tender, about eight hours. Transfer the steak to a big bowl, reserving the sauce inside the slow cooker. Shred the steak portions with 2 forks. Mix the shredded steak with 1 cup of the reserved sauce within the bowl, and stir within the chopped inexperienced olives.

Stir collectively the beans and 1/4 teaspoon of the salt in a medium saucepan, and cook over medium until heated through, about five minutes. Keep warm. Prepare the rice consistent with the bundle directions, and season with the remaining half of teaspoon salt. Serve the shredded steak combination with the rice, beans, and remaining reserved sauce from the slow cooker.

Nutrition
400 calories; 13 g is fat; 3 g is saturated fat; 700 mg is sodium. 38 g is carbohydrates; 7 g is fiber; 3 g is sugar; 33 g protein;

Afghan Beef Dumplings(Mantu)
Ingredients
- 2 teaspoons of extra-virgin olive oil, divided
- ½ medium sized onion, finely chopped
- 8 ounces of lean ground beef
- 4 teaspoons of grated garlic, divided
- 1 teaspoon of ground coriander
- ½ teaspoon of ground turmeric
- ¼ teaspoon of ground pepper
- ¼ teaspoon of kosher salt, divided
- 20 wonton wrappers
- ½ cup of no-salt-added tomato sauce
- ½ cup of labneh or whole-milk plain Greek yogurt
- 1 tablespoon of chopped fresh mint
- 1 teaspoon of dried mint

Directions
Heat 1 teaspoon oil in a huge skillet over medium heat. Add onion and cook dinner, stirring occasionally, till soft, 2 to 3 minutes. Add pork and a pair of teaspoons garlic; prepare dinner, breaking up the meat with a wooden spoon, till cooked through, about five mins. Transfer to a bowl and stir in coriander, turmeric, pepper and 1/eight teaspoon salt.

Place four wonton wrappers on a easy reducing board. Wet the edges of every wrapper with water. Place 1 scant tablespoon filling in the center of every.

For each dumpling, grab the alternative corners of a wrapper and press collectively. Grab the corners and press together, so all four corners meet inside the middle to make a four-pointed star. Press the rims of the wrapper together to seal. (Optional: Take 2 points of the star which can be subsequent to each different and press them together, the usage of greater water if needed. Repeat on the alternative side.) Place the dumplings on a baking sheet and cowl with a moist towel. Repeat with the closing wrappers and filling.

Add 1 in of water and a steamer basket to a massive pot; coat the basket with cooking spray. Arrange the dumplings within the basket without touching and cover. Bring to a boil over excessive heat. Reduce warmth to medium-low and steam for 15 minutes. Meanwhile, warmth the final 1 teaspoon oil in a small saucepan over medium-low heat. Add 1 teaspoon garlic and prepare dinner, stirring, for 30 sec. Add tomato sauce and salt; convey to a simmer and cook for five minutes. Remove from warmness and cowl to hold warm.

Combine labneh (or yogurt) with the closing 1 tsp garlic and salt in a bowl. Spread the sauce on a platter and topping with a swirl of the tomato sauce. Arrange the dumplings at the sauces and pinnacle with sparkling and dried mint.

Nutrition Facts
304 calories; 10.1 g total fat; 51 mg is cholesterol; 412 mg is sodium. 412 mg potassium; 29.3 g is carbohydrates; 2 g fiber; 3 g is sugar. 23 g protein; 4 mg vitamin c; 63 mcg folate; 80 mg is calcium; 4 mg iron; 34 mg magnesium;

Beef Rib Roast With Mushrooms & Fennel

Ingredients
- 5 teaspoons of kosher salt, divided
- ¾ ounce of dried porcini mushrooms, finely ground
- 1 (6 to 7 pound) of bone-in beef rib roast (3 bones), trimmed
- 2 medium sized fennel bulbs with fronds, divided
- 12 cloves garlic, minced
- 6 tablespoons of minced fresh rosemary
- 1 tablespoon of ground fennel
- 1 tablespoon of crushed red pepper
- Zest of 3 lemons
- 7 tablespoons of extra-virgin olive oil, divided, plus more if needed
- 2 pounds of mixed mushrooms, preferably wild, halved or quartered if large
- 2 medium sized shallots, sliced
- 6 sprigs fresh thyme, plus more for garnishing
- ⅓ cup of pine nuts, toasted
- 1 tablespoon of sherry vinegar

Directions
Combine 4 and 1/2 teaspoons salt and mushroom powder in a small bowl. Rub the mixture all over meat. Place the roast fat-aspect up on a rack in a roasting pan. Refrigerate it, uncovered, for 1 day or up to three days.

When geared up to continue, permit the roast stand at room temperature for 1 hour before cooking. Preheat oven to 325 degrees F.

Finely chop the fennel fronds to make 6 tbsp (reserve bulbs). Combine the fronds, garlic, rosemary, ground fennel, crushed purple pepper, lemon zest and 6 tablespoons oil in a small bowl. Rub the aggregate everywhere in the roast (but now not the bones). Roast the beef till an instant-study thermometer inserted inside the thickest component with out touching bone registers one hundred twenty five levels F for medium-rare, 2 to a few hours.

Transfer the roast at the rack to a reducing board, tent with foil and let relaxation for at the least 30 minutes.

Meanwhile, increase oven temperature to 450 levels. Pour half cup of the drippings from the roasting pan into a bowl. (If necessary, add oil to measure half cup total.)

Trim, center and slice the fennel bulbs. Add to the drippings in conjunction with mushrooms, shallots and thyme sprigs; toss to coat. Divide the mixture between 2 massive rimmed baking sheets. Roast, stirring, until lightly browned and tender, 20 to 30 minutes. Discard the thyme.

Combine pine nuts and vinegar with the remaining half of teaspoon salt and 1 tablespoon oil in a mini meals processor. Pulse till normally smooth.

Transfer the roasted vegetables to a serving bowl and toss with the vinaigrette. To carve the roast, dispose of the bones by cutting along their contours among the meat and the bone. Thinly slice the red meat crosswise and serve with the vegetables. Garnish with more thyme, if desired.

Nutrition
329 calories; 26.2 g total fat; 59 mg cholesterol; 498 mg is sodium. 493 mg potassium; 5.3 g is carbohydrates; 1.8 g fiber; 2 g is sugar; 18.2 g protein; 6 mg vitamin c; 20 mcg is folate; 31 mg is calcium; 2 mg iron; 30 mg magnesium;

Slow-Cooker Flank Steak Au Jus Sandwiches

Ingredients
- 1 ½ tablespoons of olive oil
- 2 tablespoons of dark brown sugar
- ¾ teaspoon of kosher salt
- 1 teaspoon of ground cumin
- 1 teaspoon of paprika
- 1 teaspoon of black pepper
- 3 garlic cloves, grated (about 1 tablespoon)
- 2 pounds of flank steak, trimmed
- 1 large sized onion (about 13 3/8 ounces), cut into thin slices
- 1 (12 ounce) of bottle beer (such as Yuengling Lager)
- 2 tablespoons of lower-sodium soy sauce
- 1 bay leaf

- 1 teaspoon of fresh thyme leaves
- 2 teaspoons of cornstarch
- 1 teaspoon of water
- 8 small whole-wheat hoagie rolls, toasted

Directions

Stir collectively the olive oil, brown sugar, salt, cumin, paprika, pepper, and garlic, forming a paste; rub the paste into both sides of the steak, the use of all of the mixture. Putthe onion slices in a 5- to 6-quart cooker; topping with the steak. Pour the beer and soy sauce on the steak. Add the bay leaf and thyme. Cover and cook dinner on LOW till the steak is tender, 7 to 8 hours.

Place the steak and onions to a platter, reserving the cooking liquid in the sluggish cooker; cowl the steak and onions with aluminum foil to hold warm.

Pour the reserved cooking liquid thru a wire-mesh strainer right ina saucepan, discarding the solids. Bring to a boil over high, and boil till the sauce is decreased to approximately 1 half cups, approximately 12 minutes. Mix together the cornstarch and water in a small bowl; drizzle into the sauce, and whisk until blended. Reduce the warmth to medium-high, and simmer, stirring often, till thickened, about 1 minute. Shred the steak with 2 forks. Divide the steak and onions a few of the toasted rolls. Pour the sauce indippingbowls, and serve with the sandwiches.

Nutrition Facts

402 calories; 12 g is fat; 3 g is saturated fat; 729 mg is sodium. is 41 g carbohydrates; 5 g is fiber; 9 g sugar; 31 g protein; 3 g added sugar;

Irish Beef Stew

Ingredients
- 2 ¼ pounds of boneless chuck roast, cut into 1 1/2-inch pieces
- ¾ teaspoon of salt
- ½ teaspoon of ground pepper
- 2 tablespoons of canola oil, divided
- 1 small sized yellow onion, chopped
- 3 medium sized carrots, diagonally sliced into 1-inch pieces
- 3 stalks celery, cut into 1-inch pieces
- 1 tablespoon of tomato paste
- 1 (12 fluid ounce)of bottle stout beer
- 2 teaspoons of chopped fresh thyme
- 4 cups of low-sodium beef broth
- 1 ½ pounds of baby Yukon Gold potatoes, halved
- 2 tablespoons of cornstarch
- 2 tablespoons of cold water
- 2 tablespoons of chopped fresh flat-leaf parsley, plus more for garnish

Directions

Sprinkle pork all over with salt and pepper. Heat 1 tablespoon oil in a massive heavy pot over medium-excessive heat. Add half of of the red meat; cook, turning to brown on 2 or 3 sides, about 3 minutes in keeping with side. Transfer the browned red meat to a bowl; repeat the technique with the remaining beef and 1 tablespoon oil.

Add ingredients onion, carrots and celery to the drippings in the pot; cook, stirring often, till the vegetables start to soften, about 4 mins. Add tomato paste; cook,mixing constantly, for 1 min. Add beer and thyme; cook, scraping the bottom of the pot to release any browned bits, till the liquid is slightly reduced, about 2 minutes. Add broth and the beef (with any collected juices in bowl); carry the aggregate to a boil over medium-excessive warmth. Reduce warmth to medium-low; cover and cook until the pork is normally tender, about 1 hour, 10 minutes. Stir in potatoes; cowl and cook until the red meat and potatoes are tender, 15 to 20 minutes. Whisk corn-starch and cold water in a small bowl. Increase heat to excessive; add the cornstarch aggregate and cook, stirring constantly, till thickened, about 2 minutes. Remove from warmth; stir in parsley. If desired, garnish with extra parsley.

Nutrition

405 calories; 11.9 g total fat; 102 mg is cholesterol; 704 mg is sodium. 904 mg is potassium; 32.1 g is carbohydrates; 3.5 g is fiber; 4 g sugar; 37.1 g is protein; 5347 IU vitamin aiu; 14 mg vitamin c; 39 mcg folate; 49 mg is calcium; 4 mg iron; 53 mg magnesium;

Slow-Cooker Barbecue Brisket Sliders

Ingredients
- 2 chipotle chiles in adobo sauce, minced
- 1 ½ tablespoons of light brown sugar
- 3 garlic cloves, grated (about 1 tablespoon)
- 1 teaspoon of ground cumin
- 1 ½ tablespoons of olive oil
- 1 teaspoon of kosher salt
- ¾ teaspoon of black pepper
- 2 pounds of beef brisket, trimmed
- ¾ cup of water
- ⅓ cup of no-salt-added ketchup
- 2 tablespoons of lower-sodium Worcestershire sauce
- 3 tablespoons of apple cider vinegar
- 4 cups of shredded multicolored coleslaw mix
- 16 whole-wheat slider buns

Directions

Stir together the minced chipotle chiles, brown sugar, garlic, cumin, 1/2 tablespoon of the olive oil, 3/four teaspoon of the salt, and 1/2 teaspoon of the pepper in a small bowl. Rub all of the combination over the brisket. Place the brisket in a 5- to 6-quart gradual cooker.

Whisk collectively the water, ketchup, Worcestershire, and a pair of tablespoons of the vinegar in a small bowl; pour over the brisket in the slow cooker. Cover and cook on LOW till the brisket is very tender, about eight hours.

Transfer the brisket to a slicing board, booking the sauce in the gradual cooker. Shred the brisket with 2 forks into bite-sized pieces. Return the shredded

meat to the reserved sauce inside the sluggish cooker, stirring to combine.
Just before serving, whisk together the ultimate 1 tablespoon every olive oil and vinegar and final 1/four teaspoon every salt and pepper in a medium bowl. Add the coleslaw mix, and toss for coating. Divide the brisket and slaw evenly among the slider buns.

Nutrition Facts
412 calories; 11 g total fat; 2 g saturated fat; 648 mg sodium. 44 g carbohydrates; 3 g fiber; 13 g sugar; 35 g protein; 3 g added sugar;

Spaghetti Squash Casserole

Ingredients
- 1 (2 1/2 to 3 pound) of spaghetti squash, cut in half lengthwise and seeds removed
- 2 tablespoons of water
- 1 pound of lean ground beef
- 1 medium sized shallot, sliced
- 2 cloves garlic, minced
- 1 ½ teaspoons of Italian seasoning
- ½ teaspoon of plus 1/8 teaspoon salt
- ½ teaspoon of ground pepper
- 1 (28 ounce) can of no-salt-added tomatoes
- 1 cup of shredded fontina cheese
- Fresh basil for garnishing

Directions
Preheat oven to 400 stages F.
Place squash, cut-aspect down, in a microwave-secure dish; upload water. Microwave, uncovered, on High till tender, approximately 10 minutes. (Alternatively, region squash halves cut-side down on a rimmed baking sheet. Bake at 400 levels F till tender, forty to 50 minutes.)
Meanwhile, prepare dinner ground red meat in a massive ovenproof skillet over medium-high warmth, breaking it up with a wood spoon, till no longer pink, five to 7 min. Add shallot, garlic, Italian seasoning, salt, pepper and cook, stirring, for 1 min. Stir in tomatoes and boil them. Reduce warmness to keep a simmer.
Use a fork to scrape the squash flesh from the shells in the sauce; stir to combine. Topping with cheese. Place the pan to the oven and bake until bubbling, approximately 15 min. Let stand for 5 min. Serve sprinkled with basil, if desired.

Nutrition Facts
470 calories; 19.8 g total fat; 118 mg cholesterol; 719 mg is sodium. 1299 mg is potassium; 27.5 g carbohydrates; 7.1 g is fiber; 13 g sugar; 42.9 g protein; 24 mg vitamin c; 31 mcg folate; 227 mg calcium; 8 mg iron; 60 mg magnesium;

Sausage-Spiked Meatloaves

Ingredients
- 2 tablespoons of extra-virgin olive oil
- 1 cup of chopped yellow onion
- 1 cup of chopped celery
- 6 cloves garlic, finely chopped
- 2 large sized eggs, lightly beaten
- 1 cup of panko breadcrumbs, preferably whole-wheat
- 12 tablespoons of ketchup, divided
- ½ cup of chopped fresh parsley, plus more for garnish
- 2 tablespoons of Worcestershire sauce
- ¼ teaspoon of salt
- 1 teaspoon of ground pepper
- 1 pound of 90%-lean ground beef
- 12 ounces of ground turkey
- 8 ounces of ground pork
- 8 ounces of Italian turkey sausage, casing removed

Directions
Preheat oven to 350 stages F. Coat 9-by-five-inch loaf pans with cooking spray.
Heat oil in a massive skillet at medium temp heat. Add onion and celery; cookig, stirring occasionally, until tender, 10 to 12 min. Add garlic and cook, stirring, for 1 min more. Transfer to a huge bowl and spread into a skinny layer. Let cool for 5 min.
Add eggs, and breadcrumbs, 6 tbsp of ketchup, parsley, Worcestershire, salt and pepper to the veggies and stir to combine. Add beef, turkey, pork and sausage; mix along with your hands until combined. Divide between the prepared pans.
Bake the meatloaves until an instant-study thermometer inserted in the center registers one hundred sixty levels F, forty to forty five mins. Brush the meatloaves with the remaining 6 tbsp ketchup. Turn the broiler to high. Broil the m eatloaves until the ketchup is bubbling, 3 to five minutes. Let stand for 15 minutes before slicing. Garnish with parsley, if desired.

Nutrition
305 calories; 15.6 g total fat; 119 mg cholesterol; 505 mg is sodium. 399 mg is potassium; 14.8 g is carbohydrates; 1.5 g fiber; 6 g sugar; 26.7 g protein; 7 mg vitamin c; 23 mcg folate; 43 mg calcium; 3 mg iron; 27 mg magnesium; 4 g added sugar;

Braised Brisket With Dried Fruit

Ingredients
- 3 whole star anise
- 4 teaspoons of unsweetened cocoa powder
- 4 teaspoons of ground sumac
- 2 teaspoons of Urfa pepper or crushed red pepper
- 1 ¼ teaspoons of ground cinnamon, preferably Vietnamese
- 4 pounds of beef brisket, trimmed
- ½ teaspoon of kosher salt
- 2 tablespoons of extra-virgin olive oil
- 4 medium sized white onions, sliced
- 8 cloves garlic, minced
- ¼ cup of dried apricots
- ¼ cup of dried cranberries
- ¼ cup of pitted prunes
- ¼ cup of golden raisins
- 1 medium sizedorange, cut into wedges
- 4 cups of low-sodium beef broth

Directions
Preheat oven to 325 levels F.
Finely grind superstar anise in a spice grinder or with a mortar and pestle. Transfer to a bowl and mix in cocoa, sumac, pepper and cinnamon.
Season brisket with salt and a pair of tablespoons of the spice blend. Heat oil in a massive ovenproof pot over high warmth. Add the brisket and cook till browned, about 4 minutes in keeping with side. Transfer the brisket to a plate.
Reduce warmness to medium, upload onions to the pot and cook, stirring often, till softened, approximately 10 minutes. Add garlic, apricots, cranberries, prunes, raisins, orange wedges and the final spice blend. Cook, stirring often, for three mins more. Stir in broth and convey to a simmer. Return the brisket to the pot.
Cover the brisket with a chunk of parchment paper and put the lid on the pot. Transfer to the oven and bake until the brisket is fork-tender, about three half of hours.
Transfer the brisket to a easy reducing board. Loosely cowl with foil and let relaxation for 10 mins. Slice the brisket in opposition to the grain and serve with the sauce.
Nutrition
290 calories; 9.3 g total fat; 98 mg cholesterol; 320 mg is sodium. 758 mg is potassium; 15.7 g is carbohydrates; 2.2 g fiber; 10 g is sugar; 35.5 g protein; 10 mg vitamin c; 31 mcg folate; 52 mg calcium; 4 mg iron; 48 mg magnesium; 2 g added sugar;

SMOOTHIES AND DRINKS

Orange Dream Smoothie
Ingredients
- 1 1/2 cups of orange juice, chilled
- 1 cup light of vanilla soy milk, chilled
- 1/3 cup of silken or soft tofu
- 1 tablespoon of dark honey
- 1 teaspoon of grated orange zest
- 1/2 teaspoon of vanilla extract
- 5 ice cubes
- 4 peeled orange segments

Directions
In a blender, combine the orange juice, soy milk, tofu, honey, orange zest, vanilla and ice cubes. Blend until smooth and frothy, about 30 seconds.
Pour into tall, chilled glasses and garnish each glass with an orange segment.
Nutrition
Total carbohydrate20 g Dietary fiber1 g Sodium40 mg Total fat1 g Cholesterol0 mg Protein3 gCalories101 Total sugars14 g

Strawberry Banana Milkshak
Ingredients
- 6 frozen strawberries, finely chopped
- 1 medium sized banana
- 1/2 cup of soy milk
- 1 cup of fat-free vanilla frozen yogurt
- 2 fresh strawberries, finely sliced

Directions
In a blender, combine the frozen strawberries, banana, soy milk and frozen yogurt. Blend until smooth.
Pour into tall, frosty glasses and garnish each with fresh strawberry slices. Serve immediately.
Nutrition
Total fat1 gCalories183 Protein6 g Cholesterol0 mg Total carbohydrate40 g Dietary fiber8 g Sodium117 mg Added sugars17

Watermelon-Cranberry Agua Fresca
Ingredients
- 2 1/2 pounds of seedless watermelon, rind removed and diced (about 7 cups)
- 1 cup of fruit-sweetened cranberry juice
- 1/4 cup of fresh lime juice
- 1 lime, cut into 6 slices

Directions
Place the melon in a blender or meals processor. Process until smooth. Pass the puree via a fine-mesh sieve positioned over a bowl to get rid of the pulp and make clear the juice. Pour the juice into a massive pitcher. Add the cranberry and lime juices and stir to combine.
Refrigerate until very cold. Pour into tall chilled glasses and garnish each with a slice of lime.
Nutrition
Total carbohydrate20 g Dietary fiber1 g Sodium9 mg Saturated fat0 g Total fat0 g Cholesterol0 mg Protein1 gCalories84 Total sugars16 g

Chocolate Berry Smoothies
Ingredients
2 tablespoons of cashews
12 ounces of cold water
¼ cup of frozen blueberries
½ of an avocado
2 tablespoons of organic cocoa powder
½ teaspoon of vanilla extract
little raw honey to sweeten it to your liking
Place all ingredients in a blender for mixing and blend on high speed for 40 - 60 seconds.
Pour serve and enjoy.
Nutritional Facts
Calories 250 • Total Fat 17.2 g • Fiber 7.7 g • Protein 6.4 g • Sugar 8 g • Sodium 55 mg

Ginger Carrot And Turmeric Smoothie
Ingredients
CARROT JUICE
- 2 cups of carrots
- 1 and 1/2 cups of water should be filtered

Make carrot juice by including carrots and filtered water to a excessive velocity blender and mixing on high till absolutely pureed and smooth. Add greater water if it has trouble blending / scrape down sides as needed. Keep juice in refrigerator and use when needed.

SMOOTHIE
- 1 large sized ripe banana, (more for a sweeter smoothie)
- 1 cup of (140 g) frozen or fresh pineapple
- 1/2 Tbsp of fresh ginger
- 1/4 tsp of ground turmeric
- 1/2 tsp of cinnamon
- 1/2 cup of (120 ml) carrot juice
- 1 Tbsp of lime juice
- 1 cup pf (240 ml) unsweetened almond milk Blend all ingredients together in a blender.

Nutrition
Calories: 144, Carbohydrates: 32g Sugar: 17.5g Sodium: 112mg Fiber: 5g Protein: 2.4g

Raspberry Green Smoothie

Ingredients
- 1 cup of water
- 1 tbsp of Chia seeds
- 1 cup of raspberries
- 1 medium sized banana
- 1/4 cup of spinach
- 1 tbsp. of almond butter
- 2 tbsp. of lemon

Instructions
Wash the raspberries and spinach in a strainer under running stream of water. Peel the banana and slice it into pieces. Pulse the raspberries inside the blender 4 or five times to interrupt them down. Add the banana and spinach to the blender and pulse a few times to interrupt down the larger pieces, after which blend until smooth (approximately a minute).

Avocado Smoothie

Ingredients
- 1/2 avocado
- 2 tbsp cacao powder
- 1/2 medium cold banana
- 1/4 cup plain coconut milk
- 1/2 teaspoon chia seeds

Directions
1. Blend all ingredients in a blender for mixing until smooth.
2. Add a little lime juice and cucumbers for additional flavoring this is 391 calories per serving, so it is a substitute for an entire meal, but it will curb your cravings for hours.

Peanut Butter & Banana Breakfast Smoothie

Ingredients
1 cup nonfat milk
- 1 tablespoon of all natural peanut butter
- 1 medium of banana, frozen or fresh
- Directions:
- Combine all ingredients in the blender, and blend until very smooth.
Banana Breakfast Smoothie

Ingredients
- ½ cup and 1% low-fat milk
- 1/2 cup of crushed ice
- 1 tablespoon of honey
- 1 large sized ripe banana, sliced and frozen
- 1 (6-ounce) of carton vanilla fat-free yogurt

Preparation:
1. Place first 4 ingredients in a blender for mixing ; process 1 minor until smooth. Add yogurt; process 20 to 30 sec or until blended. Serve immediately.

Oatmeal Smoothie For The Dash Diet Breakfast

Ingredients
- 1/2 cup of ice plus 1 banana – or just 1 frozen banana
- 1 cup of frozen mixed berries (any berries. I use the Costco mix)
- 1/2 cup of plain lowfat yogurt
- 1/2 cup of rolled oats
- 1 cup of milk (or other liquid, such as almond milk) – adjust to taste
- 1 tsp of honey or some stevia to sweeten it up

Directions:
Place ingredients in your blender for mixing, first frozen ones, then oats, then liquids.
If using frozen banana, don;t forget to peel and slice it
Blend until mixed well.

Kale And Banana Smoothie

Ingredients
- 1 banana
- 2 cups chopped kale
- 1/2 cup light unsweetened soy milk
- 1 tablespoon flax seeds
- 1 teaspoon maple syrup
- Place the banana, kale, soy milk, flax seeds, and maple syrup into a blender.
- Cover, and puree until smooth.
- Serve over ice.

Nutrition Facts
311 calories; 7.3 g fat; 56.6 g carbohydrates; 12.2 g protein; 0 mg cholesterol; 110 mg sodium.

Strawberry Banana Smoothie

Ingredients
- 1 1/2 cups vanilla yogurt
- 2 bananas, cut up
- 1/2 cup frozen strawberries
- 2 tablespoons wheat germ
- 1 tablespoon honey

Combine the yogurt, bananas, strawberries, wheat germ, and honey in a blender; blend until smooth, about 1 minute.

Nutrition
332 calories; 3.4 g fat; 68 g carbohydrates; 12.2 g protein; 9 mg cholesterol; 124 mg sodium.

Banana, Avocado, And Spinach Smoothie

Ingredients
- 1 banana, sliced
- 1/2 avocado, peeled and sliced
- 1/2 cup fresh spinach
- 1/2 cup 1% milk
- 6 ice cubes
- 2 teaspoons honey
- 1 teaspoon vanilla extract

Blend banana, avocado, spinach, milk, ice cubes, honey, and vanilla extract together in a blender until smooth.

Nutrition
190 calories; 8.2 g fat; 27.5 g carbohydrates; 4 g protein; 2 mg cholesterol; 45 mg sodium.

Strawberry Oatmeal Breakfast Smoothie
Ingredients
- 1 cup soy milk
- 1/2 cup rolled oats
- 1 banana, broken into chunks
- 14 frozen strawberries
- 1/2 teaspoon vanilla extract
- 1 1/2 teaspoons white sugar

In a blender, combine soy milk, oats, banana and strawberries. Add vanilla and sugar if desired. Blend until smooth. Pour into glasses and serve.

Nutrition Facts
236 calories; 3.7 g fat; 44.9 g carbohydrates; 7.6 g protein; 0 mg cholesterol; 65 mg sodium.

Orange Banana Smoothie
Ingredients
- 1 cup cold milk
- 2 oranges, peeled and segmented
- 1 banana
- 1/4 cup sugar
- 1 pinch salt
- 1/2 (8 ounce) container vanilla fat-free yogurt
- 4 cubes ice

In a blender, combine milk, oranges, banana, sugar, salt and yogurt. Blend for about 1 minute. Insert ice cubes, and blend until smooth. Pour into glasses and serve.

Nutrition
340 calories; 2.9 g fat; 73.7 g carbohydrates; 9.1 g protein; 11 mg cholesterol; 90 mg sodium.

Kiwi Banana Apple Smoothie
Ingredients
- 1 apple, roughly chopped
- 1 banana, broken into chunks
- 2 kiwifruit, peeled
- 1 1/4 cups milk
- 1/4 cup ice, or as desired
- 2 teaspoons chia seeds
- 1 teaspoon maca powder

Blend apple, banana, kiwifruit, milk, ice, chia seeds, and maca powder together in a blender until smooth.

Nutrition
232 calories; 4.5 g fat; 44.1 g carbohydrates; 7.6 g protein; 12 mg cholesterol; 67 mg sodium.

Spinach And Kale Smoothie
Ingredients
- 2 cups fresh spinach
- 1 cup almond milk
- 1 tablespoon peanut butter
- 1 tablespoon chia seeds (optional)
- 1 leaf kale
- 1 sliced frozen banana

Blend spinach, almond milk, peanut butter, chia seeds, and kale together in a blender until smooth. Add banana and blend until smooth.

Nutrition
325 calories; 13.9 g fat; 46.1 g carbohydrates; 10 g protein; 0 mg cholesterol; 293 mg sodium.

Banana Pina Coladasmoothie
Ingredients
- 1 large banana
- 1 cup coconut juice blend, or more to taste
- 2 pineapple spears
- 3 cubes ice
- 1 tablespoon agave nectar

Blend banana, coconut juice blend, pineapple, ice, and agave nectar together in a blender until smooth.

Nutrition
520 calories; 7.1 g fat; 121.5 g carbohydrates; 2.1 g protein; 0 mg cholesterol; 92 mg sodium.

Power Drink ***The Orange***
Ingredients
- 2 ripe bananas, peeled
- 4 carrots, scrubbed and trimmed
- 2 apples, cored
- 1 (8 ounce) container plain yogurt
- 1/2 cup orange juice
- 1 lemon, juiced
- 1 tablespoon ground flax seed
- 1 pinch salt
- 4 pitted dates, or to taste (optional)
- 8 cubes ice, or as needed (optional)

Blend the bananas, carrots, apples, yogurt, orange juice, lemon juice, flax seed, salt, dates, and ice cubes in a blender until smooth.

Nutrition
204 calories; 2.2 g fat; 44.9 g carbohydrates; 5.2 g protein; 3 mg cholesterol; 85 mg sodium.

Sissy's Frozen Banana And Pumpkin Smoothie
Ingredients
- 3 cups of vanilla-flavored almond milk
- 2 bananas, frozen
- 1/2 (15 ounce) can of pumpkin puree, frozen into small balls
- 5 tablespoons of honey, or to taste

Mix all the ingredients almond milk, bananas, pumpkin puree, and honey in a juicer blender. Cover

it and blend until thick and texture resemble a smoothie, about 3 min.
Nutrition
397 calories; 4.7 g fat; 91.6 g carbohydrates; 4.2 g protein; 0 mg cholesterol; 500 mg sodium.

Broccolicious

Ingredients
- 2 cups of chopped broccoli
- 1 cup of seedless green grapes, or more to taste
- 1 small sized cucumber, finely chopped
- ½ cup of water
- 1 lime, extract its juice

Instructions
Blend the all ingredients broccoli, cucumber, water and lime juice in the juicer blender an mix it will till become smooth.
Per Serving:
110 of calories; 1 g of total fat; 0 mg of cholesterol; 36 mg of sodium. 26.7 g of carbohydrates; 3.9 g protein;

Green Power Mojito Smoothie

Ingredients
- 3 cups of ice cubes
- 2 cups of baby spinach leaves, or to taste
- 1 (7 ounce) can of finely crushed pineapple
- 1/2 cup of water
- 1 banana, finely divided into chunks
- 1 orange, peeled it and cut it into pieces
- 10 mint leaves (fresh)
- 1 lemon, extract its juice

Blend the all ingredients ice, spinach, water, pineapple, banana, mint, lemon juice and lime juice in a juicer blender and mix till bemoce soomth.
94 calories; 0.3 g fat; 24.2 g of carbohydrates; 1.5 g protein; 0 mg of cholesterol; 19 mg sodium.

Pumpkin Smoothie

Ingredients
- 1 (16 ounce) can pumpkin puree
- 2 cups milk
- 1/4 cup brown sugar
- 2 teaspoons ground cinnamon
- Place the pumpkin puree in a freezer bag; shop in the freezer for at least 24 hours.
- Heat the container of pumpkin puree within the microwave on HIGH to soften, 1 to 2 minutes.
- Pour the milk right into a blender. Add the brown sugar, cinnamon, and pumpkin; blend until smooth.

155 calories; 2.7 g of fat; 29.3 g carbohydrates; 5.3 g of protein; 10 mg of cholesterol; 328 mg sodium.

Grapefruit Smoothie

Ingredients
- 3 grapefruit, peeled and sectioned
- 1 cup cold water
- 3 ounces fresh spinach
- 6 ice cubes
- 1 (1/2 inch) piece peeled fresh ginger
- 1 teaspoon flax seeds

Blend grapefruit, water, spinach, ice cubes, ginger, and flax seeds in a blender or NutriBullet(R) until smooth.
Per Serving: 201 calories; 1 g fat; 47.4 g carbohydrates; 4.6 g protein; 0 mg cholesterol; 39 mg sodium.

Almond Butter And Blueberry Smoothie

Ingredients
- 1 cup of almond milk
- 1 cup of blueberries
- 4 ice cubes
- 1 scoop of vanilla protein powder
- 1 tablespoon of almond butter
- 1 tablespoon of chia seeds

Blend all ingredients almond, milk, blueberries, vanilla protein powder, ice cubes, chia seeds, and almond butter in a juicer blender and mix well until become smooth.
230 calories; 8.1 g fat; 20 g carbohydrates; 21.6 g protein; 6 mg cholesterol; 225 mg sodium.

Groovy Green Smoothie

Ingredients
- 1 banana, cut in chunks
- 1 cup grapes
- 1 (6 ounce) tub vanilla yogurt
- 1/2 apple, cored and chopped
- 1 1/2 cups fresh spinach leaves

Place the banana, grapes, yogurt, apple, and spinach into a blender. Cover and blend till smooth, frequently stopping to push down something caught to the sides. Pour into glasses and serve.
205 calories; 1.9 g of fat; 45 g of carbohydrates; 6.1 g of protein; 4 mg cholesterol; 76 mg of sodium.

Green Slime Smoothie

Ingredients
- 2 cups spinach
- 2 cups frozen strawberries
- 1 banana
- 2 tablespoons honey
- 1/2 cup ice
- Add
- Place the spinach in the freezer until frozen, at least 1 hour.
- Combine the spinach, strawberries, banana, honey, and ice in a blender. Blend until smooth. Serve immediately.

Per Serving: 100 calories; 0.3 g fat; 26 g carbohydrates; 1.3 g protein; 0 mg cholesterol; 16 mg sodium.

Strawberry Blueberry Smoothies

Ingredients
- 1/2 cup almond milk
- 1/2 cup frozen strawberries
- 1/2 cup frozen blueberries
- 1/2 cup low-fat plain yogurt

- 1 teaspoon flax seed oil
- 1 teaspoon agave nectar

Blend almond milk, strawberries, blueberries, yogurt, flax seed oil, and agave nectar in a blender until smooth.
Per Serving: 231 calories; 5.3 g fat; 40 g carbohydrates; 8.7 g protein; 7 mg cholesterol; 170 mg sodium.

Red, White, And Blue Fruit Smoothie
Ingredients
- 1/2 large sized banana cut it into pieces and freeze it
- 2 large sized fresh strawberries, rinsed it well and sliced it into pieces
- 1/4 cup of blueberries
- 1/2 cup of milk
- 1 teaspoon of vanilla extract
- 2 tablespoons of vanilla yogurt
- 2 ice cubes for freezing

Blend all ingredients banana, blueberries, strawberries, vanilla extract, yogurt and ice cubes in a juicer blender and mix well till become smooth.
192 calories; 3.2 g fat; 34 g carbohydrates; 6.8 g protein; 11 mg cholesterol; 73 mg sodium.

Triple Threat Fruit Smoothie
Ingredients
- 1 kiwi, sliced
- 1 banana, peeled and chopped
- 1/2 cup blueberries
- 1 cup strawberries
- 1 cup ice cubes
- 1/2 cup orange juice
- 1 (8 ounce) container peach yogurt

In a blender, blend the kiwi, banana, blueberries, strawberries, ice, orange juice, and yogurt until smooth.
Per Serving: 134 calories; 1.1 g fat; 29.6 g carbohydrates; 3.6 g protein; 4 mg cholesterol; 41 mg sodium.

Super Healthy Fruit Smoothie
Ingredients
- 1/3 cup fresh blueberries
- 1/3 cup fresh raspberries
- 4 large fresh strawberries, hulled
- 1/3 cup pomegranate juice
- 1/3 cup mango juice
- 2/3 cup milk
- 2 tablespoons honey

Blend all ingredients pomegranate, blueberries, strawberries, mango juice, milk, honey and ice cubes in a juicer blender and mix well till become smooth.
191 calories; 1.9 g of fat; 42.7 g carbohydrates; 3.4 g of protein; 7 mg of cholesterol; 37 mg sodium.

Blueberry Mint Smoothie
Ingredients
- 2 cups frozen blueberries
- 1 cup water
- 1 cup fresh mint leaves
- 1 avocado, peeled and pitted
- 1/2 cup orange juice
- 2 teaspoons lemon juice

Blend blueberries, water, mint leaves, avocado, orange juice, and lemon juice in a blender until smooth.
Per Serving: 273 calories; 15.9 g fat; 35 g carbohydrates; 3.5 g protein; 0 mg cholesterol; 13 mg sodium.

All-Fruit Smoothies
Ingredients
- 1 cup pineapple juice
- 1 large banana, cut into chunks
- 1 cup frozen strawberries
- 1 cup frozen blueberries

Pour pineapple juice into a blender and add banana, strawberries, and blueberries. Cover and blend until smooth, about 1 minute. Pour into 2 glasses.
Per Serving: 205 calories; 1 g fat; 51.1 g carbohydrates; 2 g protein; 0 mg cholesterol; 6 mg sodium.

Lemon Berry Smoothie
Ingredients
- 1 (8 ounce) container blueberry nonfat yogurt
- 1 1/2 cups skim milk
- 1 cup ice cubes
- 1 cup fresh blueberries
- 1 cup fresh strawberries
- 1 teaspoon powdered lemonade mix

Place yogurt, milk, ice cubes, blueberries, strawberries, and lemonade mix in a blender. Pulse until smooth and creamy.

Zucchini Chocolate Banana Nut Milkshake
Ingredients
- 1 cup grated zucchini, frozen
- 2 large ripe bananas, peeled and frozen
- 2 tablespoons cocoa powder
- 1/4 cup chopped peanuts
- 1/2 cup sugar
- 1 cup half and half

Blend the zucchini, bananas, cocoa powder, peanuts, sugar, and half and half in a food processor until smooth, thick, and creamy.
Per Serving: 300 calories; 12.1 g fat; 47.6 g carbohydrates; 5.6 g protein; 22 mg cholesterol; 30 mg sodium.

Heavenly Blueberry Smoothie
Ingredients
- 1 frozen banana
- 1/2 cup of vanilla soy milk
- 1 cup of vanilla fat-free yogurt
- 1 1/2 teaspoons of flax seed meal
- 1 1/2 teaspoons of honey
- 2/3 cup of blueberries frozen

Cut the banana into small pieces and vicinity into the bowl of a blender. Add the soy milk, yogurt, flaxseed meal, and honey. Blend on lowest speed until smooth, about 5 seconds. Gradually add the blueberries while continuing to mix on low. Once the blueberries were incorporated, growth speed, and blend to preferred consistency.
250 calories; 2.6 g of fat; 50.2 g carbohydrates; 9.5 g of protein; 2 mg of cholesterol; 117 mg of sodium.

Orange Smoothie
Ingredients
- 1 (6 ounce) can frozen orange juice concentrate
- 1 cup milk
- 1 cup water
- 1 teaspoon vanilla extract
- 1/3 cup white sugar
- 10 cubes ice

In a blender, combine orange juice concentrate, milk, water, vanilla, sugar and ice. Blend until smooth. Pour into glasses and serve.
Per Serving: 183 calories; 1.3 g fat; 40 g carbohydrates; 3.3 g protein; 5 mg cholesterol; 28 mg sodium.

Mongolian Strawberry-Orange Juice Smoothie
Ingredients
- 1 cup chopped fresh strawberries
- 1 cup orange juice
- 10 cubes ice
- 1 tablespoon sugar

In a blender, combine strawberries, orange juice, ice cubes and sugar. Blend until smooth. Pour into glasses and serve.
Per Serving: 52 calories; 0.2 g fat; 12.5 g carbohydrates; 0.7 g protein; 0 mg cholesterol; 3 mg sodium.

Mango Pineapple Green Smoothie
Ingredients
- 2/3 cup frozen pineapple chunks
- 1 cup frozen mango chunks
- 1 ripe banana, sliced
- 2/3 cup fresh spinach
- 1/3 cup orange juice
- 1 cup ice

Place pineapple, mango, banana, spinach, orange juice, and ice, respectively, in a blender and blend until smooth.
Per Serving: 197 calories; 0.6 g fat; 50.3 g carbohydrates; 2 g protein; 0 mg cholesterol; 16 mg sodium.

Orange Snowman
Ingredients
- 1 (6 ounce) can of orange juice frozen
- 1/2 cup of milk
- 1/2 cup of water
- 1/2 cup of sugar
- 1/2 teaspoon of vanilla extract
- 14 cubes of ice

In a blender, mix all ingredients orange juice concentrate, milk, water, sugar, vanilla and ice. Continue to blend until smooth. Pour the juice into glasses to serve.
198 calories; 0.7 g of fat; 46.8 g carbohydrates; 2.3 g of protein; 2 mg cholesterol; 16 mg of sodium.

SOUPS

Pumpkin Soup

Ingredients
- 3/4 cup of water, divided
- 1 small sized onion, chopped
- 1 can (15 ounces) of pumpkin puree
- 2 cups of unsalted vegetable broth
- 1/2 teaspoon of ground cinnamon
- 1/4 teaspoon of ground nutmeg
- 1 cup of fat-free milk
- 1/8 teaspoon of black pepper
- 1 green onion top, finely chopped

Instructions
- In a considerable saucepan, warmth 1/four cup water over medium warmth. Add onion and cook until tender, about three minutes. Don't permit onion dry out.
- Add last water, pumpkin, broth, cinnamon, and nutmeg. Bring to a boil, reduce warmness, and simmer for 5 min. Stir in the milk and cook until hot. Don't boil.
- Ladle soup into warmed bowls and garnish with black pepper and soft onion tops. Serve immediately.

Nutrition
Total carbohydrate14 g Dietary fiber4 g Sodium57 mg Total fat1 g Cholesterol1 gCalories77 Protein3 g

Summer Vegetable Soup

Ingredients
- 1 tablespoon of olive oil
- 1 yellow color onion, finely chopped (about 1 cup)
- 3 cloves of garlic, finely chopped
- 4 plum (Roma) of tomatoes, peeled and seeded, then divided into pieces
- 1 tablespoon of chopped fresh oregano
- 1 teaspoon of ground cumin
- 4 cups of no salt added vegetable stock
- 1 bay leaf
- 1 carrot, thinly sliced (about 1 cup)
- 1 yellow bell pepper, diced (about 1 cup)
- 1 zucchini, thinly sliced (about 1 cup)
- 1 tablespoon of grated lemon zest
- 2 tablespoons of chopped fresh cilantro (fresh coriander)
- 1/4 teaspoon of salt
- 1/4 teaspoon of freshly ground black pepper

Directions
In a massive saucepan, heat the olive oil over medium warmth. Add the onion and saute until gentle and translucent, about four minutes. Add the garlic and saute for 30 seconds; do not let the garlic brown. Add the tomatoes, oregano and cumin and saute until the tomatoes are softened, about 4 minutes.Add the stock and bay leaf and bring to a boil, then lessen the warmth to medium low and convey to a simmer. Add the carrot and bell pepper and cook for 2 mins. Add the zucchini and simmer until the veggies are tender, about three mins longer. Stir within the lemon zest and cilantro. Season with the salt and pepper. Discard the bay leaf.Ladle into man or woman bowls or mugs and serve immediately.

Nutrition Info
Calories62 Total fat2 g Cholesterol0 mg Sodium156 mg Total carbohydrate9 g Dietary fiber2 g Total sugars5 g Protein2 g

Tuscan White Bean Stew

Ingredients
For the croutons:
- 1 tablespoon of extra-virgin olive oil
- 2 cloves of garlic, chopped
- 1 slice of whole-grain bread, cubes

For the soup:
- 2 cups (about 1 pound) of dried cannellini, drained
- 6 cups of water
- 1/2 teaspoon of salt
- 1 bay leaf
- 2 tablespoons of olive oil
- 1 cup of coarsely chopped yellow onion
- 3 carrots, peeled and coarsely chopped
- 6 cloves garlic, chopped
- 1/4 teaspoon of freshly ground black pepper
- 1 tablespoon of chopped fresh rosemary, plus 6 sprigs
- 1 1/2 cups of vegetable stock or broth

Instructions
To make the croutons, heat the olive oil over medium warmness in a large frying pan. Add the garlic and saute for 1 minute. Remove from the warmth and let stand for 10 mins to infuse the garlic taste into the oil. Remove the garlic pieces and discard them. Return the pan to medium heat. Add the bread cubes and saute, frequently stirring, till gently browned 3 to five minutes. Transfer to a small bowl and set aside.
To make the soup, integrate into a soup pot the white beans, water, 1/4 teaspoon of the salt, and the bay leaf. Bring to a boil over excessive heat. Reduce the heat to low, cowl partly and simmer until the beans are tender, 60 to 75 minutes. Drain the beans, reserving half a cup of the cooking liquid. Discard the bay leaf. Place the cooked beans into a big bowl and keep the cooking pot for later use.
In a small bowl, combine the reserved cooking liquid and a half cup of the cooked beans. Mash with a fork to form a paste. Stir the bean paste into the baked beans.
Return the cooking pot to the stovetop and add the olive oil. Heat over medium-excessive heat. Stir within the onion and carrots and saute until the

carrots are tender-crisp, 6 to 7 mins. Stir in the garlic and cook till softened, approximately 1 minute. Stir inside the closing 1/four teaspoon salt, the pepper, chopped rosemary, bean aggregate, and stock. Bring to a boil then lessen the heat to low and simmer until the stew is heated through, about five minutes. Ladle the stew into warmed bowls and sprinkle with the croutons. Garnish each dish with a rosemary sprig and serve immediately.

Nutrition
Total carbohydrate45 g Dietary fiber11 g Sodium334 mg Saturated fat1 g Total fat7 g Cholesterol0 mg Protein16 gCalories307 Total sugars3 g

Chicken Noodle Soup

Ingredients
- 1 teaspoon of olive oil
- 1 cup of chopped onion
- 3 cloves of garlic, finely minced
- 1 cup of chopped celery
- 1 cup of sliced, peeled carrots (2 medium)
- 4 cups of Maureen's Chicken Broth
- 4 ounces of dried linguini, broken
- 1 cup of cooked non-brined chicken breast, cut into desired size
- 2 tablespoons of snipped fresh parsley

In a big saucepan, warmness olive oil over medium warmth and saute onion and garlic until translucent. Add celery and carrots and hold to saute for another three minutes. Add Maureen's Chicken Broth. Bring to a boil; lessen heat and simmer, covered, five minutes. Stir in linguini; cook dinner and stir until combination returns to a boil. Reduce heat and simmer, covered, 10 minutes extra or until pasta and veggies are tender, stirring occasionally.
Add cooked bird and clean parsley. Heat through.

Steak And Vegetable Soup

Ingredients
- 1 lb boneless top loin steak, cut into 1-inch pieces
- 2 Tbsp of olive oil
- 2 onions, finely chopped
- 4 carrots, sliced
- 4 celery ribs, thinly sliced
- 6 garlic cloves, chopped
- 1 Tbsp of chopped thyme
- 1/2 tsp of salt, plus more to taste
- 1/2 tsp of black pepper, plus more to taste
- 1 lb Yukon Gold potatoes, cut into 1/2-inch cubes
- 2 cups of canned diced tomatoes with some juice
- 3 1/2 cups of beef broth
- 4 cups of chopped kale leaves
- 2 cups of medium egg noodles, cooked

Pat steak dry. Heat oil in a massive 4- to 5-quart pot over medium-high till it shimmers. Cook steak till browned on all aspects and medium-rare, about 3 minutes; transfer to a plate.
Cook onions, carrots, celery, garlic, thyme, 1/2 tsp salt, and 1/2 tsp pepper over medium, occasionally stirring, till softened, approximately eight minutes. Stir in potatoes, tomatoes with juice, broth, and four 1/2 cups water; simmer, partly covered, till vegetables are tender, approximately 15 minutes. Stir in kale. Cook till tender, about 5 min. Add steak with meat juices and noodles; season with salt and pepper, if needed.

Thai Red Curry Chicken Soup

Ingredients
2 tablespoons red curry paste
1 red bell pepper, thinly sliced
1 small onion, chopped
1 (14 ounce) can coconut milk
1 tablespoon fish sauce
3 cups homemade chicken stock
2 cups shredded cooked chicken
1 ½ cups cooked basmati rice
4 tablespoons chopped fresh cilantro

Directions
Cook curry paste in a large, heavy saucepan over medium-excessive heat until oils start to release, 1 to 2 minutes. Add pink pepper and onion and cook, stirring, till softened, about five minutes. Stir in coconut milk until well blended. Add fish sauce, and then bird stock.
Reduce heat to low and simmer for 15 minutes. Add cooked chicken and rice. Stir over heat until warmed through. Add chopped cilantro right before serving.

Nutrition
303 calories; 23.1 g total fat; 37 mg cholesterol; 663 mg sodium. 16.8 g carbohydrates; 16.4 g protein;

Ham And Split Pea Soup Recipe - A Great Soup

Ingredients
2 tablespoons butter
1/2 onion, diced
2 ribs celery, diced
3 cloves garlic, sliced
1 pound ham, diced
1 bay leaf
1 pound dried split peas
1 quart chicken stock
2 1/2 cups water
salt and ground black pepper to taste

Place the butter in a massive soup pot over medium-low heat. Stir in onion, celery, and sliced garlic. Cook slowly until the onions are translucent but not brown, five to 8 minutes.
Mix in ham, bay leaf, and break up peas. Pour in chicken inventory and water. Stir to combine, and simmer till the peas are smooth, and the soup is thick, about 1 hour and 15 minutes. Stir occasionally — season with salt and black pepper to serve.

374 calories; 14.4 g of fat; 37 g carbohydrates; 25.1 g of protein; 40 mg cholesterol; 1187 mg sodium.

Vegan Red Lentil Soup

Ingredients
- 1 tablespoon of peanut oil
- 1 small sized onion, finely chopped
- 1 tablespoon of minced fresh ginger root
- 1 clove of garlic, chopped
- 1 pinch of fenugreek seeds
- 1 cup of dry red lentils
- 1 cup of butternut squash, cubed
- 1/3 cup of finely chopped fresh cilantro
- 2 cups of water
- 1/2 (14 ounce) can of coconut milk
- 2 tablespoons of tomato paste
- 1 teaspoon of curry powder
- 1 pinch of cayenne pepper
- 1 pinch of ground nutmeg
- salt and pepper to your taste

Heat the oil in a large pot over medium warmth, and prepare dinner the onion, ginger, garlic, and fenugreek until onion is tender.

Mix the lentils, squash, and cilantro into the pot. Stir within the water, coconut milk, and tomato paste — season with curry powder, cayenne pepper, nutmeg, salt, and pepper. Bring to a boil, lessen heat to low, and simmer 30 minutes, or till lentils and squash are tender.

303 calories; 14.6 g fat; 34.2 g carbohydrates; 13 g protein; 0 mg cholesterol; 81 mg sodium.

Slow-Cooker Chicken Tortilla Soup

Ingredients
- 1 pound of shredded, cooked chicken
- 1 (15 ounce) can of whole peeled tomatoes, mashed
- 1 (10 ounce) can of enchilada sauce
- 1 medium sized onion, chopped
- 1 (4 ounce) can of chopped green chili peppers
- 2 cloves of garlic, minced
- 2 cups of water
- 1 (14.5 ounce) can of chicken broth
- 1 teaspoon of cumin
- 1 teaspoon of chili powder
- 1 teaspoon of salt
- ¼ teaspoon of black pepper
- 1 bay leaf
- 1 (10 ounce) package of frozen corn
- 1 tablespoon of chopped cilantro
- 7 corn tortillas
- vegetable oil

Instructions
Place chicken, tomatoes, enchilada sauce, onion, green chili, and garlic into a slow cooker. Pour in water and bird broth, and season with cumin, chili powder, salt, pepper, and bay leaf. Stir in corn and cilantro. Cover and prepare dinner on Low placing for 6 to eight hours or on High setting for three to 4 hours.

Preheat oven to 400 ranges F (200 tiers C). Lightly brush each facet of tortillas with oil. Cut tortillas into strips, then unfold on a baking sheet. Bake in the preheated oven until crisp, about 10 to 15 minutes. To serve, sprinkle tortilla strips over soup.

Nutrition
262 calories; 10.8 g total fat; 45 mg cholesterol; 893 mg sodium. 24.7 g carbohydrates; 18 g protein;

Quick And Easy Chicken Noodle Soup

Ingredients
- 1 tablespoon butter
- ½ cup chopped onion
- ½ cup chopped celery
- 4 (14.5 ounce) cans chicken broth
- 1 (14.5 ounce) can vegetable broth
- ½ pound chopped cooked chicken breast
- 1 ½ cups egg noodles
- 1 cup sliced carrots
- ½ teaspoon dried basil
- ½ teaspoon dried oregano
- salt and pepper to taste

In a big pot over medium heat, melt butter. Cook onion and celery in butter till naturally tender, 5 mins. Pour in hen and vegetable broths and stir in hen, noodles, carrots, basil, oregano, salt, and pepper. Bring to a boil, then lessen warmness and simmer 20 minutes before serving.

Nutrition
161 calories; 6.1 g total fat; 46 mg cholesterol; 1357 mg sodium. 12.1 g carbohydrates; 13.4 g protein;

Delicious Ham And Potato Soup

Ingredients
- 3 1/2 cups of peeled and diced potatoes
- 1/3 cup of diced celery
- 1/3 cup of finely chopped onion
- 3/4 cup of diced cooked ham
- 3 1/4 cups of water
- 2 tablespoons of chicken bouillon granules
- 1/2 teaspoon of salt, or to taste
- 1 teaspoon of ground white or black pepper
- 5 tablespoons of butter
- 5 tablespoons of all-purpose flour
- 2 cups of milk

Combine the potatoes, celery, onion, ham, and water in a stockpot. Bring to a boil, then prepare dinner over medium heat until potatoes are tender, about 10 to fifteen minutes. Stir in the hen bouillon, salt, and pepper.

In a separate saucepan, soften butter over medium-low heat. Whisk in flour with a fork, and cook dinner, continually stirring till thick, approximately 1 minute. Slowly stir in milk as not to permit lumps to form until all of the liquid has been added. Continue

stirring over medium-low heat until thick, 4 to five minutes.
Stir the milk combination into the stockpot, and cook dinner soup till heated through. Serve immediately.
Per Serving: 195 calories; 10.5 g fat; 19.5 g carbohydrates; 6.1 g protein; 30 mg cholesterol; 394 mg sodium.

Butternut Squash Soup
Ingredients
- 6 tablespoons chopped onion
- 4 tablespoons margarine
- 6 cups peeled and cubed butternut squash
- 3 cups water
- 4 cubes chicken bouillon
- 1/2 teaspoon dried marjoram
- 1/4 teaspoon ground black pepper
- 1/8 teaspoon ground cayenne pepper

2 (8 ounce) packages cream cheese
In a large saucepan, saute onions in margarine until tender. Add squash, water, bouillon, marjoram, black pepper, and cayenne pepper. Bring to boil; cook 20 minutes, or till squash is tender.
Puree squash and cream cheese in a blender or meals processor in batches till smooth. Return to saucepan and heat through. Do now not allow to boil.
397 calories; 33.4 g of fat; 20.2 g of carbohydrates; 7.7 g of protein; 83 mg cholesterol; 1081 mg sodium.

Geneva's Ultimate Hungarian Mushroom Soup
Ingredients
- 2 tablespoons of unsalted butter
- 2 cups of chopped onions
- 1 1/2 pounds of fresh mushrooms
- 4 1/2 teaspoons of chopped fresh dill
- 1 tablespoon of Hungarian sweet paprika
- 1 tablespoon of soy sauce
- 2 cups of low-sodium chicken broth
- 1 cup of skim milk
- 3 tablespoons of all-purpose flour
- 1/2 ripe tomatoes
- 1/2 Hungarian wax pepper
- 1 teaspoon of salt
- ground black pepper to your taste
- 1/2 cup of light sour cream

Melt the butter in a massive pot over medium heat. Cook and stir the onions in the butter until fragrant, about 5 mins. Add the mushrooms and retain cooking until the mushrooms are tender, about 5 mins more. Stir the dill, paprika, soy sauce, and fowl broth into the mushroom mixture; reduce warmness to low, cover, and simmer 15 mins.
Whisk the milk and flour together in a small bowl. Stir the mixture into the soup. Add the tomato and Hungarian wax pepper. Return cover to the pot and simmer any other 15 minutes, occasionally stirring — season with salt and pepper. Mix the buttercream into the soup and maintain cooking and stirring till the soup has thickened, five to 10 mins more. Remove the Hungarian wax pepper and tomato and discard before serving the soup.
144 calories; 7 g fat; 16.2 g of carbohydrates; 7 g of protein; 19 mg cholesterol; 573 mg sodium.

Super-Delicious Zuppa Toscana
Ingredients
- 1 pound of bulk mild Italian sausage
- 1 1/4 teaspoons of crushed red pepper flakes
- 4 slices of bacon, cut pieces
- 1 large sized onion, diced
- 1 tablespoon of minced garlic
- 5 (13.75 ounce) cans of chicken broth
- 6 medium sized potatoes, sliced
- 1 cup of heavy cream
- 1/4 bunch fresh spinach

Cook the Italian sausage and red pepper flakes in a Dutch oven over medium-excessive heat till crumbly, browned, and now not pink, 10 to 15 mins. Drain and set aside.
Cook the bacon in the same Dutch oven over medium heat until crisp, approximately 10 minutes. Drain, leaving a few tablespoons of drippings with the bacon inside the backside of the Dutch oven. Stir in the onions and garlic; cook until onions are gentle and translucent, about 5 minutes.
Pour the chook broth into the Dutch oven with the bacon and onion mixture; deliver to a boil over excessive warmness. Add the potatoes and boil till fork-tender, about 20 minutes. Reduce the warmth to medium and stir in the heavy cream and the cooked sausage; warmth through. Mix the spinach into the soup just earlier than serving.
554 calories; 32.6 g of fat; 45.8 g carbohydrates; 19.8 g of protein; 99 mg cholesterol; 2386 mg of sodium.

California Italian Soup
Ingredients
- 1/2 pound of extra-lean ground beef
- 1 egg, beaten
- 2 tablespoons of Italian-seasoned breadcrumbs
- 1 tablespoon of grated Parmesan cheese
- 2 tablespoons of shredded fresh basil leaves
- 1 tablespoon of chopped Italian flat leaf parsley
- 2 green onions, finely sliced
- 5 3/4 cups of chicken broth
- 2 cups of finely sliced escarole
- 1 lemon, zested
- 1/2 cup of orzo (rice-shaped pasta), uncooked
- grated Parmesan cheese for topping purpose

Mix the meat, egg, bread crumbs, cheese, basil, parsley, and green onions; form into 3/4 inch balls.

Pour broth into a large saucepan over high warmness. When boiling, drop in meatballs. Stir in escarole, lemon zest, and orzo. Return to a boil; lessen warmness to medium. Cook at a slow boil for 10 min, stirring frequently. Serve sprinkled with cheese.
159 calories; 5.6 g is fat; 15.4 g carbohydrates; 11.5 g is protein; 55 mg cholesterol; 99 mg sodium.

Soup Hamburger
Ingredients
- 1 1/2 pounds of ground beef
- 1 medium sized onion, finely chopped
- 3 (14.5 ounce) cans of beef consomme
- 1 (28 ounce) can of diced tomatoes
- 2 cups of water
- 1 (10.75 ounce) can of condensed tomato soup
- 4 carrots, finely chopped
- 3 stalks of celery, finely chopped
- 4 tablespoons of pearl barley
- 1/2 teaspoon of dried thyme
- 1 bay leaf

Turn on a multi-functional strain cooker (along with Instant Pot(R)) and pick Saute function. Cook and stir red meat and onion until browned, five to 10 minutes. Pour in beef consomme, tomatoes, water, and tomato soup. Add carrots, celery, barley, thyme, and bay leaf. Close and lock the lid. Select Soup function; set timer for 30 mins allow 10 to 15 minutes for stress to build. Release pressure the usage of the natural-release approach in keeping with manufacturer's instructions, about 10 mins.
251 calories; 11.2 g is fat; 17.8 g carbohydrates; 18.7 g id protein; 52 mg cholesterol; 950 mg sodium.

Broccoli Cheese Soup
Ingredients
- ½ cup of butter
- 1 onion, finely chopped
- 1 (16 ounce) package of frozen chopped broccoli
- 4 (14.5 ounce) cans of chicken broth
- 1 (1 pound) loaf of processed cheese food, cubed
- 2 cups of milk
- 1 tablespoon of garlic powder
- ⅔ cup of cornstarch
- 1 cup of water

In a stockpot, soften butter over medium heat. Cook onion in butter till softened. Stir in broccoli, and cover with chook broth. Simmer till broccoli is tender, 10 to fifteen mins.
Reduce heat, and stir in cheese cubes until melted. Mix in milk and garlic powder.
In a small bowl, stir cornstarch into water until dissolved. Stir into soup; cook, frequently stirring, till thick.
Nutrition

265 calories; 18.2 g total fat; 56 mg cholesterol; 1136 mg sodium. 15.1 g carbohydrates; 10 g protein;

Beef Noodle Soup
Ingredients
- 1 pound cubed beef stew meat
- 1 cup chopped onion
- 1 cup chopped celery
- 1/4 cup beef bouillon granules
- 1/4 teaspoon dried parsley
- 1 pinch ground black pepper
- 1 cup chopped carrots
- 5 3/4 cups water
- 2 1/2 cups frozen egg noodles

In a large saucepan over medium high heat, saute the stew meat, onion and celery for 5 minutes, or until meat is browned on all sides.
Stir in the bouillon, parsley, ground black pepper, carrots, water and egg noodles. Bring to a boil, reduce heat to low and simmer for 30 minutes.
Per Serving: 377 calories; 19.4 g fat; 24.8 g carbohydrates; 25.5 g protein; 89 mg cholesterol; 1040 mg sodium.

Soup Lentil
Ingredients
- 1 onion, finely chopped
- 1/4 cup of olive oil
- 2 carrots, finely diced
- 2 stalks of celery, finely chopped
- 2 cloves of garlic, minced

1 teaspoon of dried oregano
- 1 bay of leaf
- 1 teaspoon of dried basil
- 1 (14.5 ounce) can of crushed tomatoes
- 2 cups of dry lentils
- 8 cups of water
- 1/2 cup of spinach, rinsed and thinly sliced
- 2 tablespoons of vinegar
- salt to your taste
- ground black pepper to your taste

In a huge soup pot, warm oil over medium warmth. Add onions, carrots, and celery; cook dinner and stir till onion is tender. Stir in garlic, bay leaf, oregano, and basil; cook dinner for two minutes.
Stir in lentils, and add water and tomatoes. Bring to a boil. Reduce warmness and simmer for as a minimum of 1 hour. When ready to serve stir in spinach, and prepare dinner till it wilts. Stir in vinegar, and season to taste with salt and pepper, and more vinegar if desired.
349 calories; 10 g is fat; 48.2 g carbohydrates; 18.3 g is protein; 0 mg cholesterol; 131 mg is sodium.

Absolutely Ultimate Potato Soup
- **Ingredients**
- 1 pound of bacon, chopped
- 2 stalks of celery, diced
- 1 onion, finely chopped

- 3 cloves of garlic, minced
- 8 potatoes, peeled

4 cups of chicken stock

- 3 tablespoons of butter
- 1/4 cup of all-purpose flour
- 1 cup of heavy cream
- 1 teaspoon of dried tarragon
- 3 teaspoons of chopped fresh cilantro
- salt and pepper to your taste

In a Dutch oven, cook the bacon over medium heat until done. Remove bacon from pan and set aside. Drain off all but 1/4 cup of the bacon grease.
Cook celery and onion in reserved bacon drippings until onion is translucent, about five minutes. Stir in garlic, and retain cooking for 1 to 2 minutes. Add cubed potatoes, and toss to coat. Saute for three to 4 minutes. Return bacon to the pan, and add enough chicken stock to cover the vegetables. Cover and simmer until potatoes are tender.
In a separate pan, melt butter over medium heat. Whisk in flour. Cook, constantly stirring, for 1 to two minutes. Whisk in the heavy cream, tarragon, and cilantro. Bring the cream aggregate to a boil, and prepare dinner, continually stirring, until thickened. Stir the cream mixture into the potato combination. Puree about 1/2 the soup and go back to the pan. Adjust seasonings to taste.
594 calories; 41.5 g is fat; 44 g carbohydrates; 12.6 g is protein; 91 mg cholesterol; 879 mg sodium.

Slow Cooker Taco Soup

- **Ingredients**
- 1 pound of ground beef

1 onion, finely chopped

- 1 (16 ounce) can of chili beans, with liquid
- 1 (15 ounce) can of kidney beans with liquid
- 1 (15 ounce) can of whole kernel corn, with liquid
- 1 (8 ounce) can of tomato sauce
- 2 cups of water
- 2 (14.5 ounce) cans of diced tomatoes
- 1 (4 ounce) can of diced green chile peppers
- 1 (1.25 ounce) package of taco seasoning mix

In a medium skillet, prepare dinner the floor beef till browned over medium heat. Drain, and set aside.
Place the floor beef, onion, chili beans, kidney beans, corn, tomato sauce, water, diced tomatoes, green chile peppers, and taco seasoning blend in a sluggish cooker. Mix to blend, and cook on Low placing for eight hours.
362 calories; 16.3 g is fat; 37.8 g carbohydrates; 18.2 g is protein; 48 mg cholesterol; 1356 mg is sodium.

Moroccan Lentil Soup

Ingredients

- 2 onions, chopped
- 2 cloves garlic, minced
- 1 teaspoon grated fresh ginger
- 6 cups water
- 1 cup red lentils
- 1 (15 ounce) can garbanzo beans, drained
- 1 (19 ounce) can cannellini beans
- 1 (14.5 ounce) can diced tomatoes
- 1/2 cup diced carrots
- 1/2 cup chopped celery
- 1 teaspoon garam masala
- 1 1/2 teaspoons ground cardamom
- 1/2 teaspoon ground cayenne pepper
- 1/2 teaspoon ground cumin
- 1 tablespoon olive oil

In a big pot, saute the onions, garlic, and ginger in a little olive oil for about 5 min.
Add the water, lentils, chickpeas, white kidney beans, diced tomatoes, carrots, celery, garam masala, cardamom, cayenne pepper, and cumin. Bring to a boil for a couple of minutes, then simmer for 1 to 1 1/2 hours or longer, till the lentils are soft.
Puree half of the soup in a meals processor or blender. Return the pureed soup to the pot, stir.
329 calories; 3.6 g fat; 56.5 g carbohydrates; 18.3 g protein; 0 mg cholesterol; 317 mg sodium.

Baked Potato Soup

Ingredients

- 12 slices bacon
- 2/3 cup margarine
- 2/3 cup all-purpose flour
- 7 cups milk
- 4 large baked potatoes, peeled and cubed
- 4 green onions, chopped
- 1 1/4 cups shredded Cheddar cheese
- 1 cup sour cream
- 1 teaspoon salt
- 1 teaspoon ground black pepper

Place bacon in a large, deep skillet. Cook over medium heat till browned. Drain, crumble and set aside.
In a inventory pot or Dutch oven, soften the margarine over medium heat. Whisk in flour till smooth. Gradually stir in milk, continually whisking till thickened. Stir in potatoes and onions. Bring to a boil, stirring frequently.
Reduce heat, and simmer 10 minutes. Mix in bacon, cheese, sour cream, salt, and pepper. Continue cooking, frequently stirring, till cheese is melted.
Per Serving: 748 calories; 49.3 g fat; 49.7 g carbohydrates; 27.2 g protein; 85 mg cholesterol; 1335 mg sodium.

Turkish Red Lentil 'Bride' Soup

Ingredients

- ¼ cup butter
- 2 onions, finely chopped
- 1 teaspoon paprika
- 1 cup red lentils
- ½ cup fine bulgur

- 2 tablespoons tomato paste
- 8 cups vegetable stock
- ⅛ teaspoon cayenne pepper
- 1 tablespoon dried mint leaves
- 4 slices lemon
- ½ teaspoon chopped fresh mint

Directions

Melt the butter in a large saucepan over low heat. Cook the onions within the warm butter till they may be golden brown, about 15 minutes.
Stir the paprika, lentils, and bulgur into the onions and coat with the butter.
Add the tomato paste, vegetable stock, and cayenne pepper; bring to a boil and cook until tender and creamy, approximately 1 hour.
Crumble the dried mint leaves into the soup; stir the soup and dispose of from heat.
Ladle into bowls and garnish with lemon slices and clean mint to serve.

Nutrition

442 calories; 14 g total fat; 31 mg cholesterol; 1080 mg sodium. 64.2 g carbohydrates; 18.7 g protein;

Chicken Tortilla Soup V

Ingredients

- 2 skinless, chicken breasts, divide into cubes
- ½ teaspoon of olive oil
- ½ teaspoon of minced garlic
- ¼ teaspoon of ground cumin
- 2 (14.5 ounce) cans of chicken broth
- 1 cup of frozen corn kernels
- 1 cup of chopped onion
- ½ teaspoon of chili powder
- 1 tablespoon of lemon juice
- 1 cup of chunky salsa
- 8 ounces of corn tortilla chips
- ½ cup of shredded Monterey Jack cheese

Instructions

In a large pot over medium heat, prepare dinner and stir chicken inside the oil for five minutes. Add the garlic and cumin and blend well. Then add the broth, corn, onion, chili powder, lemon juice, and salsa. Reduce heat to low and simmer for approximately 20 to 30 minutes. Break up some tortilla chips into individual bowls and pour soup over chips. Top with the Monterey Jack cheese and a bit bitter cream.

Nutrition Info

486 calories; 19.8 g total fat; 51 mg cholesterol; 1618 mg sodium. 55.2 g carbohydrates; 25.2 g protein;

Clam Chowder

Ingredients

- 3 (6.5 ounce) cans minced clams
- 1 cup minced onion
- 1 cup diced celery
- 2 cups cubed potatoes
- 1 cup diced carrots
- 3/4 cup butter
- 3/4 cup all-purpose flour
- 1 quart half-and-half cream
- 2 tablespoons red wine vinegar
- 1 1/2 teaspoons salt

ground black pepper to taste

Drain juice from clams into a large skillet over the onions, celery, potatoes, and carrots. Add water to cover and cook dinner over medium heat until tender. Meanwhile, in a large, heavy saucepan, soften the butter over medium heat. Whisk in flour until smooth. Whisk in cream and stir continuously till thick and creamy. Stir in greens and clam juice. Heat through, but do not boil.
Stir in clams just earlier than serving. If they prepare dinner, an excessive amount of they gets tough. When clams are heated through, stir in vinegar, and season with salt and pepper.
501 calories; 32.7 g is fat; 28.4 g carbohydrates; 23.9 g is protein; 137 mg cholesterol; 712 mg is sodium.

Classic Minestrone

Ingredients

- 3 tablespoons is olive oil
- 1 leek, sliced
- 2 carrots, finely chopped
- 1 zucchini, sliced
- 4 ounces of green beans, cut into 1 inch pieces
- 2 stalks of celery, thinly sliced
- 1 1/2 quarts of vegetable stock
- 1 pound of chopped tomatoes
- 1 tablespoon of chopped fresh thyme
- 1 (15 ounce) can of cannellini beans, with liquid
- 1/4 cup of elbow macaroni
- salt and ground black pepper to your taste

Heat olive oil in a big saucepan, over medium heat. Add leek, carrots, zucchini, inexperienced beans, and celery. Cover and decrease warmness to low. Cook for 15 minutes, shaking the pan occasionally.
Stir inside the stock, tomatoes, and thyme. Bring to a boil, then update the lid, and decrease warmth to low; simmer gently for 30 minutes.
Stir within the cannellini beans with liquid and pasta. Simmer for an extra 10 minutes, or till pasta is al dente — season with salt and pepper to taste earlier than serving.
Per Serving: 320 calories; 12 g fat; 44.5 g carbohydrates; 12 g protein; 0 mg cholesterol; 471 mg sodium.

Creamy Italian White Bean Soup

Ingredients

- 1 tablespoon of vegetable oil
- 1 onion, finely chopped
- 1 stalk of celery, finely chopped
- 1 clove of garlic, minced
- 2 (16 ounce) cans of white kidney beans, drained

- 1 (14 ounce) can of chicken broth
- 1/4 teaspoon of ground black pepper
- 1/8 teaspoon of dried thyme
- 2 cups of water
- 1 bunch of fresh spinach, rinsed and thinly sliced
- 1 tablespoon of lemon juice

In a big saucepan, warm oil. Cook onion and celery in oil for 5 to eight minutes, or until tender. Add garlic, and prepare dinner for 30 seconds, always stirring. Stir in beans, hen broth, pepper, thyme, and a pair of cups water. Bring to a boil, reduce warmth, and then simmer for 15 minutes.

With a slotted spoon, do away with 2 cups of the bean and vegetable mixture from soup and set aside. In blender at low speed, blend the remaining soup in small batches till smooth (it facilitates to get rid of the centerpiece of the blender lid to allow steam to escape.) Once blended, pour soup again into inventory pot and stir in reserved beans.

Bring to a boil, sometimes stirring. Stir in spinach and cook dinner 1 minute or until spinach is wilted. Stir in lemon juice and remove from warmth and serve with fresh grated Parmesan cheese on top.

Nutrition Facts
245 calories; 4.9 g is fat; 38.1 g carbohydrates; 12 g is protein; 2 mg cholesterol; 1014 mg is sodium

Spicy Chicken Soup

Ingredients
- 2 quarts of water
- 8 skinless, chicken breast halves
- ½ teaspoon of salt
- 1 teaspoon of ground black pepper
- 1 teaspoon of garlic powder
- 2 tablespoons of dried parsley
- 1 tablespoon of onion powder
- 5 cubes of chicken bouillon
- 3 tablespoons of olive oil
- 1 onion, finely chopped
- 3 cloves of garlic, chopped
- 1 (16 ounce) jar of chunky salsa
- 2 (14.5 ounce) cans of peeled and diced tomatoes
- 1 (14.5 ounce) can of whole peeled tomatoes
- 1 (10.75 ounce) can of condensed tomato soup
- 3 tablespoons of chili powder
- 1 (15 ounce) can of whole kernel corn, drained
- 2 (16 ounce) cans of chili beans, undrained
- 1 (8 ounce) container of sour cream

In a massive pot over medium heat, integrate water, chicken, salt, pepper, garlic powder, parsley, onion powder, and bouillon cubes. Bring to a boil, then reduce warmth and simmer 1 hour, or until bird juices run clear. Remove chicken, reserve broth. Shred chicken.

In a large pot over medium warmness, prepare dinner onion and garlic in olive oil until slightly browned. Stir in salsa, diced tomatoes, whole tomatoes, tomato soup, chili powder, corn, chili beans, sour cream, shredded bird and five cups broth. Simmer 30 min.

473 calories; 15.3 g is total fat; 82 mg cholesterol; 2436 mg is sodium. 50.3 g carbohydrates; 39.6 g is protein;

Split Pea And Ham Soup I

Ingredients
- 1 cup chopped onion
- 1 teaspoon vegetable oil
- 1 pound dried split peas
- 1 pound ham bone
- 1 pinch salt and pepper to taste

In a medium pot, saute onions in oil. Add the split peas, ham bone, and enough water to cowl ingredients; season with salt and pepper. Cover and cook till there are no peas left, only a inexperienced liquid, 2 hours. While it's miles cooking, take a look at to look if water has evaporated. You may need to add higher water because the soup keeps cooking.

Once the soup is a green liquid remove from heat, and permit stand, so it's going to thicken. Once thickened, you may need to heat thru to serve.

413 calories; 2.5 g is fat; 72.2 g carbohydrates; 23.3 g is protein; 0 mg cholesterol; 19 mg sodium.

Spinach And Leek White Bean Soup

Ingredients
- 2 teaspoons of olive oil
- 4 leeks, chopped
- 2 cloves of garlic, chopped
- 2 (16 ounce) cans of fat-free chicken broth
- 2 (16 ounce) cans of cannellini beans, rinsed and drained
- 2 bay leaves
- 2 teaspoons of ground cumin
- 1/2 cup of whole wheat couscous
- 2 cups of packed fresh spinach
- salt and pepper to your taste

Heat olive oil in a big saucepan or soup pot at medium temperature. Add the leeks and garlic; saute till tender, about five minutes. Stir within the bird broth, cannellini beans, bay leaves, and cumin. Bring to a boil, then reduce the warmth to low, and stir within the couscous. Cover and simmer for 5 mins. Stir in spinach and season with salt and pepper Serve immediately.

179 calories; 2 g fat; 30.6 g carbohydrates; 9.4 g protein; 0 mg cholesterol; 432 mg sodium.

Spicy Black Bean Vegetable Soup

Ingredients
- 1 tablespoon of vegetable oil
- 1 onion, finely chopped

- 1 clove of garlic, minced
- 2 carrots, finely chopped
- 2 teaspoons of chili powder
- 1 teaspoon of ground cumin
- 4 cups of vegetable stock
- 2 (15 ounce) cans of black beans, rinsed and drained
- 1 (8.75 ounce) can of whole kernel corn
- 1/4 teaspoon of ground black pepper
- 1 (14.5 ounce) can of stewed tomatoes

In a large saucepan, warm oil over medium warmness; cook onion, garlic, and carrots, occasionally stirring, for five mins or until onion is softened. Add chili powder and cumin; prepare dinner, stirring, for 1 min. Add stock; one can of the beans, corn, and pepper; carry to boil.
Meanwhile, in meals processor or blender, puree collectively tomatoes and last can of beans; add to the pot. Reduce warmness, cover, and simmer for 10 to 15 min or till carrots are tender.
164 calories; 3.4 g is fat; 26.9 g carbohydrates; 7.6 g is protein; 0 mg cholesterol; 683 mg is sodium.

Pumpkin Black Bean Soup

Ingredients
- 3 (15 ounce) cans of black beans, rinsed and drained
- 1 (16 ounce) can of diced tomatoes
- 1/4 cup of butter
- 1 1/4 cups of chopped onion
- 4 cloves of garlic, chopped
- 1 teaspoon of salt
- 1/2 teaspoon of ground black pepper
- 4 cups of beef broth
- 1 (15 ounce) can of pumpkin puree
- 1/2 pound of cubed cooked ham
- 3 tablespoons of sherry vinegar

Pour two cans of the black beans into a meals processor or blender, together with the can of tomatoes. Puree till smooth. Set aside.
Melt butter in a soup pot over medium heat. Add the onion and garlic, and season with salt and pepper. Cook and stir until the onion is softened. Stir in the bean puree, the closing can of beans, beef broth, pumpkin puree, and sherry vinegar. Mix till properly blended, then simmer for approximately 25 min, or until thick enough to coat the lower back of a metal spoon. Stir within the ham, and warmth through before serving.
151 calories; 10.2 g fat; 7.4 g carbohydrates; 7.4 g protein; 28 mg cholesterol; 1052 mg sodium.

Spicy Slow Cooker Black Bean Soup

Ingredients
- 1 pound dry black beans, soaked overnight
- 4 teaspoons diced jalapeno peppers
- 6 cups chicken broth
- 1/2 teaspoon garlic powder
- 1 tablespoon chili powder
- 1 teaspoon ground cumin
- 1 teaspoon cayenne pepper
- 3/4 teaspoon ground black pepper
- 1/2 teaspoon hot pepper sauce
- Drainthe black beans and rinse.

Combine beans, jalapenos, and hen broth in a gradual cooker — season with garlic powder, chili powder, cumin, cayenne, pepper, and warm pepper sauce. Cook on High flame for four hours. Reduce warmth to Low, and maintain cooking for two hours, or till you are equipped to eat.
281 calories; 2 g is fat; 49.7 g carbohydrates; 17.7 g is protein; 5 mg cholesterol; 1012 mg is sodium.

Black Bean And Salsa Soup

Ingredients
- 2 (15 ounce) cans black beans, drained and rinsed
- 1 1/2 cups vegetable broth
- 1 cup chunky salsa
- 1 teaspoon ground cumin
- 4 tablespoons sour cream
- 2 tablespoons thinly sliced green onion

In an electric food processor or blender, combine beans, broth, salsa, and cumin. Blend until pretty smooth.
Heat the bean mixture in a saucepan over medium heat till thoroughly heated.
Ladle soup into four character bowls, and pinnacle each dish with one tablespoon of the sour cream and 1/2 tablespoon green onion.
240 calories; 5 g is fat; 34.5 g carbohydrates; 13.3 g is protein; 6 mg cholesterol; 1216 mg is sodium.

Split Pea Soup With Rosemary

Ingredients
- 6 slices bacon, cut into 1 inch pieces
- 1 small onion, chopped
- 1 leek, thinly sliced
- 1 large carrot, chopped
- 2 cloves garlic, minced
- 4 (10.5 ounce) cans chicken broth
- 1 1/2 cups green split peas
- 2 bay leaves
- 1 teaspoon chopped fresh rosemary

Place bacon in a large pot, and cook over medium heat until crisp. Stir in onion, leek, carrot, and garlic; cook until the vegetables are soft, about 8 minutes. Pour in chicken broth. Stir in split peas, bay leaves, and rosemary. Bring to a boil. Reduce heat to low; cover, and simmer until peas are cooked, about 1 hour, stirring occasionally.
Per Serving: 253 calories; 5 g fat; 35.5 g carbohydrates; 17 g protein; 15 mg cholesterol; 1195 mg sodium.

Split Pea Soup

Ingredients
- 2 1/4 cups dried split peas

- 2 quarts cold water
- 1 1/2 pounds ham bone
- 2 onions, thinly sliced
- 1/2 teaspoon salt
- 1/4 teaspoon ground black pepper
- 1 pinch dried marjoram
- 3 stalks celery, chopped
- 3 carrots, chopped
- 1 potato, diced

In a massive inventory pot, cowl peas with 2 quarts bloodless water and soak overnight. If you want a faster method, simmer the peas gently for two min, after which soak for l hour.

Once peas are soaked, add ham bone, onion, salt, pepper and marjoram. Cover, deliver to boil after which simmer for one-half of hours, stirring occasionally.

Remove bone; reduce off meat, dice and go back meat to soup. Add celery, carrots, and potatoes. Cook slowly, exposed for 30 to forty min, or till greens are tender.

310 calories; 1 g is fat; 57.9 g carbohydrates; 19.7 g is protein; 0 mg cholesterol; 255 mg is sodium.

Bean Soup

Ingredients

- 1 (16 ounce) package dried navy beans
- 7 cups water
- 1 ham bone
- 2 cups diced ham
- 1/4 cup minced onion
- 1/2 teaspoon salt
- 1 pinch ground black pepper
- 1 bay leaf
- 1/2 cup sliced carrots
- 1/2 cup sliced celery

Place rinsed beans into a big stockpot. Add water and bring to a boil. Boil gently for two minutes; dispose of from heat, cowl, and allow stand for 1 hour.

Add ham bone, cubed ham, onion, salt, pepper, and bay leaves. Bring to a boil; reduce heat, cover, and simmer for 1 hour and 15 mins or until beans are soft. Occasionally skim the floor of soup while it s miles cooking.

Add carrots and celery, cook until tender. Remove ham bone; scrape any meat from the bone, and location returned into the soup and serve.

246 calories; 3.8 g is fat; 36.7 g carbohydrates; 17.4 g is protein; 17 mg cholesterol; 543 mg is sodium.

Sweet Potato, Carrot, Apple, And Red Lentil Soup

Ingredients

- 1/4 cup butter
- 2 large sweet potatoes, peeled and chopped
- 3 large carrots, peeled and chopped
- 1 apple, peeled, cored and chopped
- 1 onion, chopped
- 1/2 cup red lentils
- 1/2 teaspoon minced fresh ginger
- 1/2 teaspoon ground black pepper
- 1 teaspoon salt
- 1/2 teaspoon ground cumin
- 1/2 teaspoon chili powder
- 1/2 teaspoon paprika
- 4 cups vegetable broth
- plain yogurt

Melt the butter in a large, heavy-bottomed pot over medium-excessive heat. Place the chopped sweet potatoes, carrots, apple, and onion inside the container. Stir and prepare dinner the apples and vegetables till the onions are translucent about 10 min.

Stir the lentils, ginger, floor black pepper, salt, cumin, chili powder, paprika, and vegetable broth into the pot with the apple and vegetable mixture. Bring the soup to a boil over high heat, then lessen the heat to medium-low, cover, and simmer till the lentils and greens are soft, approximately 30 min.

Working in batches, pour the soup into a blender, filling the pitcher no extra than halfway full. Hold down the lid of the blender with a folded kitchen towel, and thoroughly begin the mixer, the usage of a few quick pulses to get the soup moving before leaving it directly to puree. Puree in batches till smooth and pour right into a clean pot. Alternately, you could use a stick blender and puree the soup proper within the cooking pot.

Return the pureed soup to the cooking pot. Bring lower back to a simmer over medium-high heat, about 10 minutes. Add water as needed to skinny the soup to your chosen consistency. Serve with yogurt for garnish.

322 calories; 9 g is fat; 52.9 g carbohydrates; 9 g is protein; 22 mg cholesterol; 876 mg is sodium.

SALADS

Ambrosia With Coconut And Almonds
Ingredients
- 1/2 cup of slivered almonds
- 1/2 cup of unsweetened shredded coconut
- 1 small sized pineapple, cubed
- 5 oranges, in pieces
- 2 red apples, diced
- 1 banana, halved
- 2 tablespoons of cream sherry
- Fresh mint leaves for garnishing

Instructions
Heat the oven to 325 F. Spread the almonds on a baking sheet and bake, occasionally stirring, until golden and fragrant, about 10 minutes. A transfer without delay to a plate to cool. Add the coconut to the sheet and bake, often stirring, until gently browned, about 10 minutes — a transfer without delay to a plate to cool.
In a large bowl, integrate the pineapple, oranges, apples, banana, and sherry. Toss gently to combine well. Divide the fruit combination evenly among individual bowls. Sprinkle lightly with the toasted almonds and coconut and garnish with the mint. Serve right away.

Nutrition
Calories177 Total fat5 g Saturated fat1 g Cholesterol0 mg Sodium2 mg Total carbohydrate30 g Dietary fiber6 g Total sugars21 g Protein3 g

Quick Bean And Tuna Salad
Ingredients
- 1/2 whole-grain baguette, divide into pieces
- 2 tablespoons of olive oil
- 1 can (16 ounces) of cannellini beans, rinsed
- 2 small dill pickles, cut into pieces
- 1 small sized red onion, sliced
- 2 tablespoons of red wine vinegar
- 1/4 teaspoon of pepper
- 1 can (7 ounces) of water-packed tuna, rinsed
- 2 tablespoons of finely chopped fresh parsley

Instructions
Heat broiler. Place the baguette pieces on a massive cookie sheet and brush with one tablespoon of the oil. Place under broiler for about 1 to 2 min, till golden. Turn the bread pieces and broil for a further 1 or 2 min.
In a massive bowl, combine the final oil, beans, pickles, onion, vinegar, and pepper. Fold in the broiled baguette portions. Divide the combination among four bowls and top with the tuna and parsley.
Nutrition info
Total carbohydrate23 g Dietary fiber6 g Sodium171 mg Saturated fat1.5 g Total fat10 g Cholesterol21 mg Protein19 gCalories316 Total sugars6 g

Couscous Salad
Ingredients
- 1 cup of whole-wheat couscous
- 1 cup of zucchini, cut into 1/4-inch pieces
- 1 medium sized red bell pepper, cut into 1/4-inch pieces
- 1/2 cup of finely chopped red onion
- 3/4 teaspoon of ground cumin
- 1/2 teaspoon of ground black pepper
- 2 tablespoons of extra virgin olive oil
- 1 tablespoon of lemon juice
- Chopped parsley, basil or oregano for garnishing

Instructions
Cook couscous in step with preparation instructions on the package.
When couscous is cooked, fluff with a fork. Mix in zucchini, bell pepper, onion, cumin, and black pepper. Set aside.
In a small bowl, whisk together the olive oil and lemon juice. Pour over the couscous aggregate and toss to combine. Cover and refrigerate it. Serve chilled. Garnish with sparkling herbs.

Nutrition
Total carbohydrate21 g Dietary fiber4 g Sodium3 mg Saturated fat0.5 g Total fat4 g Protein4 gCalories136 Total sugars2 g

Steak Salad With Roasted Corn Vinaigrette
Ingredients
- 3 cups of fresh corn kernels
- 1/2 cup of water
- 2 tablespoons of fresh lime juice
- 2 tablespoons of chopped red bell pepper
- 2 tablespoons of extra-virgin olive oil
- 1/2 teaspoon of salt
- 1/2 teaspoon of freshly ground black pepper
- 1/4 cup of chopped fresh cilantro
- 1 tablespoon of ground cumin
- 2 teaspoons of dried oregano
- 1/4 teaspoon of red pepper flakes
- 3/4 pound of (12 ounces) flank steak
- 1 large head romaine lettuce,
- 4 cups of cherry tomatoes, halved
- 3/4 cup of thinly sliced red onion
- 1 1/2 cups of cooked black beans

Instructions
Place a dry, massive cast-iron or heavy nonstick frying pan over medium-excessive warmth. Add the corn and cook, often stirring, till the corn starts offevolved to brown, 4 to 5 mins. Remove from the heat and set aside.

In a meals processor, combine the water, lime juice, bell pepper, and 1 cup of the roasted corn. Pulse to puree adds the olive oil, 1/4 teaspoon of the salt, 1/four teaspoon of the black pepper, and the cilantro. Pulse to blend. Set the vinaigrette aside.

Prepare a hot fireplace in a charcoal grill or warmth a gas grill or broiler (restaurant). Away from the warmth source, gently coat the grill rack or broiler pan with cooking spray. Position the cooking rack four to 6 inches from the heat source.

In a small bowl, mix the cumin, oregano, pink pepper flakes, and the closing 1/4 teaspoon salt and 1/4 teaspoon black pepper collectively. Rub on each facet of the steak. Place the steak on the grill rack or broiler pan and grill or broil, turning once, till browned, four to 5 minutes on each side. Cut into the center to test for doneness (medium doneness is a hundred and sixty F if the usage of a meat thermometer). Let stand for 5 minutes. Cut throughout the grain into thin slices. Cut the slices into pieces 2 inches long.

In a considerable bowl, combine the lettuce, tomatoes, onion, black beans, and final roasted corn. Add the vinaigrette and toss gently to mix nicely and coat evenly.

To serve, divide the salad among person plates — top every serving with slices of grilled steak.

Nutrition
Total carbohydrate37 g Dietary fiber9 g Sodium249 mg Saturated fat2 g Total fat9 g Cholesterol36 mg Protein21 gCalories295 Total sugars7 g

Greek Salad
Ingredients
For the vinaigrette:
- 1 tablespoon of red wine vinegar
- 1 tablespoon of fresh lemon juice
- 2 teaspoons of chopped fresh oregano
- 1/4 teaspoon of salt
- 1/4 teaspoon of freshly ground black pepper
- 2 1/2 tablespoons of extra-virgin olive oil

For the salad:
- 1 large eggplant
- 1 pound of spinach, pieces
- 1 English (hothouse) cucumber, diced
- 1 tomato, diced
- 1/2 red onion, finely diced
- 2 tablespoons of pitted, chopped black Greek olives
- 2 tablespoons of crumbled feta cheese

Instructions
Position a rack within the lower 0.33 of the oven and warmth to 450 F. Lightly coat a baking sheet with olive oil cooking spray.

To make the French dressing, whisk together the vinegar, lemon juice, oregano, salt, and pepper in a small bowl. While whisking, slowly add the olive oil in a thin stream until emulsified. Set apart.

Spread the eggplant cubes in a single layer on the organized baking sheet. Spray the eggplant with olive oil cooking spray. Roast for 10 mins turn the cubes and roast until softened and lightly golden, 8 to 10 min longer. Set aside and allow cooling completely.

In a massive bowl, integrate the spinach, cucumber, tomato, onion, and cooled eggplant. Pour the vinaigrette over the salad and toss gently to mix nicely and coat evenly. Divide the mixture among serving plates. Sprinkle with the olives and feta.

Nutrition
Total carbohydrate10 g Dietary fiber4 g Sodium158 mg Saturated fat1 g Total fat5 g Cholesterol2 mg Protein3 gCalories97 Total sugars4 g

Warm Coleslaw With Honey Dressing
Ingredients
- 6 teaspoons of olive oil
- 1 medium sized yellow onion, finely chopped (about 1/2 cup)
- 1 teaspoon of dry mustard
- 1 large sized carrot, peeled
- 1/2 head napa cabbage, sliced
- 3 tablespoons of cider vinegar
- 1 tablespoon of dark honey
- 1/4 teaspoon of salt
- 1/4 teaspoon of freshly ground black pepper
- 1/2 teaspoon of caraway seed
- 1 tablespoon of chopped fresh flat-leaf (Italian) parsley

Instructions
In a massive nonstick saute pan, warm 2 teaspoons of the olive oil over medium-excessive warmth until hot but now not smoking. Add the onion and mustard and saute until the onion is soft and lightly golden about 6 mins. Transfer to a huge bowl.

Reduce the heat to medium and add two greater teaspoons of the olive oil to the pan. Add the carrot and toss and continuously stir until the carrot is tender-crisp, approximately 3 mins. Transfer to the bowl with the onion.

Add the last two teaspoons oil to the pan over medium warmth. Add the cabbage and toss and continuously stir until the cabbage begins to wilt about three minutes. Quickly switch the cabbage to the bowl with the other vegetables.

Quickly add the vinegar and honey to the pan over medium warmness, stirring till combined and bubbly, and the baby is dissolved. Pour over the slaw. Add the salt and pepper and toss well.

Nutrition
Calories74 Total fat5 g Saturated fat1 g Cholesterol0 mg Sodium117 mg Total carbohydrate8 g Dietary fiber2 g Total sugars5 g Protein1 g

Yellow Pear And Cherry Tomato Salad
Ingredients
For vinaigrette

- 2 tablespoons of sherry vinegar or red wine vinegar
- 1 tablespoon of minced shallot
- 1 tablespoon of extra-virgin olive oil
- 1/4 teaspoon of salt
- 1/8 teaspoon of freshly ground black pepper
- 1 1/2 cups of yellow pear tomatoes, halved
- 1 1/2 cups of orange cherry tomatoes, halved
- 1 1/2 cups of red cherry tomatoes, halved
- 4 large fresh basil leaves

To make the vinaigrette, in a small bowl, combine the vinegar and shallot and allow stand for 15 min. Add the olive oil, salt, and pepper and whisk till adequately blended. In a big serving or salad bowl, toss together all the tomatoes. Pour the French dressing over the vegetables, add the basil shreds and toss gently to mix correctly and coat evenly.

Nutrition
Total fat3 gCalories47 Protein1 g Cholesterol0 mg Total carbohydrate4 g Dietary fiber1 g Sodium125 mg Added sugars0 g

Chunky Spicy Egg Salad

Ingredients
- 8 large sized eggs
- 2 stalks of celery, trimmed and thinly sliced
- 1 red bell pepper, finely diced
- 1 jalapeño pepper, chopped
- 1 baby sized white onion, finely chopped
- Salt and pepper
- 1/2 cup of mayonnaise
- Juice of 1 lime
- 1/2 to 1 tsp of chili powder, to taste
- Tabasco, to your taste
- Cilantro Chopped

Instructions
1. Put the eggs in a big pot of bloodless salted water and bring to a boil. Boil 2 min, turn off the heat and allow the eggs to come to room temperature. Peel the cooled eggs, reduce them into chunks, and toss them right into a bowl. Add the celery, crimson pepper, jalapeño, and onion; season with salt and pepper.
2. Whisk the mayonnaise, lime juice, and chili powder collectively. Add Tabasco and salt and pepper. Taste and add extra chili powder or Tabasco, if you'd like more heat. Gently mix the mayo into the egg salad. If you've got time, chill before serving.
3. Sprinkle with cilantro and serve over veggies and tomatoes, or make sandwiches, using buttermilk biscuits.

Pasta Salad With Mixed Vegetables

Ingredients
- 12 ounces whole-wheat rotini (spiral-shaped) pasta
- 1 tablespoon olive oil
- 1/4 cup low-sodium chicken broth
- 1 garlic clove, chopped
- 2 medium onions, chopped
- 1 can (28 ounces) unsalted diced tomatoes in juice
- 1 pound mushrooms, sliced
- 1 red bell pepper, sliced
- 1 green bell pepper, sliced
- 2 medium zucchini, shredded
- 1/2 teaspoon basil
- 1/2 teaspoon oregano
- 8 romaine lettuce leaves

Cook pasta according to the package directions. Drain the pasta thoroughly. Place pasta in a large serving bowl. Add the olive oil and toss. Set aside.
In a large skillet, heat the chicken broth over medium heat. Add the garlic, onions and tomatoes. Saute until the onions are transparent, about 5 minutes. Add the remaining vegetables and saute until tender-crisp, about 5 minutes. Stir in the basil and oregano.
Add the vegetable mixture to the pasta. Toss to mix evenly. Cover and refrigerate until well chilled, about 1 hour.
Place lettuce leaves on individual plates. Top with the pasta salad and serve immediately.

Chicken Broccoli Salad

Ingredients
- 8 cups broccoli florets
- 3 cooked skinless, boneless chicken breast halves, cubed
- 1 cup chopped walnuts
- 6 green onions, chopped
- 1 cup mayonnaise
- ¼ cup apple cider vinegar
- ¼ cup white sugar
- ¼ cup crumbled cooked bacon

Directions
Combine broccoli, chicken, walnuts, and green onions in a large bowl.
Whisk mayonnaise, vinegar, and sugar together in a bowl until well blended.
Pour mayonnaise dressing over broccoli mixture; toss to coat.
Cover and refrigerate until chilled, if desired.
Sprinkle with crumbled bacon to serve.
341 calories; 28.7 g total fat; 28 mg cholesterol; 266 mg sodium. 12.8 g carbohydrates; 11 g protein;

Blue Cheese Broccoli Salad

Ingredients
- 2 heads of fresh broccoli, with stalks
- 2 tomatoes, seeded and coarsely chopped
- 1 cup of blue cheese dressing
- salt to your taste
- ground white pepper to your taste

Instructions
Cut the florets from the broccoli. With a vegetable peeler, peel the stalks and slice half-inch thick. Bring a big pot of water to a boil. Immerse the broccoli

florets and stalks inside the boiling water for 1 to 2 min, still brilliant green. Drain and cool.
In a bowl, mix the broccoli, tomatoes, and blue cheese dressing — season with salt and white pepper.
282 calories; 24.5 g total fat; 14 mg cholesterol; 430 mg sodium. 11.2 g carbohydrates; 3.9 g protein;

Curry Broccoli Salad

Ingredients
- ½ pound bacon
- 6 cups fresh broccoli florets
- ½ cup diced onion
- ½ cup dried cherries
- ½ cup sunflower seeds
- ¾ cup mayonnaise
- 1 teaspoon curry powder
- 2 tablespoons cider vinegar
- ¼ cup white sugar

Directions
Place bacon in a large, deep skillet. Cook over medium high heat until evenly brown. Drain, crumble and set aside.
In a large bowl, combine the bacon, broccoli, onion, dried fruit and sunflower seeds.
Whisk together the mayonnaise, curry powder, vinegar and sugar.
Pour dressing over salad; toss to coat, and marinate over night.
412 calories; 33.6 g total fat; 31 mg cholesterol; 431 mg sodium. 21.8 g carbohydrates; 6.8 g protein;

Broccoli Coleslaw

Ingredients
- 1 cup olive oil
- ⅓ cup distilled white vinegar
- ½ cup white sugar
- 1 (3 ounce) package chicken flavored ramen noodles, crushed, seasoning packet reserved
- 1 large head fresh broccoli, diced
- 2 carrots, grated
- 2 bunches green onions, chopped
- 1 cup sunflower seeds

Directions
In a small bowl, integrate oil, vinegar, sugar, and the seasoning packet from the ramen noodles. Mix well and refrigerate at the least one hour earlier than serving, or overnight.
In a massive bowl, integrate broccoli, carrots, green onions, and sunflower seeds. Crush ramen noodles and stir in. Pour dressing over salad approximately 10 min before serving.
413 calories; 31.3 g total fat; 0 mg cholesterol; 169 mg sodium. 31.8 g carbohydrates; 4.6 g protein;

Broccoli Buffet Salad

Ingredients
- 3 cups broccoli florets
- ½ cup chopped red onion
- ¼ cup sunflower seeds
- ½ cup chopped raisins
- ½ cup crumbled feta cheese
- ½ cup plain low-fat yogurt
- ¼ cup light mayonnaise
- 2 tablespoons white sugar
- 1 tablespoon lemon juice
- salt and pepper to taste

Directions
In a measuring cup, mix together yogurt, mayonnaise, sugar, and lemon juice.
In a salad bowl, stir broccoli, red onion, sunflower seeds, raisins, and crumbled feta cheese collectively. Toss with yogurt dressing and season with salt and pepper to taste. Cover and refrigerate for 2 hours.
119 calories; 5.2 g is total fat; 12 mg cholesterol; 267 mg is sodium. 20.1 g is carbohydrates; 4.6 g is protein;

Bodacious Broccoli Salad

Ingredients
- 8 slices bacon
- 2 heads fresh broccoli, chopped
- 1 ½ cups sharp Cheddar cheese, shredded
- ½ large red onion, chopped
- ¼ cup red wine vinegar
- ⅛ cup white sugar
- 2 teaspoons ground black pepper
- 1 teaspoon salt
- ⅔ cup mayonnaise
- 1 teaspoon fresh lemon juice

Directions
Place bacon in a big, deep skillet. Cook over medium excessive heat till flippantly brown. Drain and crumble.
In a big bowl, combine broccoli, cheese, bacon, and onion.
Prepare the dressing in a small bowl by whisking the purple wine vinegar, sugar, pepper, salt, mayonnaise, and lemon juice collectively. Combine dressing with salad. Cover, and refrigerate till equipped to serve.
273 calories; 24 g is total fat; 35 mg cholesterol; 543 mg is sodium. 7.3 g is carbohydrates; 8.1 g is protein;

Minnesota Broccoli Salad

Ingredients
- 3 eggs
- 1 pound broccoli, chopped
- ¼ cup finely chopped red onion
- 1 cup green olives, sliced
- 1 (4 ounce) jar diced pimentos, drained
- ¾ cup mayonnaise
- 1 teaspoon dry mustard powder
- ½ pinch salt, or to taste
- ½ teaspoon celery seed
- 1 tablespoon chopped fresh dill

Directions
Place the eggs into a saucepan in a single layer and fill with water to cover the eggs through 1 inch. Cover the pan and convey the water to a boil over high heat. Once the water is boiling, put off from the

warmth and allow the eggs to stand within the hot water for 15 min. Pour out the freshwater, then cool the eggs beneath cold running water within the sink. Peel and chop once raw.

Meanwhile, bring a large pot of lightly salted water to a boil. Add the broccoli and cook uncovered until bright green and just tender, about 2 minutes. Drain in a colander, then immediately immerse in ice water for several minutes until cold to stop the cooking process. Once the broccoli is cold, drain well and set aside.

Combine the red onion, hard-cooked eggs, green olives, pimentos, mayonnaise, mustard powder, salt, celery seed, and dill in a mixing bowl. Stir in the drained cooked broccoli. Refrigerate overnight for best flavor.

297 calories; 27.9 g total fat; 103 mg cholesterol; 793 mg sodium. 8.2 g carbohydrates; 6.3 g protein

Loaded Egg Salad

Ingredients
- 8 ounces bacon
- 4 stalks celery, minced
- 1/2 cup mayonnaise
- 1/4 cup minced yellow onion
- 1 1/2 tablespoons sweet pickle relish
- 1 1/2 tablespoons prepared yellow mustard
- 2 teaspoons chile-garlic sauce (such as Sriracha®)
- 1 1/2 teaspoons dried dill weed
- 1 teaspoon Worcestershire sauce
- 1 teaspoon ground black pepper
- 1/2 teaspoon paprika
- 1/4 teaspoon salt
- 12 hard boiled eggs, shells removed

Place the bacon in a large skillet and cook over medium-high heat, occasionally turning, until crispy, about 10 minutes. Drain the bacon slices on paper towels and crumble once cooled.

Mix bacon, celery, mayonnaise, onion, relish, mustard, chile-garlic sauce, dill, Worcestershire, black pepper, paprika, and salt in a large bowl; add eggs. Break egg whites and yolks with a potato masher into the bacon mixture. Stir broken egg pieces into the salad.

Cover the bowl with plastic wrap and refrigerate at least 60 min.

205 calories; 17.2 g is fat; 3.1 g carbohydrates; 9.8 g is protein; 209 mg cholesterol; 474 mg is sodium

Crunchy Egg Salad

Ingredients
- 4 eggs
- 1 (4 ounce) can sliced water chestnuts, drained and chopped
- 1/3 cup mayonnaise
- 1/3 cup sweet pickle relish
- 1 teaspoon dry mustard
- 1 teaspoon paprika
- salt and pepper to taste

Place the eggs right into a saucepan in a single layer and fill with water to cowl the eggs by using 1 inch. Cover the pan and bring the water to a boil over high heat. Once the water is boiling, take away from the warmth and allow the eggs to stand in the warm water for 15 min. Cool the eggs under cold running water: peel and chop.

Combine eggs, water chestnuts, mayonnaise, pickle relish, dry mustard, and paprika in a large bowl. Stir until well combined. Season to taste with salt and pepper.

Per Serving: 477 calories; 39.9 g fat; 18.9 g carbohydrates; 13.8 g protein; 384 mg cholesterol; 838 mg sodium.

Fresh Broccoli Salad

Ingredients
- 2 heads fresh broccoli
- 1 red onion
- ½ pound bacon
- ¾ cup raisins
- ¾ cup sliced almonds
- 1 cup mayonnaise
- ½ cup white sugar
- 2 tablespoons white wine vinegar

Directions
Place bacon in a deep skillet and cook over medium high heat until evenly brown. Cool and crumble.

Cut the broccoli into bite-size pieces and cut the onion into thin bite-size slices. Combine with the bacon, raisins, your favorite nuts and mix well.

To prepare the dressing, mix the mayonnaise, sugar and vinegar together until smooth. Stir into the salad, let chill and serve.

374 calories; 27.2 g total fat; 18 mg cholesterol; 353 mg sodium. 28.5 g carbohydrates; 7.3 g protein

Egg Salad I

Ingredients
- 8 eggs
- 1 tablespoon mayonnaise
- 2 tablespoons prepared Dijon-style mustard
- 1 teaspoon dried dill weed
- 1 teaspoon paprika
- 1/2 red onion, minced
- salt and pepper to taste

Place eggs in a saucepan and cover with bloodless water. Bring water to a boil; cowl, cast off from heat and permit eggs to stand in hot water for 10 to 12 min. Remove from hot water, cool, peel and chop.

In a big bowl, integrate the egg, mayonnaise, mustard, dill, paprika, onion, and salt and pepper. Mash well with a fork or timber spoon.

Serve on bread as a sandwich or over crisp lettuce as a salad.

183 calories; 12.8 g is fat; 4.2 g carbohydrates; 12.9 g is protein; 373 mg is cholesterol; 348 mg is sodium.

Broccoli And Tortellini Salad

Ingredients
- 6 slices bacon
- 20 ounces fresh cheese-filled tortellini
- ½ cup mayonnaise
- ½ cup white sugar
- 2 teaspoons cider vinegar
- 3 heads fresh broccoli, cut into florets
- 1 cup raisins
- 1 cup sunflower seeds
- 1 red onion, finely chopped

Directions
Place bacon in a large, deep skillet. Cook over medium-high heat until frivolously brown. Drain, crumble and set aside.
Bring a massive pot of lightly salted water to a boil. Cook tortellini in boiling water for 8 to 10 min or until al dente drain and rinse beneath cold water.
In a small bowl, mix mayonnaise, sugar, and vinegar collectively to make the dressing.
In a massive bowl, integrate broccoli, tortellini, bacon, raisins, sunflower seeds, and pink onion. Pour dressing over salad and toss.
322 calories; 16.1 g total fat; 20 mg cholesterol; 341 mg sodium. 38.7 g carbohydrates; 9 g protein;

Shrimp Egg Salad

Ingredients
- 1 pound cooked shrimp - peeled, deveined, and chopped
- 4 hard-cooked eggs, chopped
- 4 tablespoons mayonnaise
- 1 teaspoon Dijon mustard
- 1 sprig chopped fresh dill

4 leaves green leaf lettuce
In a medium bowl, mix together the shrimp, eggs, mayonnaise and mustard. Spoon onto lettuce leaves to serve.
Per Serving: 292 calories; 17.5 g fat; 1.6 g carbohydrates; 30.3 g protein; 439 mg cholesterol; 429 mg sodium

Broccoli And Ramen Noodle Salad

Ingredients
- 1 (16 ounce) package broccoli coleslaw mix
- 2 (3 ounce) packages chicken flavored ramen noodles
- 1 bunch green onions, chopped
- 1 cup unsalted peanuts
- 1 cup sunflower seeds
- ½ cup white sugar
- ¼ cup vegetable oil
- ⅓ cup cider vinegar

Directions
In a large salad bowl, combine the slaw, broken noodles and green onions.
Whisk together the sugar, oil, vinegar and ramen seasoning packets. Pour over salad and toss to evenly coat. Refrigerate until chilled; top with peanuts and sunflower seeds before serving.
562 calories; 34.4 g total fat; 0 mg cholesterol; 356 mg sodium. 52.3 g carbohydrates; 16.5 g protein

Delicious Egg Salad For Sandwiches

Ingredients
- 8 eggs
- 1/2 cup mayonnaise
- 1 teaspoon prepared yellow mustard
- 1/4 cup chopped green onion
- salt and pepper to taste
- 1/4 teaspoon paprika

Place egg in a saucepan and cowl with cold water. Bring water to a boil and immediately cast off from the heat. Cover and permit eggs stand in hot water for 10 to 12 min. Remove from hot water, fresh, peel, and chop.
Place the chopped eggs in a bowl, and stir within the mayonnaise, mustard and green onion. Season with salt, pepper, and paprika stir and serve on your favored bread or crackers.
344 calories; 31.9 g is fat; 2.3 g carbohydrates; 13 g is protein; 382 mg cholesterol; 351 mg is sodium.

Easy Egg Salad

Ingredients
- 8 hard-cooked eggs, chopped
- 1/4 cup plain fat-free yogurt
- 1 tablespoon parsley flakes
- 1/4 teaspoon onion powder
- 1/4 teaspoon paprika
- 1/4 teaspoon salt

Mix chopped eggs, yogurt, parsley, onion powder, paprika, and salt together in a bowl.
Per Serving: 83 calories; 5.3 g fat; 1.3 g carbohydrates; 6.8 g protein; 212 mg cholesterol; 141 mg sodium

Crisp Apples With Citrus Dressing

Ingredients
- 1 apple, cored and cut into chunks
- 2 tangerines, juiced - divided
- 1 tablespoon sour cream
- 1 tablespoon mayonnaise
- 1 teaspoon white sugar, or more to taste
- 1 pinch salt

Toss apple chunks in a bowl with 2 teaspoons tangerine juice. Whisk remaining tangerine juice, sour cream, mayonnaise, sugar, and salt in a bowl until sugar and salt have dissolved. Pour dressing over apple and toss.Per Serving: 258 calories; 14.4 g fat; 33.6 g carbohydrates; 1.4 g protein; 12 mg cholesterol; 88 mg sodium.

Green Grape Salad

Ingredients
- 4 pounds seedless green grapes
- 1 (8 ounce) package cream cheese

- 1 (8 ounce) container sour cream
- 1/2 cup white sugar
- 1 teaspoon vanilla extract
- 4 ounces chopped pecans
- 2 tablespoons brown sugar

Wash and dry grapes. In a large bowl, mix together the cream cheese, sour cream, sugar and vanilla. Add grapes and mix until evenly incorporated. Sprinkle with brown sugar and pecans, mix again and refrigerate until serving.

Per Serving: 479 calories; 27.1 g fat; 60.1 g carbohydrates; 5.8 g protein; 43 mg cholesterol; 103 mg sodium.

Colorful Winter Fruitsalad

Ingredients
- 2 red apples, cored and diced
- 2 pears, cored and diced
- 3 clementines, peeled and segmented
- 3 kiwifruit - peeled, sliced, and quartered
- 1 cup pomegranate seeds
- *Dressing:*
- 1 tablespoon honey
- 3 tablespoons lime juice
- 1 tablespoon chopped fresh mint

Combine apples, pears, clementines, kiwi, and pomegranate seeds in a massive bowl. Whisk collectively honey, lime juice, and mint. Sprinkle dressing over fruit and toss till adequately combined.

142 calories; 0.6 g is fat; 36.6 g carbohydrates; 1.5 g is protein; 0 mg cholesterol; 5 mg is sodium.

Egg Salad With Chopped Gherkins

Ingredients
- 8 eggs
- 1/2 cup mayonnaise
- 1/4 cup chopped green onion
- 2 tablespoons chopped celery, or more to taste
- 1 tablespoon chopped gherkins, or more to taste
- 1/4 teaspoon brown mustard
- 1/4 teaspoon dry mustard
- salt and ground black pepper to taste
- 1/4 teaspoon paprika

Place eggs in a big saucepan and cover with bloodless water. Bring to a boil and eliminate from heat. Cover the pan with a lid and allow sit till eggs are cooked through, 10 to 12 min. Drain and rinse with bloodless water till eggs are bloodless. Peel and chop eggs. Stir chopped eggs, mayonnaise, onion, celery, gherkins, brown mustard, and dry mustard together in a bowl. Season with salt and black pepper sprinkle paprika over the top.

347 calories; 31.9 g is fat; 3 g carbohydrates; 13.1 g is protein; 382 mg cholesterol; 356 mg is sodium.

Smoked Salmon And Egg Salad

Ingredients
- 12 eggs
- 2 stalks celery, chopped
- 1 red onion, chopped
- 5 ounces diced smoked salmon
- 1 cup mayonnaise
- 3 tablespoons chopped fresh dill
- salt and pepper to taste

Place eggs in a saucepan and cover with cold water. Bring water to a boil; cover, remove from heat, and let eggs stand in hot water for 10 to 12 minutes. Remove from hot water, cool, peel and chop. In a medium bowl, combine eggs, celery, onion, smoked salmon and mayonnaise. Season with dill, salt and pepper. Refrigerate at least 2 hours to allow flavors to combine.

Per Serving: 333 calories; 30.1 g fat; 3.1 g carbohydrates; 13.2 g protein; 294 mg cholesterol; 410 mg sodium.

Pistachio Fluff Fruit Salad

Ingredients
- 1 (20 ounce) can crushed pineapple with juice
- 1 (3 ounce) package instant pistachio pudding mix
- 1 (12 ounce) container frozen whipped topping, thawed
- 2 large bananas, sliced
- 2 cups miniature marshmallows
- 1 (15.25 ounce) can fruit cocktail, drained
- 1 (11 ounce) can mandarin oranges, drained

Dump instant pudding into a large mixing bowl. Add pineapple, and mix well. Mix in whipped topping. Stir in bananas, marshmallows, fruit cocktail, and mandarin oranges. Cover, and refrigerate until thoroughly chilled.

Per Serving: 444 calories; 14.8 g fat; 79.8 g carbohydrates; 2.5 g protein; 0 mg cholesterol; 269 mg sodium

Delicious Egg Salad For Sandwiches

Ingredients
- 8 eggs
- 1/2 cup mayonnaise
- 1 teaspoon prepared yellow mustard
- 1/4 cup chopped green onion
- salt and pepper to taste
- 1/4 teaspoon paprika

Place egg in a saucepan and cover with bloodless water. Bring water to a boil and immediately dispose of from heat. Cover and let eggs stand in hot water for 10 to 12 min. Remove from hot water, fresh, peel, and chop.

Place the chopped eggs in a bowl and stir in the mayonnaise, mustard, and green onion. Season with salt, pepper, and paprika mix and serve on your favorite bread or crackers.

344 calories; 31.9 g is fat; 2.3 g carbohydrates; 13 g is protein; 382 mg cholesterol; 351 mg is sodium

Mango Cashew Salad

Ingredients
- 1 mango - peeled, seeded, and cubed
- 1 Granny Smith apple - peeled, cored and diced
- 3/4 cup toasted cashews
- 1 tablespoon balsamic vinegar
- 1/2 teaspoon ground cinnamon
- 1/4 teaspoon ground ginger
- 1 pinch salt

In a medium bowl, toss together mango, Granny Smith apple, cashews, balsamic vinegar, cinnamon, ginger, and salt.

Per Serving: 133 calories; 8 g fat; 14.9 g carbohydrates; 2.9 g protein; 0 mg cholesterol; 111 mg sodium

Salad Frog Eye

Ingredients
- 1 cup of white sugar
- 2 tablespoons of all-purpose flour
- 2 1/2 teaspoons of salt
- 1 3/4 cups of unsweetened pineapple juice
- 2 eggs, beaten
- 1 tablespoon of lemon juice
- 3 quarts of water
- 1 tablespoon of vegetable oil
- 1 (16 ounce) package of acini di pepe pasta
- 3 (11 ounce) cans of mandarin oranges, drained
- 2 (20 ounce) cans of pineapple tidbits, drained
- 1 (20 ounce) can of crushed pineapple, drained
- 1 (8 ounce) container of frozen whipped topping, thawed
- 1 cup of miniature marshmallows
- 1 cup of shredded coconut

In a saucepan, integrate sugar, flour, half teaspoon salt, pineapple juice, and eggs. Stir and cook dinner over medium heat till thickened. Remove from heat; add lemon juice and cool to room temperature. Bring water to a boil, upload oil, remaining salt and cook pasta until al dente. Rinse below bloodless water and drain.

In a large bowl, combine the pasta, egg mixture, mandarin oranges, pineapple and whipped topping. Mix well and refrigerate overnight or until chilled before serving upload marshmallows and coconut. Toss and serve.

581 calories; 11 g is fat; 114.1 g carbohydrates; 8.6 g is protein; 37 mg cholesterol; 648 mg is sodium

Almost Eggless Egg Salad

Ingredients
- 2 tablespoons of mayonnaise
- 1 tablespoon of sweet pickle relish
- 1 teaspoon of distilled white vinegar
- 1 teaspoon of prepared mustard
- 1 teaspoon of white sugar
- 1/2 teaspoon of ground turmeric
- 1/4 teaspoon of dried dill weed
- 1 tablespoon of dried parsley
- 1 pound of firm tofu, sliced and well drained
- 1 tablespoon of minced onion
- 2 tablespoons of minced celery
- salt to your taste
- ground black pepper to your taste

In a small bowl, integrate mayonnaise, candy pickle relish, vinegar, mustard, sugar, turmeric, dill, and parsley: mix well and reserve.

Place drained tofu in a massive bowl and fall apart with a fork. Stir in onion and celery. Mix in the reserved mixture — season to flavor with salt and pepper chill for several hours to allow flavors to blend.

227 calories; 15.5 g is fat; 8.2 g carbohydrates; 18.2 g is protein; 3 mg cholesterol; 90 mg is sodium.

Peach And Berry Salad

Ingredients
- 3 peaches fresh
- 2 1/2 of pints blackberries
- 1 pint strawberries, sliced
- 1/4 cup of honey
- 1/2 teaspoon of ground cardamom

Bring a medium pot of water to boil. Add peaches and blanch for 30 sec. Drain and switch to a medium bowl. Cover with bloodless water and fresh. Drain, peel, and slice.

In a medium bowl, combine peaches, blackberries, strawberries, honey, and cardamom. Toss together and refrigerate.

190 calories; 1.2 g fat; 46.3 g carbohydrates; 3.2 g protein; 0 mg cholesterol; 7 mg sodium

Layered Deviled Egg Pasta Salad

Ingredients
- 6 eggs
- 2 1/2 tablespoons mayonnaise
- 2 teaspoons prepared yellow mustard
- salt and ground black pepper to taste
- 2 sprigs fresh dill
- *Pasta Salad:*
- 3 cups farfalle (bow-tie) pasta
- 2 tablespoons mayonnaise
- 1 pound cherry tomatoes, halved
- 2 cups chopped celery
- 2 cups diced cooked ham
- 4 cups chopped lettuce
- 4 spring onions, thinly sliced

Place eggs in a large saucepan and cover with cold water. Bring water to a boil. Remove pan from heat;

permit eggs stand in hot water for 10 minutes. Immerse eggs in a bowl of ice water and allow new, 1 to 2 min.
Peel eggs and halve them lengthwise. Scoop yolks into a bowl arrange egg whites cut-side up on a plate. Mash egg yolks into a crumbly paste with a fork. Mix in 2 1/2 tablespoons mayonnaise and mustard with the fork. Season with salt and pepper spoon egg yolk mixture into a small piping bag; pipe into the egg whites. Garnish with sparkling dill.
Bring a big pot of gently salted water to a boil. Cook bow-tie pasta at a boil, occasionally stirring, until gentle yet firm to the bite, about 12 min. Drain and permit refreshing, approximately 15 min.
Mix cooled pasta with 2 tablespoons mayonnaise in a bowl. Season with salt and pepper.
Spoon pasta into the bottom of a massive glass trifle bowl: layer tomatoes, celery, ham, and lettuce on the pinnacle. Arrange deviled eggs on crest before serving. Garnishing with spring onions.
355 calories; 22.4 g is fat; 20.9 g carbohydrates; 18.7 g is protein; 215 mg cholesterol; 797 mg is sodium.

Strawberry Spinach Salad
Ingredients
- 2 tablespoons of sesame seeds
- 1 tablespoon of poppy seeds
- 1/2 cup of white sugar
- 1/2 cup of olive oil
- 1/4 cup of distilled white vinegar
- 1/4 teaspoon of paprika
- 1/4 teaspoon of Worcestershire sauce
- 1 tablespoon of minced onion
- 10 ounces of fresh
- 1 quart of strawberries, sliced
- 1/4 cup aof lmonds, blanched and slivered

In a medium bowl, whisk the sesame seeds, poppy seeds, sugar, olive oil, vinegar, paprika, Worcestershire sauce, and onion collectively. Cover, and sit back for one hour.
In a considerable bowl, integrate the spinach, strawberries, and almonds. Pour dressing over salad and toss. Refrigerate 10 to 15 min earlier than serving.
491 calories; 35.2 g is fat; 42.9 g carbohydrates; 6 g is protein; 0 mg cholesterol; 63 mg is sodium.

Cranberry And Cilantro Quinoa Salad
Ingredients
1 1/2 cups water
1 cup uncooked quinoa, rinsed
1/4 cup red bell pepper, chopped
1/4 cup yellow bell pepper, chopped
1 small red onion, finely chopped
1 1/2 teaspoons curry powder
1/4 cup chopped fresh cilantro
1 lime, juiced
1/4 cup toasted sliced almonds
1/2 cup minced carrots
1/2 cup dried cranberries
salt and ground black pepper to taste
Pour the water right into a saucepan, and cover with a lid. Bring to a boil over high heat, then pour within the quinoa, recover, and continue to simmer over low heat until the water has been absorbed, 15 to 20 min. Scrape right into a blending bowl, and chill within the refrigerator until cold.
Once cold, stir in the purple bell pepper, yellow bell pepper, purple onion, curry powder, cilantro, lime juice, sliced almonds, carrots, and cranberries — season to flavor with salt and pepper chill earlier than serving.
176 calories; 3.9 g is fat; 31.6 g carbohydrates; 5.4 g is protein; 0 mg cholesterol; 13 mg is sodium

FISH RECIPES

Healthier Broiled Tilapia Parmesan

Ingredients
1/2 cup Parmesan cheese
1/8 cup butter, softened
3 tablespoons light mayonnaise
2 tablespoons fresh lemon juice
1/4 teaspoon dried basil
1/4 teaspoon ground black pepper
1/8 teaspoon onion powder
1/8 teaspoon celery salt
2 pounds tilapia fillets

Preheat oven broiler. Grease broiling pan or line with aluminum foil.
Mix Parmesan cheese, butter, mayonnaise, and lemon juice collectively in a small bowl. Season with dried basil, pepper, onion powder, and celery salt. Mix well and set aside. Arrange fillets in a single layer on prepared pan.
Broil a few inches from the heat for two to three minutes. Flip fillets over and broil for 2-3min more. Remove fillets from oven and cowl with Parmesan mixture on the pinnacle side. Broil until fish flakes easily with a fork, about 2 mins.
Per Serving: 180 calories; 7.7 g fat; 1.1 g carbohydrates; 25.3 g protein; 56 mg cholesterol; 231 mg sodium

Grilled Salmon

Ingredients
- 1/2 cup olive oil
- 1/4 cup lemon juice
- 4 green onions, thinly sliced
- 1 tablespoon chopped fresh parsley
- 1 teaspoon chopped fresh rosemary
- 1 teaspoon chopped fresh thyme
- 1/2 teaspoon salt
- 1/8 teaspoon black pepper
- 1/8 teaspoon garlic powder
- 3 pounds salmon fillets

Combine olive oil, lemon juice, green onions, parsley, rosemary, thyme, salt, black pepper, and garlic powder in a small bowl. Set apart 1/4 cup of the marinade. Place salmon in a shallow dish and pour the closing marinade over the top. Cover and refrigerate for 30 min. Remove the salmon and discard the used marinade.
Preheat grill for medium heat and lightly oil the grate. Place salmon at the preheated grill skin aspect down. Cook, basting on occasion with the reserved marinade, till the fish flakes without problems with a fork, 15 to 20 min.
 412 calories; 25.7 g is fat; 1.8 g carbohydrates; 41.8 g is protein; 97 mg cholesterol; 299 mg is sodium.

Veracruz-Style Red Snapper

Ingredients
- 2 tablespoons of olive oil
- 1/2 white color onion, diced
- 3 cloves of garlic, minced
- 1 tablespoon of capers
- 1 tablespoon of caper juice
- 1 cup of cherry tomatoes, halved
- 1/3 cup of pitted, sliced green olives
- 1 jalapeno pepper, chopped
- 2 teaspoons of chopped fresh oregano
- 2 teaspoons of olive oil
- 2 (7 ounce) of red snapper fillets, cut in half
- salt and pepper to your taste
- 1/2 teaspoon of cayenne pepper
- 2 limes, extract juice

Preheat oven to 425 ranges F (220 tiers C).
Heat olive oil in a skillet over medium heat. Stir in onion; prepare dinner and stir until onions begin to turn translucent, 6 to 7 min.
Cook and stir in garlic till fragrant, approximately 30 sec. Add capers and caper juice; stir to combine.
Stir in tomatoes, olives, jalapeno pepper, Cook and stir until jalapeno pepper softens and plants start to collapse about three minutes. Remove from heat; stir in oregano.
Drizzle one teaspoon olive oil right into a small baking dish. Sprinkle in 1 tablespoon of the tomato-olive mixture. Top with one snapper fillet, salt, black pepper, and cayenne pepper. Top with more fabulous filling and juice from 1 lime. Repeat with last snapper fillet, seasoning, and lime juice in a 2nd baking dish.
Bake inside the preheated oven till fish is flaky and not translucent, 15 to 20 min.
452 calories; 25.2 g is fat; 16.2 g carbohydrates; 43.1 g is protein; 73 mg cholesterol; 1034 mg is sodium.

Avocado And Tuna Tapas

Ingredients
- 1 (12 ounce) can is solid white tuna packed in water, drained
- 1 tablespoon of mayonnaise
- 3 green onions, thinly sliced
- 1/2 red bell pepper, finely chopped
1 dash balsamic vinegar
- black pepper to your taste
- 1 pinch of garlic salt, or to taste
- 2 ripe avocados, halved

Stir together tuna, mayonnaise, inexperienced onions, crimson pepper, and balsamic vinegar in a bowl. Season with pepper and garlic salt, then pack the avocado halves with the tuna mixture. Garnishing with reserved onions and a dash of black pepper before serving.
294 calories; 18.2 g is fat; 11 g carbohydrates; 23.9 g is protein; 27 mg cholesterol; 154 mg is sodium.

Quick Fish Tacos

Ingredients
- 1/4 cup reduced-fat sour cream

- 2 tablespoons lime juice
- salt and ground black pepper to taste
- 1 jalapeno pepper, halved lengthwise
- 2 1/2 cups shredded red cabbage
- 4 green onions, thinly sliced
- 2 tablespoons olive oil
- 1 pound tilapia fillets, cut into strips
- 8 (6 inch) flour tortillas
- 1/2 cup chopped fresh cilantro

Mix sour cream and lime juice collectively in a massive bowl; season with salt and black pepper — Reserve about half the aggregate in any other bowl for serving. Mince half the jalapeno pepper; save the other 1/2 for later. Toss cabbage, green onions, and minced jalapeno 1/2 in closing sour cream aggregate till slaw is mixed correctly.

Heat olive oil and last jalapeno half in a large skillet over medium heat; swirl oil to coat skillet evenly. Season tilapia fillets with salt and pepper. Pan-fry fish strips inside the skillet in 2 batches till fish is golden brown and easily flaked with a fork, five to 6 min. Discard jalapeno 1/2.

Heat tortillas in the microwave on high till warm, 20 to 30 sec.

Serve fish in warmed tortillas topped with cabbage slaw, reserved bitter cream combination, and cilantro.

416 calories; 15.2 g is fat; 38.9 g carbohydrates; 30.1 g is protein; 47 mg cholesterol; 481 mg is sodium

Classic Fish And Chips

Ingredients
- 4 large sized potatoes, peeled and cut into strips
- 1 cup of all-purpose flour
- 1 teaspoon of baking powder
- 1 teaspoon of salt
- 1 teaspoon of ground black pepper
- 1 cup of milk
- 1 egg
- 1 quart of vegetable oil for frying
- 1 1/2 pounds of cod fillets

Place potatoes in a medium-size bowl of cold water. In a separate medium-length blending bowl, mix flour, baking powder, salt, and pepper collectively. Stir inside the milk and egg; stir till the combination is smooth. Let the mixture stand for 20 min.

Preheat the oil in a massive pot or electric skillet to 350 degrees F (a hundred seventy-five ranges C). Fry the potatoes within the hot oil till they are tender. Drain them on paper towels.

Dredge the fish within the batter, one piece at a time, and location them in the warm oil. Fry until the fish is golden brown. If necessary, boom the heat to hold the 350 degrees F (one hundred seventy-five tiers C) temperature. Drain nicely on paper towels.

Fry the potatoes again for 1 to 2 min for delivered crispness.

782 calories; 26.2 g is fat; 91.9 g carbohydrates; 44.6 g is protein; 125 mg cholesterol; 861 mg is sodium

Grilled Fish Tacos With Chipotle-Lime Dressing

Ingredients
- 1/4 cup of extra virgin olive oil
- 2 tablespoons of distilled white vinegar
- 2 tablespoons of fresh lime juice
- 2 teaspoons of lime zest
- 1 1/2 teaspoons of honey
- 2 cloves of garlic, minced
- 1/2 teaspoon of cumin
- 1/2 teaspoon of chili powder
- 1 teaspoon of seafood seasoning
- 1/2 teaspoon of ground black pepper
- 1 teaspoon of hot pepper sauce, or to taste
- 1 pound of tilapia fillets, cut into chunks
- 1 (8 ounce) container of light sour cream
- 1/2 cup of adobo sauce from chipotle peppers
- 2 tablespoons of fresh lime juice
- 2 teaspoons of lime zest
- 1/4 teaspoon of cumin
- 1/4 teaspoon of chili powder
- 1/2 teaspoon of seafood seasoning
- salt and pepper to your taste
- *Toppings*
- 1 (10 ounce) package of tortillas
- 3 ripe tomatoes, seeded and diced
- 1 bunch of cilantro, chopped
- 1 small head of cabbage, cored and shredded
- 2 limes, cut in wedges

- To make the marinade, whisk **together** the olive oil, vinegar, lime juice, lime zest, honey, garlic, cumin, chili powder, seafood seasoning, black pepper, and **warm** sauce in a bowl **until** blended. Place the tilapia in a shallow dish and pour the marinade over the fish. Cover and refrigerate 6 **to eight** hours.
- To make the dressing, **combine** the **sour** cream and adobo sauce in a bowl. Stir **in the** lime juice, lime zest, cumin, chili powder, seafood seasoning. Add salt, and pepper in **preferred amounts**. Cover, and refrigerate **until** needed.
- Preheat **an outside** grill for **excessive heat** and **lightly** oil grate. Set grate **4** inches from the **warmness**.
- Remove fish from marinade, drain off any **excess** and discard marinade — grill fish pieces **until without problems** flaked with a fork, turning once, **approximately nine** min.
- Assemble tacos **by way of putting** fish pieces **within the center** of tortillas with **preferred quantities** of tomatoes, cilantro, and cabbage; drizzle with dressing. To serve, roll up tortillas **around** fillings, and garnish with lime wedges.

416 calories; 19.2 g is fat; 38.5 g carbohydrates; 22.6 g is protein; 43 mg cholesterol; 644 mg is sodium.

Hudson's Baked Tilapia With Dill Sauce

Ingredients
- 4 (4 ounce) of fillets tilapia
- salt and pepper to your taste
- 1 tablespoon of Cajun seasoning, or to taste
- 1 lemon, sliced
- 1/4 cup of mayonnaise
- 1/2 cup of sour cream
- 1/8 teaspoon of garlic powder
- 1 teaspoon of fresh lemon juice
- 2 tablespoons of chopped fresh dill

Preheat the oven to 350 F. Lightly grease a 9x13 inch baking dish.
Season the tilapia fillets with salt, pepper, and Cajun seasoning on each side. Arrange the pro fillets in a single layer in the baking dish. Place a layer of lemon slices over the fish fillets. I usually use approximately two slices on each piece so that it covers the maximum of the surface of the fish.
Bake uncovered for 15 to 20 min inside the preheated oven, or until fish flakes without difficulty with a fork.
While the fish is baking, mix the mayonnaise, bitter cream, garlic powder, lemon juice and dill in a small bowl collectively. Serve with tilapia.
Per Serving: 284 calories; 18.6 g fat; 5.7 g carbohydrates; 24.5 g protein; 59 mg cholesterol; 501 mg sodium.

Spanish Moroccan Fish

Ingredients
- 1 tablespoon of vegetable oil
- 1 onion, finely chopped
- 1 clove garlic, finely chopped
- 1 (15 ounce) can of garbanzo beans, drained and rinsed
- 2 red bell peppers
- 1 large sized carrot, thinly sliced
- 3 tomatoes, finely chopped
- 4 olives, finely chopped
- 1/4 cup of chopped fresh parsley
- 1/4 cup of ground cumin
- 3 tablespoons of paprika
- 2 tablespoons of chicken bouillon granules
- 1 teaspoon of cayenne pepper
- salt to your taste
- 5 pounds of tilapia fillets

Heat vegetable oil in a skillet over medium warmness. Mix in onion and garlic; cook and stir until the onion has softened and became translucent, approximately 5 mins. Add garbanzo beans, bell peppers, carrots, tomatoes, and olives; preserve to prepare dinner until the peppers are barely tender, about five mins more.
Sprinkle parsley, cumin, paprika, hen bouillon, and cayenne over the vegetables. Season with a salt mix to incorporate place tilapia on top of the vegetables and add sufficient water to cowl the vegetables.
Reduce warmness to the low, hood, and cook until fish flakes without difficulty with a fork and juices run clear about 40 min.
268 calories; 5.1 g is fat; 12.6 g carbohydrates; 41.7 g is protein; 70 mg cholesterol; 381 mg is sodium

Cedar Planked Salmon

Ingredients
- 3 (12 inch) is untreated cedar planks
- 1/3 cup of vegetable oil
- 1 1/2 tablespoons of rice vinegar
- 1 teaspoon of sesame oil
- 1/3 cup of soy sauce
- 1/4 cup of chopped green onions
- 1 tablespoon of grated fresh ginger root
- 1 teaspoon of minced garlic
- 2 (2 pound) of salmon fillets, skin removed

Soak the cedar planks for at least 1 hour in heat water. Soak longer if you have time.
In a shallow dish, stir the vegetable oil, rice vinegar, sesame oil, soy sauce, inexperienced onions, ginger, and garlic collectively. Place the salmon fillets within the marinade and flip to coat. Cover and marinate for at the least 15 min, or up to 1 hour.
Preheat an outdoor grill for medium heat. Place the planks on the grate. The boards are prepared when they begin to smoke and crackle just a little.
Place the salmon fillets onto the planks and discard the marinade: cover, and grill for about 20 min. Fish is completed when you can flake it with a fork. It will hold to prepare dinner after you cast off it from the grill.
678 calories; 45.8 g is fat; 1.7 g carbohydrates; 61.3 g is protein; 179 mg cholesterol; 981 mg is sodium

Blackened Tuna

Ingredients
1 1/2 pounds fresh tuna steaks, 1 inch thick
2 tablespoons Cajun seasoning
2 tablespoons olive oil
2 tablespoons butter
Generously coat tuna with Cajun seasoning.
Heat oil and butter in a big skillet over high heat. When the oil is nearly smoking, region steaks in the pan. Cook on one facet for three to four minutes, or until blackened. Turn steaks, and prepare dinner for 3 to 4 min, or desired doneness.
243 calories; 14 g fat; 1.1 g carbohydrates; 26.7 g protein; 54 mg cholesterol; 546 mg sodium

Baked Dijon Salmon

Ingredients
- 1/4 cup of butter, melted
- 3 tablespoons of Dijon mustard
- 1 1/2 tablespoons of honey
- 1/4 cup of dry bread crumbs
- 1/4 cup of finely chopped pecans
- 4 teaspoons of chopped fresh parsley
- 4 (4 ounce) of fillets salmon

- salt and pepper to your taste
- 1 lemon, for garnishing

Preheat oven to 400 ranges F.
In a small bowl, stir butter, mustard, and honey collectively. Set aside. In every other bowl, mix bread crumbs, pecans, and parsley.
Brush every salmon fillet gently with honey mustard mixture and sprinkle the tops of the fillets with the bread crumb mixture.
Bake salmon 12 to 15 min within the preheated oven, or until it flakes without difficulty with a fork. Season with salt and pepper, and garnish with a wedge of lemon.
422 calories; 29 g fat; 17.6 g carbohydrates; 24.3 g protein; 97 mg cholesterol; 480 mg sodium.

Ginger Glazed Mahi Mahi

Ingredients
- 3 tablespoons of honey
- 3 tablespoons of soy sauce
- 3 tablespoons of balsamic vinegar
- 1 teaspoon of grated fresh ginger root
- 1 clove of garlic, crushed or to taste
- 2 teaspoons of olive oil
- 4 (6 ounce) of mahi mahi fillets
- salt and pepper to your taste
- 1 tablespoon of vegetable oil

In a shallow glass dish, stir together the honey, soy sauce, balsamic vinegar, ginger, garlic, and olive oil. Season fish fillets with salt and pepper, and place them into the dish. If the fillets have skin on them, vicinity them skin side down. Cover, and refrigerate for 20 mins to marinate.
Heat vegetable oil in a big skillet over medium-excessive heat. Remove fish from the dish, and reserve marinade. Fry fish for four to 6 mins on each side, turning simplest once, until fish flakes effortlessly with a fork. Remove fillets to a serving platter and keep warm.
Pour reserved marinade into the skillet, and heat over medium heat till the combination reduces to a glaze consistently. Spoon glaze over fish and serve immediately.
259 calories; 7 g fat; 16 g carbohydrates; 32.4 g protein; 124 mg cholesterol; 830 mg sodium.

Pretzel Coated Fried Fish

Ingredients
- 1 quart of oil for frying
- 3/4 cup of all-purpose flour
- 1 teaspoon of salt
- 1/2 teaspoon of ground black pepper
- 1 pound of frozen cod fillets, thawed
- 2 eggs
- 3/4 cup of crushed pretzels

Heat the oil in a deep fryer to 350 stages F.
Mix the flour, salt, and pepper in a large resealable plastic bag. Place cod within the bag, and lightly shake to coat. Place eggs and crushed pretzels in two separate shallow dishes. Dip lined cod in the eggs, then within the overwhelmed pretzels.
Fry coated fish 10 min inside the preheated oil, turning once, till golden brown and effortlessly flaked with a fork.
469 calories; 26 g fat; 30.8 g carbohydrates; 27.2 g protein; 142 mg cholesterol; 949 mg sodium.

Spanish Cod

Ingredients
- 1 tablespoon of butter
- 1 tablespoon of olive oil
- 1/4 cup of finely chopped onion
- 2 tablespoons of chopped fresh garlic
- 1 cup of tomato sauce
- 15 cherry tomatoes, halved
- 1/2 cup of chopped green olives
- 1/4 cup of deli marinated Italian vegetable salad, drained and coarsely chopped
- 1 dash of black pepper
- 1 dash of cayenne pepper
- 1 dash of paprika
- 6 (4 ounce) of fillets cod fillets

Heat butter and olive oil in a big skillet over medium warmness. Cook and stir onions and garlic till onions are barely tender, being careful now not to burn the garlic. Add tomato sauce and cherry tomatoes, and bring to a simmer. Stir in inexperienced olives and marinated vegetables, and season with black pepper, cayenne pepper, and paprika. Cook fillets in sauce over medium warmness for five to 8 min, or until without problems flaked with a fork. Serve immediately.
170 calories; 6.6 g is fat; 6.5 g carbohydrates; 21.3 g is protein; 46 mg cholesterol; 597 mg is sodium.

Baked Cod In Foil

Ingredients
- 2 tomatoes
- 1 red bell pepper, cubed
- 1 onion, minced
- 2 tablespoons of olive oil
- 2 tablespoons of chopped fresh basil
- 1 clove of garlic, minced
- aluminum foil

4 (5 ounce) of cod fillets
- lemon, juiced
- salt and ground black pepper to your taste

Preheat the oven to 400 stages F.
Combine tomatoes, bell pepper, onion, olive oil, basil, and garlic in a bowl and mix well.
Lay four sheets of aluminum foil on a work floor and area 1 cod fillet within the middle of each. Spoon tomato mixture evenly on the pinnacle of the four fillets. Drizzle with lemon juice and season with salt and pepper. Place a second sheet of foil on the crest and seal the edges to make a parcel. Repeat with the remaining fillets and tomato mixture.

Bake within the preheated oven until cod flakes easily with a fork, approximately 20 mins. Remove from the oven and thoroughly unwrap the parcels. Spoon onto warmed plates and serve immediately.
216 calories; 8 g fat; 10.4 g carbohydrates; 27 g protein; 52 mg cholesterol; 146 mg sodium

Coast Cod And Shrimp

Ingredients
- 2 cups of water
- 1 cup of uncooked long-grain white rice
- 1 teaspoon of olive oil
- 2 tablespoons of butter
- 1/4 cup of minced onion
- 1 tablespoon of minced garlic
- 1 1/2 cups of heavy cream
- 1/4 cup of milk
- 1 1/2 tablespoons of cornstarch
- 1/2 pound of fresh shrimp, peeled and deveined
- 1 cup of sliced fresh mushrooms
- 1 tablespoon of chopped fresh dill
- seasoning salt to your taste
- pepper to your taste
- 1 pound of cod fillets
- 1 tablespoon of grated Parmesan cheese
- 1 tablespoon of chopped fresh parsley

In a medium saucepan, bring water to a boil. Stir within the rice, lessen the heat, and cover. Simmer 20 minutes, till the water has been absorbed.
Preheat oven to 350 stages F. Coat a medium baking dish with the olive oil.
Melt the butter in a medium saucepan over medium heat, and saute the onion and garlic until tender. Stir within the heavy cream. In a small bowl, mix the milk and cornstarch, and stir into the saucepan to thicken the heavy cream combination. Remove from heat, stir within the shrimp and mushrooms, and season with dill, seasoning salt, and pepper.
Arrange cod within the prepared baking dish. Pour the heavy cream combination over the cod. Sprinkle with Parmesan cheese and parsley.
Cover, and bake 30 min within the preheated oven, till sauce is bubbly and fish is without difficulty flaked with a fork. Serve over the rice
730 calories; 42.8 g is fat; 46.3 g carbohydrates; 39 g is protein; 275 mg cholesterol; 309 mg is sodium

Perfect Ten Baked Cod

Ingredients
- 2 tablespoons of butter
- 1/2 sleeve of buttery round crackers (such as Ritz®), crushed
- 2 tablespoons of butter
- 1 pound of thick-cut cod loin
- 1/2 lemon, juiced
- 1/4 cup of dry white wine
- 1 tablespoon of chopped fresh parsley
- 1 tablespoon of chopped green onion
- 1 lemon, cut into wedge

Preheat oven to 400 tiers F.
Place two tablespoons butter in a microwave-secure bowl; melt in the microwave on high, approximately 30 sec. Stir buttery spherical crackers into melted butter.
Place closing two tablespoons butter in a 7x11-inch baking dish. Melt within the preheated oven, 1 to three minutes. Remove the plate from the oven. Coat each facet of cod in melted butter inside the baking dish.
Bake cod in the preheated oven for 10 min. Remove from oven; top with lemon juice, wine, and cracker mixture. Place again in the oven and bake till fish is opaque and flakes without problems with a fork, approximately ten extra min.
Garnish baked cod with parsley and inexperienced onion. Serve with lemon wedges.
280 calories; 16.1 g is fat; 9.3 g carbohydrates; 20.9 g is protein; 71 mg cholesterol; 282 mg is sodium.

Moroccan Fish Tagine

Ingredients
- 1/2 cup of olive oil
- 1/2 cup of chopped fresh cilantro
- 1/2 cup of chopped fresh parsley
- 1/2 lemon, juiced
- 6 cloves of garlic, minced
- 1 teaspoon of ground paprika
- 1/2 teaspoon of ground ginger
- 1/2 teaspoon of ground cumin
- 1/2 teaspoon of salt
- 1/4 teaspoon of ground saffron (optional)
- *Fish Tagine:*
- 1 1/2 pounds of cod fillets, cut into bite-sized pieces
- 1 tablespoon of olive oil
- 1 large sized onion, cut into rings
- 1 large sized carrot, peeled and cut into matchsticks
- 2 potatoes, peeled and sliced 1/4-inch thick
- 1 large sized green bell pepper, sliced into rings
- 3 tomatoes, seeded and cut into strips
- 1/4 cup of chopped fresh cilantro

Mix half cup olive oil, half of the cup cilantro, parsley, lemon juice, garlic, paprika, ginger, cumin, salt, and saffron in a big glass or ceramic bowl. Add cod and blend well. Cover and marinate within the fridge for 2 hours.
Heat 1 tablespoon olive oil in a large pot or tagine. Layer onion earrings, carrot matchsticks, and potato slices in the pan in that order. Remove cod from marinade and unfold calmly over potatoes. Cover cod with green bell pepper jewelry and tomato strips sprinkle 1/four cup cilantro on top. Pour marinade over cilantro.

Cover pot tightly and prepare dinner over low heat till potatoes are smooth and cod flakes easily with a fork, approximately 1 hour.

368 calories; 21.4 g is fat; 22 g carbohydrates; 23.1 g is protein; 41 mg cholesterol; 289 mg is sodium

Crispy Beer Batter Fish & Chips

Ingredients
- 1 cup of self-rising flour
- 2 tablespoons of rice flour
- 1/4 teaspoon of baking powder
- *For the Fish:*
- 4 (6 ounce) of cod fillets, fully thawed if frozen
- 2 tablespoons of rice flour, or as needed
- salt to your taste
- 1 cup of lager-style beer, or more as needed
- vegetable oil for frying

Whisk self-growing flour, rice flour, and baking powder collectively in a bowl. Freeze till equipped to use.

Pat fish as dry as possible. Cut pieces lengthwise to get eight 1-inch thick strips. Place rice flour on a plate and season with salt. Dust fish lightly with the aggregate and shake off excess. Cover a dish with crinkled foil to make a brief drying rack; vicinity fish on top.

Heat oil in a deep-fryer to 375 tiers F.

Pour beer into the flour combination and whisk, adding greater as needed, till batter is the consistency of thick pancake batter. Dip fish pieces into the mixture to coat; elevate out and let extra drip off.

Fry fish in batches till golden brown, dunking now and again if needed, 3 to 4 min. Drain on paper towels. Serve immediately.

Cod Grilled

Ingredients
- 2 (8 ounce) of fillets cod, cut in half
- 1 tablespoon of Cajun seasoning
- 1/2 teaspoon of lemon pepper
- 1/4 teaspoon of salt
- 1/4 teaspoon of ground black pepper
- 2 tablespoons of butter
- 1 lemon, juiced
- 2 tablespoons of chopped green onion (white part only)

Stack about 15 charcoal briquettes right into a grill in a pyramid shape. If desired, drizzle coals lightly with lighter fluid and permit to soak for 1 minute earlier than lighting coals with a match. Allow the fire to spread to all fuels, about 10 mins, earlier than spreading briquettes out into the grill; permit coals burn until a skinny layer of white ash covers the coals — lightly oil the grates.

Season each side of cod with Cajun seasoning, lemon pepper, salt, and black pepper. Set fish apart on a plate. Heat butter in a small saucepan over medium heat, stir in lemon juice and inexperienced onion and cook till onion is softened about 3 mins.

Place cod onto oiled grates and grill till fish is browned and flakes easily, about three minutes per side; baste with butter combination regularly at the same time as grilling. Allow cod to rest off the warmth for approximately five minutes earlier than serving.

Per Serving: 152 calories; 6.6 g fat; 2.2 g carbohydrates; 20.3 g protein; 63 mg cholesterol; 661 mg sodium.

Crispy Fish

Ingredients
- 2 cups of dry potato flakes
- 1 cup of all-purpose flour
- 1 tablespoon of garlic powder
- 1 tablespoon of seasoning salt
- 1 tablespoon of ground black pepper
- 2 teaspoons of cayenne pepper, or to taste
- 4 (6 ounce) of fillets cod
- 2 cups of butter flavored shortening, for frying

Instructions

In a medium bowl, combine the potato flakes, flour, garlic powder, seasoning salt, black pepper, and cayenne pepper.

Soak fish fillets in a bowl of bloodless water.

In a deep skillet or deep fryer, melt and heat the shortening to 350 levels F.

Dredge fish fillets in dry mixture and fry inside the hot oil for 5 mins or till fish flakes aside quickly.

Remove from oil and vicinity on paper towels to take in extra fat.

446 calories; 12.3 g total fat; 62 mg cholesterol; 835 mg sodium. 47.2 g carbohydrates; 36 g protein

Sardines With Sun-Dried Tomato And Capers

Ingredients
- 1 (3.75 ounce) can of sardines packed in olive oil, drained (such as King Oscar®)
- 1/2 fresh lemon
- 1 pinch of salt and ground black pepper to taste
- 1/4 teaspoon of cayenne pepper
- 1/2 teaspoon of dried oregano
- 1/2 teaspoon of dried thyme
- 1 pinch of crushed red pepper flakes, or to taste
- 2 garlic cloves, chopped
- 2 tablespoons of chopped sun-dried tomatoes
- 1 tablespoon of capers

Place the sardines on a small plate. Squeeze the lemon half of over the sardines; season with salt, black pepper, cayenne pepper, oregano, thyme, and beaten pink pepper flakes. Scatter the garlic, sun-dried tomatoes, and capers over the mixture.

234 calories; 11.2 g is fat; 9.9 g carbohydrates; 24.6 g is protein; 131 mg cholesterol; 864 mg sodium.

Fresh Sardines

Ingredients
- 2 pounds of fresh sardines
- 1 cup of all-purpose flour
- 3/4 cup of olive oil
- 2 cloves of garlic, chopped
- 1 cup of white vinegar
- 1 cup of white wine
- 1/2 cup of fresh mint leaves

Prepare the sardines by getting rid of the heads and lower backbones. Rinse and pat dry. Dredge in flour, shaking off any excess.

Heat olive oil in a large skillet over medium-excessive heat. When the oil is hot, fry the sardines a few at a time till brown and crispy. Remove to a large serving plate, and hold warm.

In another skillet over medium heat, heat a chunk of the oil. Add garlic, and cook dinner for approximately half a minute. Add the wine and vinegar, and permit the aggregate to simmer, stirring occasionally. When the liquid has reduced by about half of, pour the sauce over the sardines and sprinkle with clean mint. Let stand for about 1 hour before serving to allow the fish to marinate.

1011 calories; 72.2 g is fat; 26.1 g carbohydrates; 47.1 g is protein; 0 mg cholesterol; 5 mg is sodium.

Pasta Con Sarde (Pasta with Sardines)

Ingredients
- 1 (16 ounce) package of spaghetti
- 3/4 cup of olive oil, divided
- 6 cloves of garlic, minced
- 2 (4 ounce) cans of sardines packed in olive oil, drained
- 1 cup of seasoned bread crumbs
- 1/3 cup of freshly grated Parmesan cheese
- 1/4 cup of chopped fresh parsley
- 1 teaspoon of ground black pepper
- Parmesan cheese for serving

Bring a large pot of gently salted water to a boil. Add the spaghetti, and prepare dinner till al dente, or 8 to 10 minutes. Drain, and rinse below cold water. Toss with 1/four cup olive oil, cowl, and preserve warm. Place another 1/four cup olive oil in a skillet, and warmth over medium heat. Stir within the garlic, and prepare dinner just until golden, 2 to a few mins. Add the sardines, and cook 1 min more. Mix inside the bread crumbs and 1/3 cup Parmesan cheese. If essential to present the mixture a crumbly texture, stir within the last 1/4 cup of olive oil. Stir within the parsley and pepper, and put off from the heat. If desired, serve with additional Parmesan cheese.

1046 calories; 52.4 g fat; 106.5 g carbohydrates; 35.9 g protein; 87 mg cholesterol; 930 mg sodium.

Quick Sardine Curry

Ingredients
- 1 tablespoon canola oil
- 1 tablespoon Thai red curry paste, or more to taste
- 1 clove garlic, minced
- 1 shallot, minced
- 1 tablespoon unsweetened coconut cream
- 1 (3.75 ounce) can sardines in oil, drained

Heat the canola oil in a skillet. Stir the pink curry paste into the hot oil; cook dinner and stir for some sec before including the garlic and shallot. Cook and stir the garlic and shallot till fragrant. Add the sardines; toss around within the pan to brown the skin a touch bit and cowl it nicely with the paste combination. Gently stir the coconut cream into the aggregate and retain to toss to coat the sardines. Allow mixture to come back to a boil till the sauce thickens, about 5 mins.

Per Serving: 416 calories; 29.8 g fat; 12.5 g carbohydrates; 24.6 g protein; 131 mg cholesterol; 760 mg sodium.

Island-Style Sardines and Rice

Ingredients
- 1 tablespoon of coconut oil
- 1 roma (plum) tomato, diced
- 1/4 cup of sliced white onion
- 1 small garlic clove, finely minced
- 1/8 teaspoon of minced scotch bonnet chile pepper
- 2 (3.75 ounce) cans of sardines packed in soybean oil
- salt and ground black pepper to your taste
- 2 cups of cooked white rice

Melt coconut oil in a skillet at medium heat; upload tomato, onion, garlic, and scotch bonnet chile pepper. Cook and stir tomato combination till onion is translucent about 5 min.

Pour sardines and soybean oil in tomato-onion mixture; mash fish with a fork till incorporated. Cover the skillet, reduce to low and cook until sardines are heated through, about 3 min. Seasoning with salt and pepper.

235 calories; 9 g is fat; 23.8 g is carbohydrates; 13.7 g is protein; 65 mg cholesterol; 234 mg is sodium.

Pasta Sardine

Ingredients
8 ounces dry fettuccine pasta
2 tablespoons olive oil
1 medium yellow onion, chopped
3 cloves garlic, crushed
1 lemon, juiced
1 (3.75 ounce) can sardines in tomato sauce
1 pinch of red pepper flakes
1/4 cup freshly grated Parmesan cheese

Bring a large bowl of gently salted water to a boil. Add pasta, and cook dinner for about eight minutes, or till nearly tender.

While the pasta is cooking, heat olive oil in a skillet over medium warmness, add the onion and cook for a few minutes until soft, then upload the garlic, and cook till fragrant. Stir within the sardines with their sauce. When the sardines warmth through, reduce heat to low and simmer until the pasta is ready. When the pasta is ready, then add it to the sardine sauce. Stir, cover, and turn the warmth off. Let stand for a few mins to absorb the flavors of the sauce. Squeeze juice from the lemon over the pasta. Divide onto serving plates, and pinnacle with red pepper flakes and grated Parmesan cheese.
350 calories; 12.8 g fat; 47.3 g carbohydrates; 14.5 g protein; 21 mg cholesterol; 192 mg sodium

Miso & Tofu

Ingredients
2 tablespoons sesame seeds
½ cup dried Asian-style whole sardines
2 ½ tablespoons red miso paste
½ cup boiling water
1 (16 ounce) package silken tofu, cubed
4 green onions, thinly sliced
crushed red pepper flakes

In a dry heavy skillet at medium tempreture, stir the sesame seeds and dried sardines till they provide off their fragrance; however, do not burn, approximately 2 min. Place the sesame seeds and dried sardines inside the paintings bowl of a small food processor and pulse till floor to a exceptional powder.
Place the dried sardine combination in a big bowl and stir inside the miso to make a thick paste. Add boiling water and mix it to a smooth, creamy consistency, and stir in the cubed tofu, green onions, and red pepper flakes.
82 calories; 4.5 g total fat; 6 mg cholesterol; 358 mg sodium. 4.6 g carbohydrates; 7.4 g protein

MediterraneanCasserole

Ingredients
1 pound potatoes
3 tablespoons extra-virgin olive oil
4 (4.375 ounce) cans sardines, drained
1/2 pound cherry tomatoes, diced
2 cloves garlic, chopped
1 tablespoon dried basil
2 tablespoons bread crumbs

Place the potatoes in a bowl and then add salted water. Bring it to a boil; reduce heat to medium-low, cover, and simmer until tender, about 20 min. Drain. Cover with cold water and allow to sit until cool, draining and replacing the cold water as needed. Peel and slice the potatoes thinly.
Preheat an oven to 350 degrees F.
Grease a casserole dish with the olive oil. Line the casserole dish with an even layer of potato slices; top with a layer of sardine fillets. Scatter the diced tomatoes over the sardines. Sprinkle the garlic, basil, and bread crumbs over the tomatoes.
Bake in the preheated oven until heated through, about 20 minutes.
Per Serving: 466 calories; 24.8 g fat; 25.7 g carbohydrates; 34 g protein; 176 mg cholesterol; 663 mg sodium

Avocado Salsa and Sardine Frenchy

Ingredients
1 avocado, finely mashed
2 romaine lettuce leaves, finely chopped
1/4 green bell pepper, chopped
1 teaspoon of lemon juice
4 slices of French bread
2 teaspoons of extra-virgin olive oil
1 (4.375 ounce) can of canned sardines in water, well drained
1 can of tomatoes finely diced with basil, garlic, and oregano - drained

Preheat oven to 350 degrees F.
Mix avocado, chopped lettuce, chopped inexperienced pepper, lemon juice in a bowl.
Grease extra-virgin olive oil on bread slices and toast in the preheated oven till browned, about five mins on each side.
Remove bread slices from oven. Spread with avocado mixture; pinnacle with sardines and canned tomatoes
Per Serving: 275 calories; 14.1 g fat; 26 g carbohydrates; 12.9 g protein; 25 mg cholesterol; 924 mg sodium.

Vegetale Sardina

Ingredients
3 tablespoons coconut oil, divided
1/2 eggplant, cut into cubes
2 zucchini, cut into cubes
1 cup garbanzo beans
1 yellow squash, cut into cubes
1/4 onion, sliced
1/4 cup kalamata olives
3 cloves garlic, sliced
4 teaspoons dried rosemary, divided
8 ounces sardines
1/2 teaspoon garlic powder
1 cup feta cheese

Preheat oven to 375 stages F.
Spread one teaspoon coconut oil into the lowest of a solid iron skillet or baking dish. Add eggplant, zucchini, garbanzo beans, yellow squash, onion, kalamata olives, and garlic to forged iron skillet. Sprinkle two teaspoons rosemary over vegetable mixture and toss to coat veggies in oil.
Bake greens within the preheated oven on the lowest rack till barely tender, about 20 min.
Heat the final coconut oil in a frying pan over medium-excessive heat; place sardines in the hot oil and sprinkle with garlic powder and the ultimate rosemary. Fry sardines till heated through, approximately five min. Top roasted vegetables with sardines and feta cheese.

335 calories; 22.5 g fat; 15.9 g carbohydrates; 18.4 g protein; 91 mg cholesterol; 877 mg sodium.

Bagna Calda

Ingredients
1 1/2 cups of vegetable oil
3/4 cup of minced garlic
4 (2 ounce) cans of anchovy fillets packed in olive oil, drained
3 (4 ounce) cans of sardines packed in olive oil, drained
1 cup of butter

Place the canola oil in a skillet and heat over medium heat. Stir in the garlic, and cook till golden brown, about 5 min. Add the butter, anchovies, and sardines. Cook and stir till nicely blended, 10 to 15 min. Serve warm.

99 calories; 8.6 g fat; 1.1 g carbohydrates; 4.5 g protein; 35 mg cholesterol; 301 mg sodium.

Solo Spaghetti Dinner

Ingredients
2 ounces dry spaghetti or capellini
2 tablespoons olive oil
1/2 onion, chopped
1 (4 ounce) can rolled sardines with capers
1 fresh tomato, chopped
2 teaspoons crushed red pepper flakes
1/3 cup Italian bread crumbs
grated Parmesan cheese to taste, for serving

Bring a bowl of salted water to a boil. Then add the spaghetti, and cook until al dente, or 8 to 10 min. Drain, and rinse under cold water. Toss with a drizzle of olive oil, cover, and keep warm.
Place 2 tablespoons olive oil in a skillet at medium tempreature. Stir in the onion, and cook till soft and transparent, about 5 minutes. Add the sardines; cook and stir 5 to 8 minutes until the sardines start to break apart. Mix in the tomatoes, and cook until mixture is heated through. Stir in the bread crumbs. Serve over spaghetti, and top with desired amount of grated Parmesan cheese.

Per Serving: 920 calories; 44.5 g fat; 87.6 g carbohydrates; 43.7 g protein; 162 mg cholesterol; 869 mg sodium

Sandwich Toast (Sardines and Pineapple)

Ingredients
4 slices bread
1 tablespoon mayonnaise
1 pinch salt and ground black pepper
2 teaspoons marmalade
4 potato chips, crushed
2 pieces pineapple, thinly sliced
4 sardines, drained, or to taste

Preheat your sandwich maker in line with the manufacturer's instructions.
Spread mayonnaise over two slices of bread. Cover with marmalade. Spread potato chips over jam. Lay pineapple over chips.
Break aside sardines in a bowl the use of a fork. Spread on the pinnacle of the pineapple slices.
Season with salt and pepper; cover with the closing two slices of bread.
Toast inside the preheated sandwich maker until brown and crispy, about 5 min.

271 calories; 10.8 g fat; 33.3 g carbohydrates; 10.1 g protein; 37 mg cholesterol; 595 mg sodium.

Iana's Pasta con le Sarde

Ingredients
1 tablespoon of olive oil
1 bulb of fennel - thinly sliced, fronds lightly chopped, stems discarded
1 onion, finely diced
4 cloves of garlic, minced
2 (4.5 ounce) cans of sardines packed in oil
1/3 cup of raisins
1/4 cup of pine nuts
1 teaspoon of chopped fresh basil
1 teaspoon of fennel seeds
salt and ground black pepper to your taste
1 pinch of red pepper flakes, or to taste
1 (28 ounce) can of crushed tomatoes
1 (16 ounce) package of spaghetti
Mudica (Seasoned Bread Crumbs):
2 tablespoons of olive oil
2 cloves ofo garlic, or more to taste, minced
1 cup of bread crumbs
1/2 teaspoon of chopped fresh basil
1 tablespoon of grated Parmesan cheese, or to taste

Heat olive oil in a saucepan over medium warmth. Add fennel bulb, fronds, and onion. Cook until gentle, approximately five minutes. Add garlic; prepare dinner for 1 minute. Add sardines with oil; stir till crumbled. Stir in raisins, pine nuts, basil, fennel seeds, salt, pepper, and crimson pepper flakes; cook until toasted. Pour in tomatoes. Let sauce simmer.
Bring a bowl of salted water to a boil. Cook spaghetti in the boiling water, stirring occasionally, until soft yet corporation to the bite, approximately 12 minutes.
Meanwhile, heat oil in another pan over medium warmth. Add garlic and saute till fragrant, about 1 minute. Add bread crumbs and basil. Cook, stirring occasionally, until browned, about three minutes. Remove from heat.
Drain pasta; serve topped with the sauce, pro bread crumbs, and Parmesan cheese.

468 calories; 13.1 g fat; 68.5 g is carbohydrates; 20.7 g is protein; 46 mg cholesterol; 439 mg is sodium

Crab Stuffed Flounder

Ingredients
1 1/2 pounds of flounder fillets
1 cup of crabmeat - drained, flaked and cartilage removed
1 tablespoon of chopped green bell pepper
1/4 teaspoon of ground dry mustard
1/4 teaspoon of Worcestershire sauce

1/4 teaspoon of salt
ground white pepper, to taste
3 crushed saltine crackers
1 egg white
1 tablespoon of mayonnaise
1/4 cup of butter, melted
1 egg yolk
5 tablespoons of mayonnaise
1/2 teaspoon of paprika
1 tablespoon of dried parsley
Preheat oven to 400 ranges F (200 ranges C). Rinse the fillets and dry with paper towels.
Mix crab meat, inexperienced pepper, mustard powder, Worcestershire sauce, salt, white pepper and the beaten saltines. Mix the egg white and 1 tbsp mayonnaise. Stir this into the crab meat combination. Grease the flounder fillets with melted butter. Place in a greased, shallow baking dish. Spoon the crab aggregate over the fillets and drizzle with any last butter.
Bake the fillets at 400 stages for 15 minutes.
While the fish is baking, gently beat the egg yolk in a small bowl. Stir in five tablespoons of mayonnaise. Remove fish from oven and unfold this aggregate over the stuffing; sprinkle with paprika and parsley. Increase oven temperature to 450 stages and bake till golden and bubbly, about 6 minutes.
 308 calories; 21.2 g is fat; 2.2 g is carbohydrates; 26.5 g is protein; 127 mg cholesterol; 408 mg is sodium

Italian Style Flounder

Ingredients
2 pounds flounder fillets
1/2 tablespoon butter
salt and pepper to taste
1 tablespoon lemon juice
1/2 cup diced fresh tomato
2 teaspoons dried basil
1 teaspoon garlic powder
Preheat oven at 350 degrees F.
Arrange flounder in a medium baking dish. Add butter, and season with salt & pepper, and sprinkle with lemon juice. Top with tomato, basil, and garlic powder.
Cover, and bake 30 min in the preheated oven, or until fish is easily flaked with a fork.
Per Serving: 228 calories; 4.2 g fat; 1.9 g carbohydrates; 43.2 g protein; 113 mg cholesterol; 196 mg sodium.
Condiments and condiments for sauces

Blueberry Sauce

Ingredients
2 cups fresh or frozen blueberries
1/4 cup water
1 cup orange juice
3/4 cup white sugar
1/4 cup cold water
3 tablespoons cornstarch
1/2 teaspoon almond extract
1/8 teaspoon ground cinnamon
In a saucepan at medium warm, integrate the blueberries, 1/4 cup of water, orange juice, and sugar. Stir gently, and produce to a boil.
In a cup or small bowl, mix together the cornstarch and 1/four cup cold water. Gently stir the cornstarch aggregate into the blueberries so as no longer to mash the berries. Simmer gently till thick enough to coat the again of a steel spoon, 3 to four minutes. Remove from heat and stir inside the almond extract and cinnamon. Thin sauce with water if it's far too thick on your liking.
 119 calories; 0.2 g fat; 30 g carbohydrates; 0.5 g protein; 0 mg cholesterol; 1 mg sodium.

EZ Red Pesto Sauce

Ingredients
1 1/2 cups fresh basil leaves
1 cup sun-dried tomatoes, or to taste
1 cup grated Parmesan cheese
2/3 cup olive oil
1/2 cup pine nuts
1 clove garlic, minced
1/2 lemon, juiced
salt and ground black pepper to taste
Blend basil leaves, tomatoes, Parmesan cheese, olive oil, pine nuts, and garlic together in a blender until a smooth paste forms. Stir in lemon juice; season with salt and black pepper.
Per Serving: 282 calories; 27.2 g fat; 5.2 g carbohydrates; 6.9 g protein; 9 mg cholesterol; 210 mg sodium.

Easy Pesto

Ingredients
1/4 cup almonds
3 cloves garlic
1 1/2 cups fresh basil leaves
1/2 cup olive oil
1 pinch ground nutmeg
salt and pepper to taste
Preheat oven to 450 degrees F. Place almonds on a cookie sheet, and bake for 10 minutes, or until lightly toasted.
In a food processor, combine toasted almonds, garlic, basil, olive oil, nutmeg, salt and pepper. Process until a coarse paste is formed.
Per Serving: 199 calories; 21.1 g fat; 2 g carbohydrates; 1.7 g protein; 0 mg cholesterol; 389 mg sodium

Quick Alfredo Sauce

Ingredients
1/2 cup butter
1 (8 ounce) package cream cheese
2 teaspoons garlic powder
2 cups milk
6 ounces grated Parmesan cheese
1/8 teaspoon ground black pepper

Melt butter in a non-stick saucepan at medium warmth. Then add cream cheese and garlic powder, mixing with twine whisk till smooth. Add milk, a bit at a time, whisking to smooth out lumps. Stir in Parmesan and pepper. Remove from warmth when sauce reaches desired consistency. Sauce will thicken rapidly, thin with milk if cooked too long. Toss with hot pasta to serve.

648 calories; 57.1 g fat; 10 g is carbohydrates; 25.1 g is protein; 170 mg cholesterol; 1030 mg is sodium

Cilantro-Lime Dressing

Ingredients
1 jalapeno pepper, seeded and coarsely chopped
1 clove garlic
3/4 teaspoon minced fresh ginger root
1/4 cup lime juice
1/3 cup honey
2 teaspoons balsamic vinegar
1/2 teaspoon salt, or to taste
1/4 cup packed cilantro leaves
1/2 cup extra-virgin olive oil

Place the jalapeno pepper, garlic clove, and ginger into a food processor or blender; pulse till the jalapeno and garlic are finely chopped. Pour within the lime juice, honey, balsamic vinegar, and salt, upload the cilantro leaves; pulse a few instances to blend. Turn the food processor or blender on, and slowly drizzle in the olive oil until integrated into the dressing. Season to taste with salt earlier than serving.

Per Serving: 87 calories; 7 g fat; 6.4 g carbohydrates; 0.1 g protein; 0 mg cholesterol; 74 mg sodium.

Yummy Honey Mustard Dipping Sauce

Ingredients
1/2 cup mayonnaise
2 tablespoons prepared yellow mustard
1 tablespoon Dijon mustard
2 tablespoons honey
1/2 tablespoon lemon juice

Mix the mayonnaise, yellow mustard, Dijon mustard, honey, and lemon juice together in a bowl. Cover and chill in refrigerator overnight.

Per Serving: 159 calories; 14.8 g fat; 7.3 g carbohydrates; 0.4 g protein; 7 mg cholesterol; 225 mg sodium

Bill's Blue Cheese Dressing

Ingredients
3/4 cup sour cream
1 1/3 cups mayonnaise
1 teaspoon Worcestershire sauce
1/2 teaspoon dry mustard
1/2 teaspoon garlic powder
1/2 teaspoon salt
1/2 teaspoon ground black pepper
4 ounces blue cheese, crumbled

In a bowl, mix the sour cream, mayonnaise and Worcestershire sauce. Season with mustard, garlic powder, salt and pepper. Stir in blue cheese. Cover, and refrigerate for 24 hours before serving.

Per Serving: 241 calories; 25.2 g fat; 1.9 g carbohydrates; 2.8 g protein; 23 mg cholesterol; 380 mg sodium.

Proper Pesto

Ingredients
4 cloves garlic, peeled
1/4 teaspoon kosher salt
1 large bunch fresh basil
3 tablespoons pine nuts
2 ounces finely grated Parmigiano-Reggiano cheese
1/2 cup mild extra-virgin olive oil

Crush garlic and pinch of kosher salt in a mortar with the pestle till garlic is mashed and paste-like, 1 or 2 minutes. Add basil in 3 or four additions, crushing and pounding down the leaves till they shape a fairly excellent paste, about 8 minutes or more relying on size of leaves and thickness of stems. Add and pound in pine nuts.

Transfer a handful of grated cheese to mortar and pound into the sauce. Add another handful of cheese and comprise into the mixture. Continue adding cheese a handful at a time till completely incorporated, about five min.

Drizzle in olive oil 1 tablespoon at a time, pounding it into the sauce. When all of the olive oil has been brought and emulsified into the mixture, transfer pesto to a bowl and drizzle floor with olive oil.

Per Serving: 181 calories; 17.8 g fat; 1.7 g carbohydrates; 4.1 g protein; 6 mg cholesterol; 169 mg sodium.

Cilantro Jalapeno Pesto with Lime

Ingredients
1 bunch fresh cilantro
2 1/2 tablespoons toasted pine nuts
1/4 cup extra virgin olive oil
5 cloves garlic
1 tablespoon fresh lime juice
1/2 fresh jalapeno pepper, seeded
1/4 cup grated Parmesan cheese

Combine the cilantro, pine nuts, olive oil, garlic, lime juice, jalapeno pepper, and Parmesan cheese in a blender; pulse until the mixture reaches a soft, paste-like consistency.

Per Serving: 129 calories; 12.4 g fat; 1.9 g carbohydrates; 2.8 g protein; 4 mg cholesterol; 69 mg sodium.

Garlic Scape Pesto

Ingredients
1 pound garlic scapes, cut into 2-inch pieces
1 1/4 cups grated Parmesan cheese
1 cup olive oil
1 tablespoon lemon juice
ground black pepper to taste

Blend the garlic scapes, Parmesan cheese, olive oil, lemon juice, and pepper together in a food processor until smooth.
Per Serving: 108 calories; 8.8 g fat; 5.6 g carbohydrates; 2.4 g protein; 3 mg cholesterol; 58 mg sodium

Cranberry, Apple, and Fresh Ginger Chutney

Ingredients
4 cups fresh cranberries
1 cup raisins
1/2 cup white sugar
3/4 cup packed brown sugar
2 teaspoons ground cinnamon
1 teaspoon minced fresh ginger root
1/4 teaspoon ground cloves
1 cup water
1/2 cup minced onion
1/2 cup chopped Granny Smith apple
1/2 cup finely chopped celery

Combine the cranberries, raisins, white sugar, brown sugar, cinnamon, ginger, cloves and water in a saucepan. Bring to a boil, then simmer over low heat until berries start to pop, about 5 minutes. Add the onion, apple, and celery; continue to cook, stirring occasionally, until the mixture begins to thicken, 5 to 10 more minutes. Transfer to a container and cool slightly. Refrigerate overnight to allow the flavors to blossom.
Per Serving: 224 calories; 0.2 g fat; 58.5 g carbohydrates; 1.1 g protein; 0 mg cholesterol; 17 mg sodium

Alfredo Sauce

Ingredients
1/4 cup butter
1 cup heavy cream
1 clove garlic, crushed
1 1/2 cups freshly grated Parmesan cheese
1/4 cup chopped fresh parsley

Melt butter in a medium saucepan over medium low heat. Add cream and simmer for 5 minutes, then add garlic and cheese and whisk quickly, heating through. Stir in parsley and serve.
Per Serving: 439 calories; 42.1 g fat; 3.4 g carbohydrates; 13 g protein; 138 mg cholesterol; 565 mg sodium

Homemade Mayonnaise

Ingredients
2 egg yolks
1 tablespoon fresh lemon juice
1 tablespoon white wine vinegar
1 teaspoon Dijon mustard
3/4 teaspoon salt
1/8 teaspoon white sugar
1 cup vegetable oil
1/2 cup olive oil

Pour egg yolks, lemon juice, white wine vinegar, Dijon mustard, salt, sugar, vegetable oil, and olive oil, respectively, into a tall, narrow bowl. Set a immersion blender into the oil mixture and hold against the bottom of the bowl; pulse until a thick, pale mixture begins to form, about 3 to 6 pulses. Continue blending until smooth and creamy.
Per Serving: 188 calories; 21.1 g fat; 0.3 g carbohydrates; 0.3 g protein; 26 mg cholesterol; 118 mg sodium.

Spinach Basil Pesto

Ingredients
1 1/2 cups baby spinachleaves
3/4 cup fresh basil leaves
1/2 cup toasted pine nuts
1/2 cup grated Parmesan cheese
4 cloves garlic, peeled and quartered
3/4 teaspoon kosher salt
1/2 teaspoon freshly ground black pepper
1 tablespoon fresh lemon juice
1/2 teaspoon lemon zest
1/2 cup extra-virgin olive oil

Blend the spinach, basil, pine nuts, Parmesan cheese, garlic, salt, pepper, lemon juice, lemon zest, and 2 tablespoons olive oil in a food processor until nearly smooth, scraping the sides of the bowl with a spatula as necessary. Drizzle the remaining olive oil into the mixture while processing until smooth.
Per Serving: 67 calories; 6.6 g fat; 0.8 g carbohydrates; 1.5 g protein; 1 mg cholesterol; 87 mg sodium

Spiced Apple Chutney

Ingredients
1 1/2 cups white vinegar
1 1/2 cups white sugar
4 tart apples - peeled, cored, and cut into 1/2-inch cubes
1/4 cup diced dried apricots
1/4 cup golden raisins
1/4 cup diced shallots
5 thick slices fresh ginger
1/4 teaspoon Aleppo pepper flakes, or to taste
1 whole star anise
2 cloves garlic, minced
1 teaspoon kosher salt, or to taste
1/2 teaspoon yellow mustard seed

Whisk vinegar and sugar together in a large saucepan; add apples, apricots, raisins, shallots, ginger, Aleppo pepper flakes, and star anise. Bring to a simmer, reduce heat to medium-low; stir in garlic, salt, and mustard.
Simmer mixture, stirring occasionally, until fruit is soft and liquid is reduced, 40 to 45 minutes. Remove from heat and cool to room temperature. Remove ginger pieces and star anise, transfer mixture to a bowl, and refrigerate until chilled. Season with salt and pepper flakes

Per Serving: 107 calories; 0.1 g fat; 27.6 g carbohydrates; 0.4 g protein; 0 mg cholesterol; 121 mg sodium

Sweet Tamarind Chutney

Ingredients
1 tablespoon canola oil
1 teaspoon cumin seeds
1 teaspoon ground ginger
1/2 teaspoon cayenne pepper
1/2 teaspoon fennel seeds
1/2 teaspoon asafoetida powder
1/2 teaspoon garam masala
2 cups water
1 1/8 cups white sugar
3 tablespoons tamarind paste

Heat the oil in a saucepan over medium heat. Add the cumin seeds, ginger, cayenne pepper, fennel seeds, asafoetida powder, and garam masala; cook and stir for about 2 minutes to release the flavors.

Stir the water into the pan with the spices along with the sugar and tamarind paste. Bring to a boil, then simmer over low heat until the mixture turns a deep chocolaty brown and is thick enough to coat the back of a metal spoon. This should take 20 to 30 minutes. The sauce will be thin, but it will thicken upon cooling.

Per Serving: 113 calories; 1.5 g fat; 25.7 g carbohydrates; 0.2 g protein; 0 mg cholesterol; 3 mg sodium

Hot Pepper Jelly

Ingredients
2 1/2 cups finely chopped red bell peppers
1 1/4 cups finely chopped green bell peppers
1/4 cup finely chopped jalapeno peppers
1 cup apple cider vinegar
1 (1.75 ounce) package powdered pectin
5 cups white sugar

Sterilize 6 (8 ounce) canning jars and lids according to manufacturer's instructions. Heat water in a hot water canner.

Place red bell peppers, green bell peppers, and jalapeno peppers in a large saucepan over high heat. Mix in vinegar and fruit pectin. Stirring constantly, bring mixture to a full rolling boil. Quickly stir in sugar. Return to full rolling boil, and boil exactly 1 minute, stirring constantly. Remove from heat, and skim off any foam.

Quickly ladle jelly into sterile jars, filling to within 1/4 inch of the tops. Cover with flat lids, and screw on bands tightly.

Place jars in rack, and slowly lower jars into canner. The water should cover the jars completely, and should be hot but not boiling. Bring water to a boil, and process for 5 minutes.

Per Serving: 88 calories; 0 g fat; 22.5 g carbohydrates; 0.1 g protein; 0 mg cholesterol; 3 mg sodium

Chimichurri Sauce

Ingredients
1/2 cup olive oil
4 cloves garlic, chopped, or more to taste
3 tablespoons white wine vinegar, or more to taste
1/2 teaspoon salt, or to taste
1/4 teaspoon ground cumin
1/4 teaspoon red pepper flakes
1/4 teaspoon freshly ground black pepper
1/2 cup fresh cilantro leaves
1/4 cup fresh oregano leaves
1 bunch flat-leaf Italian parsley, stems removed

Combine oil, garlic, vinegar, salt, cumin, red pepper flakes, black pepper, cilantro, oregano, and parsley in a blender.

Pulse blender 2 to 3 times; scrape down the sides using a rubber spatula. Repeat pulsing and scraping process until a thick sauce forms, about 12 times.

Per Serving: 255 calories; 27.3 g fat; 3 g carbohydrates; 1 g protein; 0 mg cholesterol; 304 mg sodium

Bar-B-Q Sauce

Ingredients
2 cups ketchup
2 cups tomato sauce
1 1/4 cups brown sugar
1 1/4 cups red wine vinegar
1/2 cup unsulfured molasses
4 teaspoons hickory-flavored liquid smoke
2 tablespoons butter
1/2 teaspoon garlic powder
1/2 teaspoon onion powder
1/4 teaspoon chili powder
1 teaspoon paprika
1/2 teaspoon celery seed
1/4 teaspoon ground cinnamon
1/2 teaspoon cayenne pepper
1 teaspoon salt
1 teaspoon coarsely ground black pepper

In a large saucepan over medium heat, mix together the ketchup, tomato sauce, brown sugar, wine vinegar, molasses, liquid smoke and butter. Season with garlic powder, onion powder, chili powder, paprika, celery seed, cinnamon, cayenne, salt and pepper.

Reduce heat to low, and simmer for up to 20 minutes. For thicker sauce, simmer longer, and for thinner, less time is needed. Sauce can also be thinned using a bit of water if necessary. Brush sauce onto any kind of meat during the last 10 minutes of cooking.

Per Serving: 46 calories; 0.9 g fat; 9.9 g carbohydrates; 0.3 g protein; 1 mg cholesterol; 219 mg sodium

Spicy Cranberry Chutney

Ingredients
1/4 cup dried apricots, finely chopped
1/2 cup brown sugar
1/2 cup raisins
1 cup water

3 cups fresh cranberries
1 Granny Smith apple - peeled, cored and chopped
1 teaspoon grated lemon zest
1/4 cup fresh lemon juice
1/4 cup chopped crystallized ginger
1/2 teaspoon red pepper flakes
In a saucepan, combine apricots, brown sugar, raisins and water; bring to a boil. Reduce heat to simmer and stir while simmering for 5 minutes. Stir in cranberries, apple and lemon zest; simmer for 10 minutes more.
Stir lemon juice, ginger and pepper flakes into the mixture before removing from heat. Serve chilled or at room temperature.
 Per Serving: 97 calories; 0.1 g fat; 25.3 g carbohydrates; 0.5 g protein; 0 mg cholesterol; 6 mg sodium.
Snacks and fruit recipes

MINI BELL PEPPER TURKEY "NACHOS"
INGREDIENTS
- olive oil spray
- lb 93% lean ground turkey
- 1 clove garlic, minced
- 1/4 onion, minced
- 1 tbsp chopped fresh cilantro or parsley
- 1 tsp garlic powder
- 1 tsp cumin powder
- 1 tsp kosher salt
- 1/4 cup tomato sauce
- 1/4 cup chicken broth
- 21 mini rainbow peppers, halved and seeded (about 13 oz seeded)
- 1 cup sharp shredded Cheddar cheese
- 2 tbsp light sour cream, thinned with 1 tbsp water
- 2 tbsp sliced black olives
- 1 jalapeno, sliced thin (optional)
- chopped cilantro, for garnish

INSTRUCTIONS
Preheat oven to 400F and line a large baking try with parchment or aluminum foil. Lightly spray with oil.
Spray oil in a medium nonstick skillet over medium heat.
Add onion, garlic and cilantro and saute about 2 minutes, add ground turkey, salt, garlic powder, cumin and cook meat for 4 to 5 minutes until meat is completely cooked through. Add 1/4 cup of tomato sauce and chicken broth, mix well and simmer on medium for about 5 minutes, remove from heat.
Meanwhile, arrange mini peppers in a single layer, cut-side up close together.
Fill each with cooked ground turkey mixture, then top with shredded cheese and jalapeno slices, if using. Bake 8 to 10 minutes, until cheese is melted.
Remove from oven and top with black olives, sour cream and cilantro. Serve immediately.
Serving: 7nachos, Calories: 187kcal, Carbohydrates: 6.5g, Protein: 18g, Fat: 11g, Saturated Fat: 4.5g,
Cholesterol: 62mg, Sodium: 418mg, Fiber: 1g, Sugar: 0.5g

ROAST CHICKPEAS
INGREDIENTS
2 cans chickpeas (low-sodium or no-salt-added)
oil for misting
spices (i use paprika and cayenne pepper)
INSTRUCTIONS
Drain and rinse the chickpeas.
Line a baking sheet with paper towels. Pour the chickpeas on top and use more paper towels to dry them off as well as possible.
Remove the paper towels.
Mist the chickpeas with oil, sprinkle with spices and shake pan gently until all the chickpeas are well coated.
Place pan in a cold oven.
Set oven to 425 degrees F and let roast for 25-30 minutes, shaking the pan halfway thru. The timer starts as soon as you put them in a cold oven and turn it on.
When the timer goes off, stir once more, turn the oven off and leave pan in the oven for 3-4 hours. Remove and let cool completely before transferring to a storage container.

Strawberry Corn Salsa
Ingredients
2 cups fresh strawberries, chopped
2 cups grape tomatoes, chopped
1 package (10 ounces) frozen corn, thawed
2 green onions, chopped
3 tablespoons minced fresh cilantro
1/3 cup olive oil
2 tablespoons raspberry vinegar
2 tablespoons lime juice
1/2 teaspoon salt
Baked tortilla chips
In a large bowl, combine the first 5 ingredients. In a small bowl, whisk the oil, vinegar, lime juice and salt. Drizzle over strawberry mixture; toss to coat. Refrigerate for 1 hour. Serve with chips.
Nutrition Facts
1/4 cup: 49 calories, 3g fat (0 saturated fat), 0 cholesterol, 56mg sodium, 5g carbohydrate (1g sugars, 1g fiber), 1g protein.

Balsamic-Goat Cheese Grilled Plums
Ingredients
1 cup balsamic vinegar
2 teaspoons grated lemon zest
4 medium firm plums, halved and pitted
1/2 cup crumbled goat cheese
For glaze, in a small saucepan, combine vinegar and lemon zest; bring to a boil. Cook 10-12 minutes or until mixture is thickened and reduced to about 1/3 cup (do not overcook).

Grill plums, covered, over medium heat 2-3 minutes on each side or until tender. Drizzle with glaze; top with cheese.
Nutrition Facts
1 plum half with 1 tablespoon cheese and 2 teaspoons glaze: 58 calories, 2g fat (1g saturated fat), 9mg cholesterol, 41mg sodium, 9g carbohydrate (8g sugars, 1g fiber), 2g protein. Diabetic Exchanges: 1/2 starch, 1/2 fat.

Berry White Ice Pops
Ingredients
1-3/4 cups whole milk, divided
1 to 2 tablespoons honey
1/4 teaspoon vanilla extract
1-1/2 cups fresh raspberries
1 cup fresh blueberries
10 freezer pop molds or 10 paper cups (3 ounces each) and wooden pop sticks
In a microwave, warm 1/4 cup milk; stir in honey until blended. Stir in remaining 1-1/2 cups milk and vanilla.
Divide berries among molds; cover with milk mixture. Top molds with holders. If using cups, top with foil and insert sticks through foil. Freeze until firm.
Nutrition Facts
1 pop: 51 calories, 2g fat (1g saturated fat), 4mg cholesterol, 19mg sodium, 8g carbohydrate (6g sugars, 2g fiber), 2g protein. Diabetic Exchanges: 1/2 starch.

Strawberry Lime Smoothies
Ingredients
1 cup strawberry yogurt
1/2 cup 2% milk
2 to 4 tablespoons lime juice
2 tablespoons honey
1/4 teaspoon ground cinnamon
2 cups fresh strawberries, hulled
Process all ingredients in a covered blender until smooth.
Nutrition Facts
1 cup: 172 calories, 2g fat (1g saturated fat), 7mg cholesterol, 61mg sodium, 36g carbohydrate (32g sugars, 2g fiber), 5g protein

Mixed Fruit with Lemon-Basil Dressing
Ingredients
2 tablespoons lemon juice
1/2 teaspoon sugar
1/4 teaspoon salt
1/4 teaspoon ground mustard
1/8 teaspoon onion powder
Dash pepper
6 tablespoons olive oil
4-1/2 teaspoons minced fresh basil
1 cup cubed fresh pineapple
1 cup sliced fresh strawberries
1 cup sliced peeled kiwifruit
1 cup seedless watermelon balls
1 cup fresh blueberries
1 cup fresh raspberries
Place the lemon juice, sugar, salt, mustard, onion powder and pepper in a blender; cover and pulse until blended. While processing, gradually add oil in a steady stream. Stir in basil.
In a large bowl, combine the fruit. Drizzle with dressing and toss to coat. Refrigerate until serving.
Nutrition Facts
3/4 cup: 145 calories, 11g fat (1g saturated fat), 0 cholesterol, 76mg sodium, 14g carbohydrate (9g sugars, 3g fiber), 1g protein. Diabetic exchanges: 2 fat, 1 fruit.

Crunchy Peanut Butter Apple Dip
Ingredients
1 carton (8 ounces) reduced-fat spreadable cream cheese
1 cup creamy peanut butter
1/4 cup fat-free milk
1 tablespoon brown sugar
1 teaspoon vanilla extract
1/2 cup chopped unsalted peanuts
Apple slices
In a small bowl, beat the first five ingredients until blended. Stir in peanuts. Serve with apple slices. Refrigerate leftovers.
Nutrition Facts
2 tablespoons (calculated without apples): 126 calories, 10g fat (3g saturated fat), 5mg cholesterol, 115mg sodium, 5g carbohydrate (3g sugars, 1g fiber), 5g protein.

Citrusy Fruit Kabobs
Ingredients
1/3 cup orange juice
2 tablespoons lemon juice
4-1/2 teaspoons honey
2 teaspoons cornstarch
1-1/2 teaspoons grated lemon zest
1/4 teaspoon ground allspice
24 fresh strawberries
16 cubes fresh pineapple
2 small bananas, cut into 1-inch pieces
2 teaspoons minced fresh mint
In a small saucepan, combine the first six ingredients. Bring to a boil; cook and stir for 2 minutes or until thickened. Remove from the heat; cool to room temperature.
Thread fruit onto eight metal or soaked wooden skewers. Brush with half of glaze. Lightly oil grill rack. Grill, covered, over medium heat until lightly browned, 5-7 minutes, turning occasionally and basting frequently with remaining glaze. Just before serving, sprinkle with mint. Serve warm.
Nutrition Facts
1 kabob: 83 calories, 0 fat (0 saturated fat), 0 cholesterol, 2mg sodium, 21g carbohydrate (15g sugars, 2g fiber), 1g protein. Diabetic Exchanges: 1 fruit.

Frozen Pops (Pineapple-Kiwi)
Ingredients
3 cups cubed fresh pineapple
1 cup water, divided
8 teaspoons sugar, divided
12 paper cups (3 ounces each) and wooden pop sticks
2 cups sliced peeled kiwifruit (about 6 medium)
Place pineapple, 1/2 cup water and 4 teaspoons sugar in a food processor; pulse until combined. Divide among cups. Top cups with foil and insert sticks through foil. Freeze until firm, about 2 hours. Place kiwi and remaining water and sugar in food processor; pulse until combined. Spoon over pineapple layer. Freeze, covered, until firm.
Nutrition Facts
1 pop: 50 calories, 0 fat (0 saturated fat), 0 cholesterol, 1mg sodium, 13g carbohydrate (10g sugars, 1g fiber), 1g protein. Diabetic Exchanges: 1 fruit.

Grilled Stone Fruits with Balsamic Syrup
Ingredients
1/2 cup balsamic vinegar
2 tablespoons brown sugar
2 medium peaches, peeled and halved
2 medium nectarines, peeled and halved
2 medium plums, peeled and halved
In a small saucepan, combine vinegar and brown sugar. Bring to a boil; cook until liquid is reduced by half.
On a lightly oiled grill rack, grill peaches, nectarines and plums, covered, over medium heat or broil 4 in. from the heat until tender, 3-4 minutes on each side or until tender.
Slice fruits; arrange on a serving plate. Drizzle with sauce.
Nutrition Facts
1 serving: 114 calories, 1g fat (0 saturated fat), 0 cholesterol, 10mg sodium, 28g carbohydrate (24g sugars, 2g fiber), 2g protein. Diabetic Exchanges: 1 starch, 1 fruit.

Avocado Fruit Salad with Tangerine Vinaigrette
Ingredients
 3 medium ripe avocados, peeled and thinly sliced
3 medium mangoes, peeled and thinly sliced
1 cup fresh raspberries
1 cup fresh blackberries
1/4 cup minced fresh mint
1/4 cup sliced almonds, toasted
DRESSING:
1/2 cup olive oil
1 teaspoon grated tangerine or orange peel
1/4 cup tangerine or orange juice
2 tablespoons balsamic vinegar
1/2 teaspoon salt
1/4 teaspoon freshly ground pepper
Arrange avocados and fruit on a serving plate; sprinkle with mint and almonds. In a small bowl, whisk dressing ingredients until blended; drizzle over salad.
Nutrition Facts
1 cup salad with 4 teaspoons dressing: 321 calories, 23g fat (3g saturated fat), 0 cholesterol, 154mg sodium, 29g carbohydrate (20g sugars, 8g fiber), 3g protein.

Chili-Lime Grilled Pineapple
Ingredients
1 fresh pineapple
3 tablespoons brown sugar
1 tablespoon lime juice
1 tablespoon olive oil
1 tablespoon honey or agave nectar
1-1/2 teaspoons chili powder
Dash salt
Peel pineapple, removing any eyes from fruit. Cut lengthwise into 6 wedges; remove core. In a small bowl, mix remaining ingredients until blended. Brush pineapple with half of the glaze; reserve remaining mixture for basting.
Grill pineapple, covered, over medium heat or broil 4 in. from heat 2-4 minutes on each side or until lightly browned, basting occasionally with reserved glaze.
Nutrition Facts
1 serving: 97 calories, 2g fat (0 saturated fat), 0 cholesterol, 35mg sodium, 20g carbohydrate (17g sugars, 1g fiber), 1g protein. Diabetic Exchanges: 1/2 starch, 1/2 fruit, 1/2 fat.

Italian Sausage-Stuffed Zucchini
Ingredients
6 medium zucchini (about 8 ounces each)
1 pound Italian turkey sausage links, casings removed
2 medium tomatoes, seeded and chopped
1 cup panko (Japanese) bread crumbs
1/3 cup grated Parmesan cheese
1/3 cup minced fresh parsley
2 tablespoons minced fresh oregano or 2 teaspoons dried oregano
2 tablespoons minced fresh basil or 2 teaspoons dried basil
1/4 teaspoon pepper
3/4 cup shredded part-skim mozzarella cheese
Additional minced fresh parsley, optional
Preheat oven to 350°. Cut each zucchini lengthwise in half. Scoop out pulp, leaving a 1/4-in. shell; chop pulp. Place zucchini shells in a large microwave-safe dish. In batches, microwave, covered, on high 2-3 minutes or until crisp-tender.
In a large skillet, cook sausage and zucchini pulp over medium heat 6-8 minutes or until sausage is no longer pink, breaking sausage into crumbles; drain. Stir in tomatoes, bread crumbs, Parmesan cheese, herbs and pepper. Spoon into zucchini shells.

Place in 2 ungreased 13x9-in. baking dishes. Bake, covered, 15–20 minutes or until zucchini is tender. Sprinkle with mozzarella cheese. Bake, uncovered, 5-8 minutes longer or until cheese is melted. If desired, sprinkle with additional minced parsley.

Nutrition Facts
2 stuffed zucchini halves: 206 calories, 9g fat (3g saturated fat), 39mg cholesterol, 485mg sodium, 16g carbohydrate (5g sugars, 3g fiber), 17g protein. Diabetic Exchanges: 2 lean meat, 2 vegetable, 1/2 starch.

Frozen Berry & Yogurt Swirls

Ingredients
10 plastic or paper cups (3 ounces each)
2-3/4 cups fat-free honey Greek yogurt
1 cup mixed fresh berries
1/4 cup water
2 tablespoons sugar
10 wooden pop sticks

Fill each cup with about 1/4 cup yogurt. Place berries, water and sugar in a food processor; pulse until berries are finely chopped. Spoon 1-1/2 tablespoons berry mixture into each cup. Stir gently with a pop stick to swirl.
Top cups with foil; insert pop sticks through foil. Freeze until firm.
For Frozen Clementine & Yogurt Swirls Substitute 1 cup seeded clementine segments (about 5 medium) and 1/4 cup orange juice for berries, water and sugar; proceed as directed.

Nutrition Facts
1 pop: 60 calories, 0 fat (0 saturated fat), 0 cholesterol, 28mg sodium, 9g carbohydrate (8g sugars, 1g fiber), 6g protein. Diabetic Exchanges: 1 starch.

Tomato Green Bean Soup

Ingredients
1 cup chopped onion
1 cup chopped carrots
2 teaspoons butter
6 cups reduced-sodium chicken or vegetable broth
1 pound fresh green beans, cut into 1-inch pieces
1 garlic clove, minced
3 cups diced fresh tomatoes
1/4 cup minced fresh basil or 1 tablespoon dried basil
1/2 teaspoon salt
1/4 teaspoon pepper

In a large saucepan, saute onion and carrots in butter for 5 minutes. Stir in the broth, beans and garlic; bring to a boil. Reduce heat; cover and simmer for 20 minutes or until vegetables are tender.
Stir in the tomatoes, basil, salt and pepper. Cover and simmer 5 minutes longer.

Nutrition Facts
1 cup: 58 calories, 1g fat (1g saturated fat), 2mg cholesterol, 535mg sodium, 10g carbohydrate (5g sugars, 3g fiber), 4g protein. Diabetic Exchanges: 2 vegetable

Avocado Fruit Salad

Ingredients
1/2 cup plain yogurt
2 tablespoons honey
1 teaspoon grated lemon zest
1 teaspoon plus 2 tablespoons lemon juice, divided
3 medium ripe avocados, peeled and cubed
1 medium apple, chopped
1 cup halved seedless grapes
1 can (11 ounces) mandarin oranges, drained
1 medium firm banana, cut into 1/4-inch slices

For dressing, mix yogurt, honey, lemon zest and 1 teaspoon lemon juice. Toss avocados with remaining lemon juice.
In a large bowl, combine remaining ingredients; gently stir in avocados. Serve with dressing.

Nutrition Facts
3/4 cup: 231 calories, 11g fat (2g saturated fat), 3mg cholesterol, 22mg sodium, 35g carbohydrate (25g sugars, 6g fiber), 3g protein.

Double-Nut Stuffed Figs

Ingredients
36 dried Calimyrna figs
2/3 cup finely chopped pecans
2/3 cup finely chopped walnuts
7 tablespoons agave nectar, divided
3 tablespoons baking cocoa
1/4 teaspoon ground cinnamon
1/8 teaspoon ground cloves
1/2 cup pomegranate juice
4-1/2 teaspoons lemon juice

Preheat oven to 350°. Remove stems from figs. Cut an "X" in the top of each fig, about two-thirds of the way down.
In a small bowl, combine pecans, walnuts, 3 tablespoons agave nectar, cocoa, cinnamon and cloves; spoon into figs. Arrange in a 13x9-in. baking dish coated with cooking spray.
In a small bowl, mix pomegranate juice, lemon juice and remaining agave nectar; drizzle over figs. Bake, covered, 20 minutes. Bake, uncovered, 8-10 minutes longer or until heated through, basting occasionally with cooking liquid.

Nutrition Facts
1 stuffed fig: 98 calories, 3g fat (0 saturated fat), 0 cholesterol, 3mg sodium, 17g carbohydrate (13g sugars, 3g fiber), 1g protein. Diabetic Exchanges: 1 starch, 1/2 fat.

Frosty Watermelon Ice

Ingredients
1 teaspoon unflavored gelatin
2 tablespoons water
2 tablespoons lime juice
2 tablespoons honey
4 cups cubed seedless watermelon, divided

In a microwave-safe bowl, sprinkle gelatin over water; let stand 1 minute. Microwave on high for 40 seconds. Stir and let stand 1-2 minutes or until gelatin is completely dissolved.

Place lime juice, honey and gelatin mixture in a blender. Add 1 cup watermelon; cover and process until blended. Add remaining watermelon, 1 cup at a time, processing after each addition until smooth. Transfer to a shallow dish; freeze until almost firm. In a chilled bowl, beat with an electric mixer until mixture is bright pink. Divide among 4 serving dishes; freeze, covered, until firm. Remove from freezer 15-20 minutes before serving.

Nutrition Facts
3/4 cup: 81 calories, 0 fat (0 saturated fat), 0 cholesterol, 3mg sodium, 21g carbohydrate (18g sugars, 1g fiber), 1g protein. Diabetic Exchanges: 1 fruit, 1/2 starch.

Apple-Nut Blue Cheese Tartlets

Ingredients
1 large apple, peeled and finely chopped
1 medium onion, finely chopped
2 teaspoons butter
1 cup (4 ounces) crumbled blue cheese
4 tablespoons finely chopped walnuts, toasted, divided
1/2 teaspoon salt
1 package (1.9 ounces) frozen miniature phyllo tart shells

In a small nonstick skillet, saute apple and onion in butter until tender. Remove from the heat; stir in the blue cheese, 3 tablespoons walnuts and salt. Spoon a rounded tablespoonful into each tart shell.

Place on an ungreased baking sheet. Bake at 350° for 5 minutes. Sprinkle with remaining walnuts; bake 2-3 minutes longer or until lightly browned.

Freeze option: Freeze cooled pastries in a freezer container, separating layers with waxed paper. To use, reheat pastries on a <u>baking sheet</u> in a preheated 350° oven until crisp and heated through.

Nutrition Facts
1 tartlet: 76 calories, 5g fat (2g saturated fat), 7mg cholesterol, 200mg sodium, 5g carbohydrate (2g sugars, 0 fiber), 3g protein. Diabetic Exchanges: 1 fat, 1/2 starch.

Dessert Recipes

Ambrosia With Coconut And Toasted Almonds

Ingredients
1/2 cup slivered almonds
1/2 cup unsweetened shredded coconut
1 small pineapple, cubed (about 3 cups)
5 oranges, segmented
2 red apples, cored and diced
1 banana, halved lengthwise, peeled and sliced crosswise
2 tablespoons cream sherry
Fresh mint leaves for garnish

Directions
Heat the oven to 325 F. Spread the almonds on a baking sheet and bake, stirring occasionally, until golden and fragrant, about 10 minutes Transfer immediately to a plate to cool. Add the coconut to the sheet and bake, stirring often, until lightly browned, about 10 minutes. Transfer immediately to a plate to cool.
In a large bowl, combine the pineapple, oranges, apples, banana and sherry. Toss gently to mix well. Divide the fruit mixture evenly among individual bowls. Sprinkle evenly with the toasted almonds and coconut and garnish with the mint. Serve immediately.

Nutrition
Calories177 Total fat5 g Saturated fat1 gTransfatTraceMonounsaturated fat2 g Cholesterol0 mg Sodium2 mg Total carbohydrate30 g Dietary fiber6 g Total sugars21 g Protein3 g

Apple-Berry Cobbler

Ingredients
For the filling:
1 cup fresh raspberries
1 cup fresh blueberries
2 cups chopped apples
2 tablespoons turbinado or brown sugar
1/2 teaspoon ground cinnamon
1 teaspoon lemon zest
2 teaspoons lemon juice
1 1/2 tablespoons cornstarch
For the topping:
Egg white from 1 large egg
1/4 cup soy milk
1/4 teaspoon salt
1/2 teaspoon vanilla
1 1/2 tablespoons turbinado or brown sugar
3/4 cup whole-wheat pastry flour

Directions
Preheat the oven to 350 F. Lightly coat 6 individual ovenproof ramekins with cooking spray.
In a medium bowl, add the raspberries, blueberries, apples, sugar, cinnamon, lemon zest and lemon juice. Stir to mix evenly. Add the cornstarch and stir until the cornstarch dissolves. Set aside.
In a separate bowl add the egg white and whisk until lightly beaten. Add the soy milk, salt, vanilla, sugar and pastry flour. Stir to mix well.
Divide the berry mixture evenly among the prepared dishes. Pour the topping over each. Arrange the ramekins on a large baking pan and place in oven. Bake until the berries are tender and the topping is golden brown, about 30 minutes. Serve warm.

Nutrition
Calories136 Total fatTrace Saturated fatTrace Cholesterol0 mg Sodium111 mg Total carbohydrate31 g Dietary fiber4 g Protein3 g

Apple-Blueberry Cobbler

Ingredients
2 large apples, peeled, cored and thinly sliced
1 tablespoon lemon juice
2 tablespoons sugar
2 tablespoons cornstarch
1 teaspoon ground cinnamon
12 ounces fresh or frozen blueberries
For the topping
3/4 cup all-purpose flour
3/4 cup whole-wheat flour
2 tablespoons sugar
1 1/2 teaspoons baking powder
1/4 teaspoon salt
4 tablespoons cold trans-free margarine, cut into pieces
1/2 cup fat-free milk
1 teaspoon vanilla extract

Directions
Heat the oven to 400 F. Lightly coat a 9-inch square baking dish with cooking spray.
In a large bowl, add the apple slices. Sprinkle with lemon juice. In a small bowl, combine the sugar, cornstarch and cinnamon. Add the mixture to the apples and toss gently to mix. Stir in the blueberries. Spread the apple-blueberry mixture evenly in the prepared baking dish. Set aside.
In another large bowl, combine the flours, sugar, baking powder and salt. Using a fork, cut the cold margarine into the dry ingredients until the mixture resembles coarse crumbs. Add the milk and vanilla. Stir just until a moist dough forms. Turn the dough onto a generously floured work surface and, with floured hands, knead gently 6 to 8 times until the dough is smooth and manageable. Using a rolling pin, roll the dough into a rectangle 1/2-inch thick. Use a cookie cutter to cut out shapes. Cut close together for a minimum of scraps. Gather the scraps and roll out to make more cuts.
Place the dough pieces over the apple-blueberry mixture until the top is covered. Bake until the apples are tender and the topping is golden, about 30 minutes. Serve warm.

Nutrition

Calories222 Total fat6 g Saturated fat1 g Sodium202 mg Total carbohydrate38 g Dietary fiber4 g Protein4 g

Baked Apples, Cherries And Almonds
Ingredients
- 1/3 cup dried cherries, coarsely chopped
- 3 tablespoons chopped almonds
- 1 tablespoon wheat germ
- 1 tablespoon firmly packed brown sugar
- 1/2 teaspoon ground cinnamon
- 1/8 teaspoon ground nutmeg
- 6 small Golden Delicious apples, about 1 3/4 pounds total weight
- 1/2 cup apple juice
- 1/4 cup water
- 2 tablespoons dark honey
- 2 teaspoons walnut oil or canola oil

Preheat the oven to 350 F.
In a small bowl, toss the cherries, almonds, wheat germ, brown sugar, cinnamon, and nutmeg collectively until all of the elements are calmly distributed. Set aside.
The apples can be left unpeeled, in case you like. To peel the apples decoratively, with a vegetable peeler or a sharp knife, cast off the peel from each apple in a round motion, skipping each other row so that rows of peel alternate with rows of apple flesh. Working from the stem end, core every apple, stopping 3/four inches from the bottom.
Divide the cherry combination evenly some of the apples, urgent the mixture gently into every cavity. Arrange the apples upright in a heavy ovenproof frying pan or small baking dish just massive sufficient to hold them. Pour the apple juice and water into the pan. Drizzle the honey and oil calmly over the apples, and cover the pan snugly with aluminum foil. Bake till the apples is soft when pierced with a knife, 50 to 60 mins.
Transfer the apples to person plates and drizzle with the pan juices. Serve heat or at room temperature.
Nutrition
Calories200 Total fat4 g Saturated fat0 g Cholesterol0 mg Sodium7 mg Total carbohydrate39 g Dietary fiber5 g Total sugars31 g Protein2 g

Grilled Food Cake
Ingredients
- 1 1/2 cup strawberries, chopped
- 3/4 cup chopped rhubarb
- 1/2 cup sugar
- 6 tablespoons water
- 1 3/4 teaspoons vanilla
- 1/8 teaspoon cinnamon
- 1 prepared angel food cake, cut into 6 pieces
- 3/4 cup reduced-fat whipped topping

Prepare a fire in a charcoal grill or warmth a gas grill or broiler. Away from the heat source, lightly coat the grill rack or broiler pan with cooking spray. Position the cooking rack 4 to 6 inches from the warmth source.
To make the sauce, in a saucepan, integrate the strawberries, rhubarb, sugar, water, vanilla, and cinnamon. Cook on medium heat until the aggregate starts to boil, about five min. Remove the saucepan from the heat and set aside.
Place the angel food cake closer to the edge of the grill rack where there is less warmness or on the broiler pan. Grill or broil till every facet turns brown, approximately 1 to 3 min.
Place the angel meals cake on the person serving plates. Top every piece with 1/four cup of the strawberry-rhubarb sauce and a couple of tablespoons of the whipped topping. Serve immediately.
Nutrition
Cholesterol0 mgCalories180 Sodium214 mg Total fat1 g Total carbohydrate40 g Saturated fat1 g Dietary fiber1 g Protein2 g

Balls Buckeye
Ingredients
- 1 1/2 cups creamy peanut butter
- 1/2 cup butter, softened
- 1 teaspoon vanilla extract
- 4 cups sifted confectioners' sugar
- 6 ounces semi-sweet chocolate chips
- 2 tablespoons shortening

Line a baking sheet with waxed paper; set aside.
In a medium bowl, mix peanut butter, butter, vanilla, and confectioners' sugar with hands to form a smooth, stiff dough. Shape into balls the usage of 2 teaspoons of money for each shot. Place on prepared pan, and refrigerate.
Melt shortening and chocolate together in a metallic bowl over a pan of lightly simmering water. Stir occasionally until smooth, and put off from the heat. Remove balls from the refrigerator. Insert a timber toothpick into a ball, and dip into melted chocolate. Return to wax paper, chocolate side down, and cast off the toothpick. Repeat with ultimate balls. Refrigerate for a half-hour to set.
204 calories; 12 g fat; 22.8 g carbohydrates; 3.7 g protein; 8 mg cholesterol; 81 mg sodium

Toffee Honeycomb
Ingredients
- 1 teaspoon baking soda
- 1/2 cup white sugar
- 2 tablespoons corn syrup
- 1 tablespoon honey
- 2 tablespoons water

Line a baking dish with parchment paper, measure out baking soda in a small bowl, and feature a heat-evidence spatula equipped before starting.
Whisk sugar, corn syrup, honey, and water collectively in a saucepan with a sweet thermometer

attached. Heat over medium heat till mixture is thinner however nevertheless cloudy. Let bubble till mixture is apparent, and thermometer registers 300 levels F (149 ranges C).

Remove from heat. Whisk in baking soda till just incorporated. Switch to a spatula and very cautiously pour into the covered dish. Do not spread it out with your spatula or compress mixture at all, or the bubbles will deflate. Let cool completely, at the least 30 mins.

Remove sweet from the pan by lifting out the parchment paper. Rap in opposition to the counter and use your fingers to interrupt it into individual pieces.

71 calories; 0 g fat; 18.6 g carbohydrates; 0 g protein; 0 mg cholesterol; 161 mg sodium.

Peanut Brittle

Ingredients
- 1 cup white sugar
- 1/2 cup light corn syrup
- 1/4 teaspoon salt
- 1/4 cup water
- 1 cup peanuts
- 2 tablespoons butter, softened
- 1 teaspoon baking soda

Grease a big cookie sheet. Set aside.

In a heavy 2 quart saucepan, over medium heat, convey to a boil sugar, corn syrup, salt, and water. Stir until sugar is dissolved. Stir in peanuts. Set a sweet thermometer in place, and keep cooking. Stir frequently till the temperature reaches 300 tiers F (150 levels C), or until a small quantity of aggregate dropped into icy water separates into delicate and brittle threads.

Remove from heat; straight away stir in butter and baking soda; pour at once onto cookie sheet. With two forks, elevate and pull peanut aggregate into a rectangle about 14x12 inches; cool — Snap candy into pieces.

143 calories; 6 g fat; 22.3 g carbohydrates; 2.2 g protein; 4 mg cholesterol; 132 mg sodium

Caramel

Ingredients
- 2 cups white sugar
- 1 cup packed brown sugar
- 1 cup corn syrup
- 1 cup evaporated milk
- 1 pint heavy whipping cream
- 1 cup butter
- 1 1/4 teaspoons vanilla extract

Grease a 12x15 inch pan.

In a medium-length pot, combine sugar, brown sugar, corn syrup, evaporated milk, whipping cream, and butter. Monitor the heat of the combination with a sweet thermometer, even as stirring. When the thermometer reaches 250 tiers, F (120 degrees C) dispose of the pot from the heat.

Stir in vanilla. Transfer combination to the organized pan and let the aggregate cool completely. When cooled, reduce the Carmel into small squares and wrap them in wax paper for storage.

115 calories; 6.3 g fat; 14.8 g carbohydrates; 0.5 g protein; 20 mg cholesterol; 30 mg sodium.

Pineapple Grilled

Ingredients
For the marinade
- 2 tablespoons dark honey
- 1 tablespoon olive oil
- 1 tablespoon fresh lime juice
- 1 teaspoon ground cinnamon
- 1/4 teaspoon ground cloves
- 1 firm, ripe pineapple
- 8 wooden skewers, soaked in water for 30 minutes, or metal skewers
- 1 tablespoon dark rum (optional)
- 1 tablespoon grated lime zest

Prepare a hot hearth in a charcoal grill or warmness a fuel grill or broiler (grill). Away from the heat source, lightly coat the grill rack or broiler pan with cooking spray. Position the cooking rack 4 to six inches from the heat source.

To make the marinade, in a small bowl, combine the honey, olive oil, lime juice, cinnamon, and cloves and whisk to blend. Set aside.

Cut off the crown of leaves and the bottom of the pineapple. Stand the pineapple upright and, using a large, sharp knife, pare off the skin, cutting downward just below the floor in long, vertical strips and leaving the small brown "eyes" on the fruit. Lay the pineapple on its side. Aligning the knife blade with the diagonal rows of eyes, reduce a shallow furrow, following a spiral pattern around the pineapple, to take away all of the eyes. Stand the peeled pineapple upright and cut it in half of lengthwise. Place each pineapple half reduce-aspect down and reduce it lengthwise into four lengthy wedges; slice away the core. Cut every wedge crosswise into three portions. Thread the three pineapple portions onto every skewer.

Lightly brush the pineapple with the marinade. Grill or broil, turning once and basting once or twice with the remaining marinade, till soft and golden, about five mins on each side.

Remove the pineapple from the skewers and place them on a platter or character serving plates. Brush with the rum, if using, and sprinkle with the lime zest. Serve hot or warm.

Nutrition
Total carbohydrate13 g Dietary fiber1 Sodium1 mg Total fat2 g Cholesterol0 mgCalories70

Mixed Berry Whole-Grain Coffee-Cake

Ingredients
- 1/2 cup skim milk
- 1 tablespoon vinegar

- 2 tablespoons canola oil
- 1 teaspoon vanilla
- 1 egg
- 1/3 cup packed brown sugar
- 1 cup whole-wheat pastry flour
- 1/2 teaspoon baking soda
- 1/2 teaspoon ground cinnamon
- 1/8 teaspoon salt
- 1 cup frozen mixed berries, such as blueberries, raspberries and blackberries (do not thaw)
- 1/4 cup low-fat granola, slightly crushed

Heat oven to 350 F. Sprays an 8-inch round cake pan with cooking spray and coat with flour.

In a massive bowl, blend the milk, vinegar, oil, vanilla, egg, and brown sugar until smooth. Stir in flour, baking soda, cinnamon, and salt just till moistened. Gently fold half the berries into the batter. Spoon into the organized pan. Sprinkle with ultimate seeds and pinnacle with the granola.

Bake 25 to 30 min or till golden brown and top springs returned while touched in center. Cool in pan on a cooling rack for 10 min. Serve warm.

Nutrition

Cholesterol23 mgCalories144 Sodium139 mg Total fat4 g Total carbohydrate23 g Saturated fat0.5 g Dietary fiber3 g Protein4 g

Orange Smoothie

Ingredients
- 1 1/2 cups orange juice, chilled
- 1 cup light vanilla soy milk, chilled
- 1/3 cup silken or soft tofu
- 1 tablespoon dark honey
- 1 teaspoon grated orange zest
- 1/2 teaspoon vanilla extract
- 5 ice cubes
- 4 peeled orange segments (about half an orange)

In a blender, combine the orange juice, soy milk, tofu, honey, orange zest, vanilla, and ice cubes. Blend till smooth and frothy, about 30 sec.

Pour into tall, chilled glasses and garnish each glass with an orange segment.

Nutrition

Total carbohydrate20 g Dietary fiber1 g Sodium40 mg Saturated fat< 1 g Total fat1 g Cholesterol0 mg Protein3 gCalories101 Total sugars14 g

Orange Slices

Ingredients
- 4 oranges
- Zest (outermost skin) of 1 orange, cut into thin strips 4 inches long and 1/8 inch wide
- For syrup:
- 1 1/2 cups fresh orange juice, strained
- 2 tablespoons dark honey
- For garnish:
- 2 tablespoons orange liqueur, such as Grand Marnier or Cointreau (optional)
- 4 fresh mint sprigs

Preheat the oven to 375 F. Lightly coat a 9-inch pie pan with cooking spray.

Arrange peach slices inside the organized pie plate. Sprinkle with lemon juice, cinnamon, and nutmeg.

In a small bowl, whisk together flour and brown sugar. With your fingers, collapse the margarine into the flour-sugar aggregate. Add the raw oats and stir to combine evenly. Sprinkle the flour aggregate on the pinnacle of the peaches.

Bake till peaches are gentle, and the topping is browned about 30 mins. Cut into eight even slices and serve warm. Working with one orange at a time, cut a thin slice off the top and the bottom, exposing the flesh. Stand the orange upright and the use of a sharp knife, cut off the peel, following the contour of the fruit and removing all of the white pith and membrane. Cut the orange crosswise into slices half-inch thick. Transfer to a shallow nonaluminum bowl or dish. Repeat with the closing oranges. Set aside.

In a small saucepan over medium-high heat, combine the strips of zest with water to cover. Bring to a boil and boil for 1 min. Drain and right away, plunge the punch right into a bowl of cold water. Set aside.

To make the syrup, integrate the orange juice and honey in a large saucepan over medium-high heat. Bring to a boil, stirring to dissolve the honey. Reduce the heat to medium-low and simmer, uncovered, until the combination thickens to a mild syrup, about 5 mins. Drain the orange zest and upload it to the sugar. Cook till the taste is translucent, 3 to five mins. Pour the aggregate over the oranges. Cover and refrigerate till well-chilled, or for up to a few hours.

To serve, divide the orange slices and syrup among man or woman plates. Drizzle every serving with 1 1/2 teaspoons of the orange liqueur, if using. Garnish with the mint and serve without delay.

Nutrition

Total carbohydrate39 g Dietary fiber4 g Sodium3 mg Saturated fat0 Cholesterol0 mg Protein2 gCalories183 Total sugars33 g

Crumble Peach

Ingredients
- 8 ripe peaches, peeled, pitted and sliced
- Juice from 1 lemon (about 3 tablespoons)
- 1/3 teaspoon ground cinnamon
- 1/4 teaspoon ground nutmeg
- 1/2 cup whole-wheat flour
- 1/4 cup packed dark brown sugar
- 2 tablespoons trans-free margarine, cut into thin slices
- 1/4 cup quick-cooking oats (uncooked)

Preheat the oven to 375 F. Lightly coat a 9-inch pie pan with cooking spray.

Arrange peach slices inside the organized pie plate. Sprinkle with lemon juice, cinnamon, and nutmeg.

In a small bowl, whisk together flour and brown sugar. With your fingers, collapse the margarine into the flour-sugar aggregate. Add the raw oats and stir to combine evenly. Sprinkle the flour aggregate on the pinnacle of the peaches.

Bake till peaches are gentle, and the topping is browned about 30 mins. Cut into eight even slices and serve warm.

Nutrition

Total fat4 gCalories152 Protein3 g Cholesterol0 mg Total carbohydrate26 g Dietary fiber3 g Sodium41 mg Added sugars4 g

Pumpkin-Hazelnut Cake

Ingredients
- 3 tablespoons canola oil
- 3/4 cup homemade or unsweetened canned pumpkin puree
- 1/2 cup honey
- 3 tablespoons firmly packed brown sugar
- 2 eggs, lightly beaten
- 1 cup whole-wheat (whole-meal) flour
- 1/2 cup all-purpose (plain) flour
- 2 tablespoons flaxseed
- 1/2 teaspoon baking powder
- 1/2 teaspoon ground allspice
- 1/2 teaspoon ground cinnamon
- 1/2 teaspoon ground nutmeg
- 1/4 teaspoon ground cloves
- 1/4 teaspoon salt
- 2 tablespoons chopped hazelnuts (filberts)

Instructions

Heat the oven to 350 F. Lightly coat an 8-by-4-inch loaf pan with cooking spray.

In a massive bowl, using an electric powered mixer on low speed, beat the canola oil, pumpkin puree, honey, brown sugar, and eggs collectively until adequately blended.

In a small bowl, whisk the flours, flaxseed, baking powder, allspice, cinnamon, nutmeg, cloves, and salt collectively. Add the flour aggregate to the pumpkin mixture and the usage of the electric mixer on medium speed beat until nicely blended.

Pour the batter into the prepared pan. Sprinkle the hazelnuts calmly over the pinnacle and press down lightly to inn the nuts into the mixture. Bake until a toothpick inserted into the middle of the loaf comes out clean, about 50 to fifty-five mins. Let calm within the pan on a cord rack for 10 mins. Turn the dough out of the pan onto the frame and permit cool ultimately. Cut into 12 slices to serve.

Nutrition

Calories166 Total fat6 g Saturated fat1 gTransfatTraceMonounsaturated fat3 g Cholesterol31 mg Sodium73 mg Total carbohydrate28 g Dietary fiber2.5 g Total sugars15 Added sugars15 Protein4 g

Marshmallows

Ingredients
- 3/4 cup water, divided
- 3 (.25 ounce) packages unflavored gelatin
- 2/3 cup light corn syrup
- 2 cups white sugar
- 2 teaspoons vanilla extract
- 2 teaspoons peppermint extract
- 1/4 cup cornstarch
- 1/4 cup confectioners' sugar

Line a 9x9 inch baking dish with lightly greased foil or plastic wrap. Grease every other piece of foil or plastic wrap to cover the top, and set aside.

Place half a cup of water within the bowl of an electric mixer and sprinkle gelatin on top of the water to soak.

While gelatin is soaking, combine 1/four cup of water, corn syrup, and sugar in a saucepan, and produce to a boil over medium heat. Boil the mixture hardened for 1 minute.

Pour the new sugar combination into the gelatin mixture and beat on excessive for 12 mins with electric powered mixer, until the mix is fluffy and bureaucracy stiff peaks. Add vanilla and peppermint extracts, and beat just until blended.

Pour the marshmallow mixture into the prepared baking dish, using a greased spatula to easy the pinnacle of the sweet. Cover the candy with the reserved greased foil or wrap, and press down gently to seal the covering to the crest of the delicious. Allow the marshmallow sweet to rest for four hours or overnight. Mix cornstarch and confectioner's sugar collectively in a shallow dish. Using oiled scissors or an oiled kitchen knife, cut the marshmallow sweet into strips, then into 1-inch squares. Dredge the marshmallows lightly in the cornstarch aggregate and save in an airtight container.

63 calories; 0 g is fat; 15.7 g carbohydrates; 0.5 g is protein; 0 mg cholesterol; 5 mg sodium

Oreo Truffles

Ingredients
- 1 (16 ounce) package OREO Chocolate Sandwich Cookies, divided
- 1 (8 ounce) package PHILADELPHIA Cream Cheese, softened
- 2 (8 ounce) packages BAKER'S Semi-Sweet Baking Chocolate, melted

Crush 9 of the cookies to satisfactory crumbs in meals processor; reserve for later use. (Cookies can also be finely overwhelmed in a resealable plastic bag using a rolling pin.) Crush ultimate 36 cookies to satisfactory crumbs; region in a medium bowl. Add cream cheese; mix until well blended. Roll cookie combination into 42 balls, approximately 1-inch in diameter.

Dip balls in chocolate; place on a wax paper-included baking sheet. (Any leftover chocolate may be saved at room temperature for any other use.) Sprinkle with reserved cookie crumbs.

Refrigerate till firm, approximately 1 hour. Store leftover truffles, blanketed, in the refrigerator.

Chocolate Fudge

Ingredients
- 1 (7 ounce) jar marshmallow creme

- 1 1/2 cups white sugar
- 2/3 cup evaporated milk
- 1/4 cup butter
- 1/4 teaspoon salt
- 2 cups milk chocolate chips
- 1 cup semisweet chocolate chips
- 1/2 cup chopped nuts
- 1 teaspoon vanilla extract

Line an 8x8 inch pan with aluminum foil. Set aside. In a big saucepan over medium warmth, combine marshmallow cream, sugar, evaporated milk, butter, and salt. Bring to a complete boil, and prepare dinner for five min, stirring constantly.
Remove from warmth and pour in semisweet chocolate chips and milk chocolate chips. Stir until chocolate is melted and the mixture is smooth. Stir in nuts and vanilla. Pour into an organized plan. Chill in the fridge for 2 hours or until firm.
 124 calories; 5.5 g is fat; 18.2 g carbohydrates; 1.4 g is protein; 5 mg cholesterol; 26 mg sodium

Easiest Peanut Butter Fudge

Ingredients
1/2 cup butter
1 (16 ounce) package brown sugar
1/2 cup milk
3/4 cup peanut butter
1 teaspoon vanilla extract
3 1/2 cups confectioners' sugar

Melt butter in a medium saucepan over medium heat. Stir in brown sugar and milk. Bring to a boil and boil for 2 minutes, stirring frequently. Remove from heat. Stir in peanut butter and vanilla. Pour over confectioners' sugar in a large mixing bowl. Beat until smooth; pour into an 8x8 inch dish. Chill until firm and cut into squares.
Per Serving: 357 calories; 12.8 g fat; 60.1 g carbohydrates; 3.6 g protein; 17 mg cholesterol; 115 mg sodium.

Ice Pops Like Rainbow

Ingredients
- 1 1/2 cups diced strawberries, cantaloupe and watermelon
- 1/2 cup blueberries
- 2 cups 100% apple juice
- 6 paper cups (6-8 ounces each)
- 6 craft sticks

Instructions
Mix the fruit and divide flippantly into the paper cups.
Pour 1/3 cup of juice into each paper cup.
Place the cups on a level surface in the freezer.
Freeze until partially frozen, about 1 hour. Insert a stick into the center of every cup. Freeze until firm.
Nutrition
 Total carbohydrate14 g Dietary fiber1 g Sodium6 mg Cholesterol0 mg Protein0.5 gCalories60 Added sugars0 g Total sugars11 g

Bananas Sautéed

Ingredients
- For the sauce:
- 1 tablespoon butter
- 1 tablespoon walnut oil
- 1 tablespoon honey
- 2 tablespoons firmly packed brown sugar
- 3 tablespoons 1 percent low-fat milk
- 1 tablespoon dark raisins or golden raisins (sultanas)
- For the saute:
- 4 firm bananas, about 1 pound total weight
- 1/2 teaspoon canola oil
- 2 tablespoons dark rum

Instructions
Start through making the sauce. In a small saucepan, soften the butter over medium heat. Whisk inside the walnut oil, honey, and brown sugar. Stirring continuously, cook till the sugar is dissolved, about 3 minutes. Add the milk one tablespoon at a time, and then cook, stirring continuously till the sauce thickens slightly approximately 3 minutes. Remove from the warmth and awaken within the raisins. Set apart and preserve warm.
Peel the bananas, after which cut every crosswise into three sections. Cut each phase in half of lengthwise. Lightly coat a large nonstick frying pan with the canola oil and area over medium-excessive heat. Add the bananas and saute until they begin to brown, 3 to four minutes. Transfer to a plate and preserve warm.
Add the rum to the pan, carry to a boil and deglaze the pan, stirring with a timber spoon to scrape up any browned bits from the lowest of the pan. Cook till reduced by half of, about 30 to 45 sec. Return the bananas to the pan to rewarm.
To serve, divide the bananas among character bowls or plates. Drizzle with the warm sauce and serve immediately.
Nutrition
 Total carbohydrate27 g Dietary fiber2 g Sodium21 mg Saturated fat2 g Total fat5 gTrans fatTrace Cholesterol5 mg Protein1 gMonounsaturated fat1 gCalories145 Added sugars8 g Total sugars18 g

Fruit Gratin For Summer

Ingredients
For the filling:
- 1 pound of cherries, pitted and halved
- 4 cups of peeled, pitted and sliced mixed summer stone fruits, such as nectarines, peaches and apricots
- 1 tablespoon whole-wheat flour
- 1 tablespoon turbinado sugar or firmly packed light brown sugar
- For the topping:
- 1/2 cup old-fashioned rolled oats
- 1/4 cup sliced (flaked) almonds
- 3 tablespoons whole-wheat flour
- 2 tablespoons turbinado sugar or firmly packed light brown sugar
- 1/4 teaspoon of ground cinnamon
- 1/8 teaspoon ground nutmeg
- 1/8 teaspoon salt
- 2 tablespoons walnut oil or canola oil
- 1 tablespoon dark honey

Instructions

Heat the oven to 350 F. Lightly coat a 9-inch (23-cm) square baking dish with cooking spray. In a bowl, integrate the cherries and stone fruits. Sprinkle with the flour and turbinado sugar and toss lightly to mix. To make the topping, in any other bowl, integrate the oats, almonds, flour, turbinado sugar, cinnamon, nutmeg, and salt. Whisk to blend. Stir within the oil and honey and mix until well-blended.

Spread the fruit aggregate calmly inside the organized baking dish. Sprinkle the oat-almond total lightly over the fruit. Bake until the fruit is bubbling and the topping is gently browned forty-five to fifty-five mins. Serve warm or at room temperature.

Nutrition

Total carbohydrate39 Dietary fiber5 g Sodium56 mg Saturated fat0.5 g Total fat7 g Cholesterol0 mg Protein4 gCalories235 Total sugars25 g Added sugars9 g

Chocolate Souffles

Ingredients

- 1/2 cup of unsweetened cocoa powder
- 6 tablespoons of hot water
- 1 tablespoon of unsalted butter
- 1 tablespoon of canola oil
- 3 tablespoons of all-purpose (plain) flour
- 1 tablespoon of ground hazelnuts (filberts) or almonds
- 1/4 teaspoon of ground cinnamon
- 3 tablespoons of firmly packed dark brown sugar
- 2 tablespoons of honey
- 1/8 teaspoon of salt
- 3/4 cup of 1 percent low-fat milk
- 4 egg whites
- 3 tablespoons of granulated sugar
- 1 teaspoon of powdered (confectioner's) sugar
- 1 cup of raspberries

Instructions

Heat the oven to 375 F. Lightly coat six 1-cup man or woman souffle dishes or ramekins with cooking spray or coat a 6-cup souffle dish with the spray.

In a small bowl, combine the cocoa and hot water, stirring until smooth. Set aside.

In a small, heavy saucepan over medium heat, soften the butter. Add the canola oil and stir to integrate. Add the flour, floor hazelnuts, and cinnamon and prepare dinner for 1 minute, continually stirring with a whisk. Stir inside the brown sugar, honey, and salt. Gradually add the milk and cook, frequently stirring, until thickened, about three minutes. Remove from the warmth and stir into the cocoa mixture. Let cool slightly.

In a large, thoroughly cleaned bowl, using an electric mixer on excessive speed, beat the egg whites until foamy. Add the granulated sugar one tablespoon at a time and beat till stiff peaks form. Using a rubber spatula, lightly fold 1/3 of the egg whites into the cocoa combination to lighten it. Then fold the ultimate egg whites into the cocoa mixture, blending gently beat until no white streaks remain.

Gently scoop the cocoa egg white mixture into the prepared dishes (or dish). Bake until the souffle rises above the rim and is set in the center, 15 to twenty mins for man or woman shuffles or forty to forty-five mins for the massive souffle.

Cool the souffles on a cord rack for 10 to 15 mins. Using a fine-mesh sieve, dirt the top with the powdered sugar. Garnish with raspberries and serve immediately.

Nutrition

Calories203 Total fat7 g Saturated fat2 g Cholesterol7 mg Sodium106 mg Total carbohydrate29 g Dietary fiber4 g Total sugars22 g Added sugars19 g Protein6 g

Decadent Truffles

Ingredients

- 1 (8 ounce) of package cream cheese, softened
- 3 cups of confectioners' sugar, sifted
- 3 cups of semisweet chocolate chips, melted
- 1 1/2 teaspoons of vanilla

In a large bowl, beat cream cheese till smooth. Gradually beat in confectioners' sugar till nicely blended. Stir in melted chocolate and vanilla till no streaks remain. Refrigerate for about 1 hour. Shape into 1 inch balls. In a considerable bowl, beat cream cheese until smooth. Gradually beat in confectioners' sugar until adequately blended. Stir in melted chocolate and vanilla till no streaks remain. Refrigerate for about 1 hour. Shape into 1 inch balls.

Per Serving: 78 calories; 3.8 g fat; 11.7 g carbohydrates; 0.6 g protein; 4 mg cholesterol; 12 mg sodium.

Cookie Ball

Ingredients

- 1 pound of chocolate sandwich cookies, crushed
- 1 (8 ounce) of package cream cheese, softened
- 1 pound of vanilla-flavored candy coating, melted

In a large blending bowl, combine beaten cookies and cream cheese to shape the stiff dough. Roll into balls and dip with a fork in a melted sweet coating. Let rest on waxed paper until set.

Appendix : Recipes Index

A

Absolutely Ultimate Potato Soup 78
Afghan Beef Dumplings(Mantu) 64
Alfredo Sauce 104
All American Tuna 13
All-Fruit Smoothies 72
Almond And Apricot Biscotti 29
Almond Butter And Blueberry Smoothie 71
Almond Butter Berry Smoothie 10
Almost Eggless Egg Salad 91
Ambrosia With Coconut And Almonds 84
Ambrosia With Coconut And Toasted Almonds 111
Ambrosia With Coconut And Toasted Almonds 30
Antipasto Baked Smothered Chicken 54
Apple-Berry Cobbler 111
Apple-Berry Cobbler 30
Apple-Blueberry Cobbler 111
Apple-Blueberry Cobbler 30
Apple-Cherry Pork Medallions 18
Apple-Nut Blue Cheese Tartlets 110
Apricot Jam And Almond Butter Sandwich 14
Asian-Style Chicken Salad Bowls 54
Asparagus Turkey Stir-Fry 18
Asparagus With Horseradish Dip 24
Avocado And Tuna Tapas 93
Avocado Egg Cups 10
Avocado Fruit Salad 109
Avocado Fruit Salad with Tangerine Vinaigrette 108
Avocado Salsa and Sardine Frenchy 100
Avocado Smoothie 69

B

Bacon In The Microwave 26
Bagna Calda 101
Baked Apples With Cherries And Almonds 30
Baked Apples, Cherries And Almonds 112
Baked Butternut-Squash Rigatoni 13
Baked Cod In Foil 96
Baked Dijon Salmon 95
Baked Lemon-Pepper Chicken 53
Baked Lemon-Pepper Chicken 55
Baked Potato Soup 79
Bali Bowls With Peanut Tofu 44
Balls Buckeye 112
Balsamic Marinated Chicken 54
Balsamic-Goat Cheese Grilled Plums 106
Banana Pina Coladasmoothie 70
Banana, Avocado, And Spinach Smoothie 69
Bananas Sautéed 116
Bar-B-Q Sauce 105
Bart's Black Bean Soup For Two 28
Basic Scrambled Eggs 12
Bean Soup 83
Beef And Blue Cheese Penne With Pesto 18
Beef Noodle Soup 78
Beef Rib Roast With Mushrooms & Fennel 65
Beef Tenderloin With Pomegranate Sauce &Farro Pilaf 63
Berry White Ice Pops 107
Bill's Blue Cheese Dressing 103
Black Bean & Sweet Potato Rice Bowls 19
Black Bean And Salsa Soup 82
Black Pepper Tofu With Bok Choy 39
Blackened Tempeh With Avocado, Kale, Vegan Cajun Ranch 41
Blackened Tuna 95
Blue Cheese Broccoli Salad 86
Blueberry Mint Smoothie 72
Blueberry Sauce 102
Bodacious Broccoli Salad 87
Bow Ties With Sausage & Asparagus 19
Braised Brisket With Dried Fruit 67
Breakfast Fruit Pizzas 9
Breakfast In a Jar 10
Broccoli And Ramen Noodle Salad 89
Broccoli And Tortellini Salad 89
Broccoli Buffet Salad 87
Broccoli Cheese Soup 78
Broccoli Coleslaw 87
Broccolicious 71
Brunch Banana Splits 26
Bucatini Pasta With Arugula Pesto & Heirloom Tomatoes 46
Buffalo-Style Bistro Lunch Box 56
Butternut Squash Soup 77
Butternut Turkey Soup 19

C

California Italian Soup 77
California Quinoa 24
Caramel 113
Carrot And Hummus Snack 14
Cast-Iron Cornmeal Cake With Buttermilk Cream 35
Cauliflower Chicken Fried "Rice" 56
Cauliflower Rice Bowls With Grilled Asparagus And Chicken Sausage 53
Cedar Planked Salmon 95
Chicken & Goat Cheese Skillet 17
Chicken & Shiitake Dumplings In Tangy Chile-Oil Sauce 57
Chicken Breasts With Mushroom Cream Sauce 56
Chicken Broccoli Salad 86
Chicken Club Wraps 57
Chicken Cutlets And Zucchini Noodles With Creamy Tomato Sauce 60
Chicken Kurma 59
Chicken Noodle Soup 75
Chicken Paillards With Blood Orange Pan Sauce 60
Chicken Scampi Pasta 16
Chicken Tortilla Soup V 80
Chicken Veggie Packets 17
Chicken With Celery Root Puree 18
Chili Garlic Tofu With Sesame Broccolini 47
Chili-Lime Grilled Pineapple 108
Chili-Lime Grilled Pineapple 22
Chimichurri Sauce 105
Chinese Eggplant With Spicy Szechuan Sauce 37

Chipotle Portobello Tacos (Vegan!) 37
Chocolate Berry Smoothies 68
Chocolate Chip Pecan Mug Cake 27
Chocolate Fudge 115
Chocolate Souffles 117
Chunky Spicy Egg Salad 86
Cilantro Jalapeno Pesto with Lime 103
Cilantro-Lime Dressing 103
Citrus-Herb Pork Roast 26
Citrusy Fruit Kabobs 107
Clam Chowder 80
Classic Fish And Chips 94
Classic Minestrone 80
Coast Cod And Shrimp 97
Coconut Acorn Squash 28
Coconut Oil Fat Bombs 14
Cod Grilled 98
Colorful Winter Fruitsalad 90
Cookie Ball 117
Cottage Cheese Honey Toast 15
Couscous Salad 84
Crab Stuffed Flounder 101
Cranberry And Cilantro Quinoa Salad 92
Cranberry, Apple, and Fresh Ginger Chutney 104
Creamy Italian White Bean Soup 80
Creamy Lemon Chicken Parmesan 60
Creamy Mushroom, Chicken & Asparagus Bake 58
Crisp Apples With Citrus Dressing 89
Crispy Beer Batter Fish & Chips 98
Crispy Fish 98
Crispy Sheet Pan Jackfruit Tacos 47
Crispy Vegan Quinoa Cakes With Tomato-Chickpea Relish 38
Crock-Pot Pineapple Chicken 59
Crumble Peach 114
Crunchy Egg Salad 88
Crunchy Peanut Butter Apple Dip 107
Cucumber & Hummus 14
Cucumber Tomato Salad With Tuna 15
Curry Broccoli Salad 87

D

Decadent Truffles 117
Delicious Egg Salad For Sandwiches 89
Delicious Egg Salad For Sandwiches 90
Delicious Ham And Potato Soup 76
Deviled Egg Toast 12
Double-Nut Stuffed Figs 109

E

Easiest Peanut Butter Fudge 116
Easy Egg Salad 89
Easy Pesto 102
Egg Salad I 88
Egg Salad With Chopped Gherkins 90
Escarole And Bean Soup 21
EZ Red Pesto Sauce 102

F

Fastest Ever Lemon Pudding 29
Filipino Pancitbihon 58
Fresh Broccoli Salad 88
Fresh Sardines 99

Fresh Spring Rolls With Peanut Sauce 46
Frosty Watermelon Ice 109
Frozen Berry & Yogurt Swirls 109
Frozen Pops (Pineapple-Kiwi) 108
Fruit & Almond Bites 24
Fruit Gratin For Summer 116

G

Garden Vegetable Beef Soup 23
Garlic Scape Pesto 103
Geneva's Ultimate Hungarian Mushroom Soup 77
Ginger Carrot And Turmeric Smoothie 68
Ginger Glazed Mahi Mahi 96
Granola Cereal Bars 28
Grapefruit Smoothie 71
Greek Salad 85
Green Curry Salmon With Green Beans 17
Green Grape Salad 89
Green Power Mojito Smoothie 71
Green Slime Smoothie 71
Grilled Angel Food Cake 31
Grilled Fish Tacos With Chipotle-Lime Dressing 94
Grilled Food Cake 112
Grilled Fruit With Balsamic Vinegar Syrup 31
Grilled Pineapple 31
Grilled Salmon 93
Grilled Stone Fruits with Balsamic Syrup 108
Groovy Green Smoothie 71

H

Ham And Split Pea Soup Recipe - A Great Soup 75
Healthier Broiled Tilapia Parmesan 93
Heavenly Blueberry Smoothie 72
Hemp Crusted Tofu With Celeriac Puree 51
Homemade Mayonnaise 104
Hot Pepper Jelly 105
How To Make Tlayudas 42
Hudson's Baked Tilapia With Dill Sauce 95

I

Iana's Pasta con le Sarde 101
Ice Pops Like Rainbow 116
Instant Pot 'Corned" Beef & Cabbage 62
Instant Pot Brisket 61
Instant Pot Goulash 63
Instant Pot Mujadara 39
Irish Beef Stew 66
Island-Style Sardines and Rice 99
Italian Sausage-Stuffed Zucchini 108
Italian Sausage-Stuffed Zucchini 22
Italian Style Flounder 102

J

Jade Noodles 45

K

Kale And Banana Smoothie 69
Kiwi Banana Apple Smoothie 70

L

Layered Deviled Egg Pasta Salad 91
Layered Hummus Dip 23
Lemon & Dill Chicken 54
Lemon Berry Smoothie 72
Lentil Dal With Sweet Potatoes 47

Loaded Egg Salad 88
Lola Beef Kebabs 61
Low Sodium Sheet Pan Chicken Fajitas 9

M

Macaroni And Cheese 26
Make Life Simple Instant Pot Lentil Soup 49
Mango Cashew Salad 91
Mango Pineapple Green Smoothie 73
Mango Rice Pudding 23
Marshmallows 115
MediterraneanCasserole 100
Microwave Egg Sandwich 28
Microwave Parmesan Chicken 28
Microwave Peanut Butter And Jam Brownies 29
Microwavecinnamonmaple Breakfast Quinoa 27
Middle Eastern Eggplant Wrap 46
Middle Eastern Salad Tacos 42
Mimi's Lentil Medley 22
MINI BELL PEPPER TURKEY "NACHOS" 106
Minnesota Broccoli Salad 87
Minute Microwave Cheesecake 28
Miso & Tofu 100
Mixed Berry Whole-Grain Coffee-Cake 113
Mixed Berry Whole-Grain Coffeecake 32
Mixed Fruit with Lemon-Basil Dressing 107
Mongolian Strawberry-Orange Juice Smoothie 73
Moroccan Chicken Tagine With Apricots & Olives 55
Moroccan Fish Tagine 97
Moroccan Lentil Soup 79
Mug Banana Bread 27

O

Oatmeal Smoothie For The Dash Diet Breakfast 69
Orange Banana Smoothie 70
Orange Dream Smoothie 32
Orange Dream Smoothie 68
Orange Slices 114
Orange Slices With Citrus Syrup 32
Orange Smoothie 114
Orange Smoothie 73
Orange Snowman 73
Oreo Truffles 115
Oven-Roasted Whole Chicken 53

P

Pasta Con Sarde (Pasta with Sardines) 99
Pasta Salad With Mixed Vegetables 86
Pasta Sardine 99
Peach And Berry Salad 91
Peach Crumble 33
Peanut Brittle 113
Peanut Butter & Banana Breakfast Smoothie 69
Peanut Butter & Carrots 15
Peanut Butter And Honey Toast 14
Peanut Butter And Jelly 15
Peanut Butter Overnight Oats 9
Peanut Butter Yogurt 15
Pepper Ricotta Primavera 19
Peppered Tuna Kabobs 20
Peppered Tuna Kabobs 24
Perfect Ten Baked Cod 97
Pimento Cheese Sandwich 14
Pimento Cheese Sandwich 15
Pineapple Protein Smoothie 10
Pineapple Grilled 113
Pistachio Fluff Fruit Salad 90
Pomegranate And Peaches Avocado Toast 10
Pork And Balsamic Strawberry Salad 19
Power Drink ***The Orange*** 70
Pretzel Coated Fried Fish 96
Proper Pesto 103
Pumpkin Black Bean Soup 82
Pumpkin Smoothie 71
Pumpkin Soup 74
Pumpkin-Hazelnut Cake 115
Pumpkin-Hazelnut Tea Cake 33

Q

Quick Alfredo Sauce 102
Quick And Easy Chicken Noodle Soup 76
Quick And Easy Vegetarian Biryani Recipe 36
Quick Bean And Tuna Salad 84
Quick Buffalo Chicken Salad 13
Quick Fish Tacos 93
Quick Sardine Curry 99

R

Rainbow Ice Pops 33
Raspberry Green Smoothie 69
Raspberry Peach Puff Pancake 24
Red Pepper, Kale, And Cheddar Frittata 12
Red, White, And Blue Fruit Smoothie 72
ROAST CHICKPEAS 106
Roasted Chicken Thighs With Peppers & Potatoes 21
Roasted Chiles Rellenos With Black Beans 43
Roasted Eggplant With Zaatar 45
Roasted Portobello Mushrooms With Walnut Coffee Sauce 43
Roasted Spaghetti Squash w/ Eggplant Puttanesca 44

S

Salad Frog Eye 91
Salmon With Tarragon Sauce 28
Sandwich Toast (Sardines and Pineapple) 101
Sardines With Sun-Dried Tomato And Capers 98
Sausage-Spiked Meatloaves 67
Sautéed Bananas 33
Scrambled Eggs With Bell Pepper And Feta 12
Second English Muffin 27
Sesame Brussel Sprouts, Mushrooms & Tofu 49
Shepherd's Pie With Cauliflower Topping 62
Shrimp Egg Salad 89
Shrimp Orzo With Feta 23
Simple Asparagus Soup 25
Simple Baked Sheet-Pan Ratatouille! 40
Simple Caprese Sandwich 14
Sissy's Frozen Banana And Pumpkin Smoothie 70
Skillet Apple-Ginger Crisp 35
Skillet Lemon Chicken & Potatoes With Kale 59

Skinny Quinoa Veggie Dip 25
Slow Cooker Taco Soup 79
Slow-Cooker Barbecue Brisket Sliders 66
Slow-Cooker Chicken Tortilla Soup 76
Slow-Cooker Flank Steak Au Jus Sandwiches 65
Slow-Cooker Honey-Orange Chicken Drumsticks 56
Slow-Cooker Ropavieja 64
Smoked Salmon And Egg Salad 90
Smoky Chipotle Black Bean Burger Recipe 51
Solo Spaghetti Dinner 101
Soup Hamburger 78
Soup Lentil 78
Southwest Black-Bean Pasta Salad Bowls 57
Spaghetti Squash Casserole 67
Spanish Cod 96
Spanish Moroccan Fish 95
Spiced Apple Chutney 104
Spiced Pumpkin Molten Mug Cake 27
Spiced Split Pea Soup 21
Spicy Almonds 22
Spicy Black Bean Vegetable Soup 81
Spicy Chicken Soup 81
Spicy Cranberry Chutney 105
Spicy Mexicanoaxacan Bowl 38
Spicy Miso Portobello Mushroom Burger (Vegan) 40
Spicy Slow Cooker Black Bean Soup 82
Spinach And Kale Smoothie 70
Spinach And Leek White Bean Soup 81
Spinach Basil Pesto 104
Spinach Sunshine Smoothie Bowl 10
Spinach-Orzo Salad With Chickpeas 21
Split Pea And Ham Soup I 81
Split Pea Soup 82
Split Pea Soup With Rosemary 82
Steak And Vegetable Soup 75
Steak Salad With Roasted Corn Vinaigrette 84
Strawberry Banana Milkshak 68
Strawberry Banana Smoothie 69
Strawberry Blueberry Smoothies 71
Strawberry Corn Salsa 106
Strawberry Lime Smoothies 107
Strawberry Microwave Breakfast Bowl 26
Strawberry Oatmeal Breakfast Smoothie 70
Strawberry Spinach Salad 92
Sugar Break Apple And Peanut Butter Oatmeal 11
Summer Fruit Gratin 34
Summer Vegetable Soup 74
Super Healthy Fruit Smoothie 72
Super-Delicious Zuppa Toscana 77
Sweet & Spicy Popcorn 29
Sweet Onion & Sausage Spaghetti 17
Sweet Potato Toast 11
Sweet Potato, Carrot, Apple, And Red Lentil Soup 83
Sweet Tamarind Chutney 105
Szechuan Tofu And Veggies 41

T

Thai Chicken Pasta Skillet 20
Thai Red Curry Chicken Soup 75
Toffee Honeycomb 112
Tofu Stir-Fry With Broccoli And Mushrooms 48
Tofu Turmeric Scramble 11
Tomato And Cheese Wrap 15
Tomato Green Bean Soup 109
Tomato Green Bean Soup 22
Tomato Salad 15
Triple Threat Fruit Smoothie 72
Turkey Medallions With Tomato Salad 25
Turkish Red Lentil 'Bride' Soup 79
Tuscan White Bean Stew 74

U

Ulli'Sgranelli 11

V

Vegan Collard Green Wraps 52
Vegan Lentil Cakes With Zhoug Sauce 50
Vegan Mashed Potatoes 52
Vegan Mushroom Pasta With Roasted Sun Chokes 45
Vegan Ramen With Miso Shiitake Broth 36
Vegan Red Lentil Soup 76
Vegan Stuffed Poblanos With Avocado Crema 49
Vegan Tikka Masala With Cauliflower 51
Vegetale Sardina 100
Veggie Lo Mien 41
Veracruz-Style Red Snapper 93

W

Warm Chocolate Souffles 34
Warm Coleslaw With Honey Dressing 85
Watermelon-Cranberry Agua Fresca 35
Watermelon-Cranberry Agua Fresca 68
Wedge Salad Skewers 9
Weeknight Chicken Chop Suey 20
Whole Grain Cheese Pancakes 11
Whole Roasted Cauliflower With Tahini Sauce 36

Y

Yellow Pear And Cherry Tomato Salad 85
Yogurt With Almonds & Honey 13
Yogurt With Walnuts & Honey 14
Yummy Honey Mustard Dipping Sauce 103

Z

Zaatar Roasted Cauliflower Steaks With Sauce 48
Zucchini Chocolate Banana Nut Milkshake 72

www.ingramcontent.com/pod-product-compliance
Lightning Source LLC
Chambersburg PA
CBHW081116080526
44587CB00021B/3614